Lipids in the Ocean 2021

Lipids in the Ocean 2021

Editors

Maria do Rosário Domingues
Philippe Soudant

MDPI • Basel • Beijing • Wuhan • Barcelona • Belgrade • Manchester • Tokyo • Cluj • Tianjin

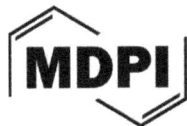

Editors
Maria do Rosário Domingues
University of Aveiro
Portugal

Philippe Soudant
Institut Universitaire
Européen de la Mer (IUEM)
France

Editorial Office
MDPI
St. Alban-Anlage 66
4052 Basel, Switzerland

This is a reprint of articles from the Special Issue published online in the open access journal *Marine Drugs* (ISSN 1660-3397) (available at: https://www.mdpi.com/journal/marinedrugs/special_issues/lipids_in_the_ocean_2020).

For citation purposes, cite each article independently as indicated on the article page online and as indicated below:

LastName, A.A.; LastName, B.B.; LastName, C.C. Article Title. *Journal Name* **Year**, *Volume Number*, Page Range.

ISBN 978-3-0365-4623-0 (Hbk)
ISBN 978-3-0365-4624-7 (PDF)

© 2022 by the authors. Articles in this book are Open Access and distributed under the Creative Commons Attribution (CC BY) license, which allows users to download, copy and build upon published articles, as long as the author and publisher are properly credited, which ensures maximum dissemination and a wider impact of our publications.

The book as a whole is distributed by MDPI under the terms and conditions of the Creative Commons license CC BY-NC-ND.

Contents

About the Editors vii

Preface to "Lipids in the Ocean 2021" ix

Kristaps Berzins, Reinis Muiznieks, Matiss R. Baumanis, Inese Strazdina, Karlis Shvirksts, Santa Prikule, Vytautas Galvanauskas, Daniel Pleissner, Agris Pentjuss, Mara Grube, Uldis Kalnenieks and Egils Stalidzans
Kinetic and Stoichiometric Modeling-Based Analysis of Docosahexaenoic Acid (DHA) Production Potential by *Crypthecodinium cohnii* from Glycerol, Glucose and Ethanol
Reprinted from: *Mar. Drugs* **2022**, *20*, 115, doi:10.3390/md20020115 1

Elina Didrihsone, Konstantins Dubencovs, Mara Grube, Karlis Shvirksts, Anastasija Suleiko, Arturs Suleiko and Juris Vanags
Crypthecodinium cohnii Growth and Omega Fatty Acid Production in Mediums Supplemented with Extract from Recycled Biomass
Reprinted from: *Mar. Drugs* **2022**, *20*, 68, doi:10.3390/md20010068 19

Marine Remize, Frédéric Planchon, Matthieu Garnier, Ai Ning Loh, Fabienne Le Grand, Antoine Bideau, Christophe Lambert, Rudolph Corvaisier, Aswani Volety and Philippe Soudant
A $^{13}CO_2$ Enrichment Experiment to Study the Synthesis Pathways of Polyunsaturated Fatty Acids of the Haptophyte *Tisochrysis lutea*
Reprinted from: *Mar. Drugs* **2022**, *20*, 22, doi:10.3390/md20010022 35

Po-Kai Chang, Ming-Fong Tsai, Chun-Yung Huang, Chien-Liang Lee, Chitsan Lin, Chwen-Jen Shieh and Chia-Hung Kuo
Chitosan-Based Anti-Oxidation Delivery Nano-Platform: Applications in the Encapsulation of DHA-Enriched Fish Oil
Reprinted from: *Mar. Drugs* **2021**, *19*, 470, doi:10.3390/md19080470 53

Luísa Marques, Maria Rosário Domingues, Elisabete da Costa, Maria Helena Abreu, Ana Isabel Lillebø and Ricardo Calado
Screening for Health-Promoting Fatty Acids in Ascidians and Seaweeds Grown under the Influence of Fish Farming Activities
Reprinted from: *Mar. Drugs* **2021**, *19*, 469, doi:10.3390/md19080469 67

Megumu Fujibayashi, Osamu Nishimura and Takashi Sakamaki
The Negative Relationship between Fouling Organisms and the Content of Eicosapentaenoic Acid and Docosahexaenoic Acid in Cultivated Pacific Oysters, *Crassostrea gigas*
Reprinted from: *Mar. Drugs* **2021**, *19*, 369, doi:10.3390/md19070369 81

Tomomi Yamazaki, Dongyang Li and Reina Ikaga
Fish Oil Increases Diet-Induced Thermogenesis in Mice
Reprinted from: *Mar. Drugs* **2021**, *19*, 278, doi:10.3390/md19050278 93

Marine Vallet, Tarik Meziane, Najet Thiney, Soizic Prado and Cédric Hubas
Laminariales Host Does Impact Lipid Temperature Trajectories of the Fungal Endophyte *Paradendryphiella salina* (Sutherland.)
Reprinted from: *Mar. Drugs* **2020**, *18*, 379, doi:10.3390/md18080379 109

Diana Lopes, Felisa Rey, Miguel C. Leal, Ana I. Lillebø, Ricardo Calado and Maria Rosário Domingues
Bioactivities of Lipid Extracts and Complex Lipids from Seaweeds: Current Knowledge and Future Prospects
Reprinted from: *Mar. Drugs* **2021**, *19*, 686, doi:10.3390/md19120686 . . . . **123**

Alessandro Colletti, Giancarlo Cravotto, Valentina Citi, Alma Martelli, Lara Testai and Arrigo F. G. Cicero
Advances in Technologies for Highly Active Omega-3 Fatty Acids from Krill Oil: Clinical Applications
Reprinted from: *Mar. Drugs* **2021**, *19*, 306, doi:10.3390/md19060306 . . . . **147**

About the Editors

Maria do Rosário Domingues

Maria do Rosário Domingues graduated in Pharmaceutical Sciences, University of Coimbra (1990), received her PhD degree in Chemistry (1998) and Habilitation in Biochemistry (2014) at University of Aveiro (UA). Since 2016, she has served as Associate Professor with habilitation at the Department of Chemistry, UA. She is an expert in lipidomics and is the leader of the Marine Lipidomic Laboratory at CESAM-UA. She is the author of one book, seven book chapters, and 360 articles. She has coordinated and participated in research projects funded by national and European programs (25 in total). At present, she is the coordinator of Cost Action CA19105 Pan-European Network in Lipidomics and EpiLipidomics.

Philippe Soudant

Philippe Soudant (PhD, Marine Biology and Biochemistry) is Director of Research at the National Center for Scientific Research (CNRS). His research is focused on studying the lipid composition of marine organisms as well as the physiological mechanisms regulating lipid synthesis, dietary acquisition, and allocation. He is interested in various marine organisms (microalgae, bivalves, copepods, and fish, among others) in all their complexity and diversity and at various scales from the subcellular to the ecosystem level. More recently, his research has extended toward compound-specific isotope analysis of fatty acids applied to microalgae fluxomics, trophic ecology, and seafood and oil traceability.

Preface to "Lipids in the Ocean 2021"

From a chemical viewpoint, lipids are biological molecules that are insoluble in water but soluble in organic solvents. Within this broad definition, lipids are divided in a large number of types, including the most common categories of "oil", "fatty acid", "cholesterol", and "lecithin". Lipids are vital to life and are thus present in all living organisms from animals to plants as well as fungi and bacteria, where they serve as energy reserve and functional molecules.

Scientific interest for lipids in environmental sciences has rapidly increased in the last two decades. Recent research has provided evidence that some lipids (and not only the well-known omega-3 EPA (eicosapentaenoic acid) and DHA (docosahexaenoic acid)) play essential roles in maintaining vital biological functions that are related to the fitness components of marine organisms. In particular, lipids are key players in an organism's ability to respond to and cope with environmental changes (temperature, light, salinity, nutrients, and pH). Yet, sources, the biosynthetic pathways and functions of many lipids in marine organisms remain poorly described and understood.

Lipids also allow shedding light over the recurrent question of "who is eating what" and revealing local to regional adaptations of marine organisms to shifting biotic and abiotic conditions, a feature of extreme relevance if one considers the changes ongoing in the oceans of today and tomorrow.

From a conceptual and methodological viewpoint, investigations on marine lipids are based on resolutely interdisciplinary approaches that include specialists in analytical chemistry, biochemistry, cell biology, molecular biology, physiology, ecology, and biogeochemistry. Marine lipids allow researchers to work at multiple organizational levels, from unicellular marine organisms to the functioning of entire ecosystems.

From a more applied perspective, framed by blue growth opportunities, a better understanding of lipids from the ocean is paramount to fostering new biotechnological solutions as well as more sustainable fisheries and aquaculture practices. Lipid fingerprints can be used to pinpoint the geographic origin of seafood, either harvested from the wild or farmed under different aquaculture practices, as well as to fight illegal, unreported, and unregulated fishing. The growing interest on the smart valorization of "green lipids" produced by microalgae, seaweeds, and other salt-tolerant macrophytes must also be highlighted, as only now, with the advent of lipidomics, can one truly start to understand the remarkable chemical diversity of marine lipids present in these and other marine taxa.

Multidisciplinary projects on marine lipids are now essential to develop groundbreaking and integrative research programs and to acquire relevant concepts on biological mechanisms associated with lipids. Such knowledge is necessary to address broader scientific questions related to climate change, conservation, and human health.

Maria do Rosário Domingues and Philippe Soudant
Editors

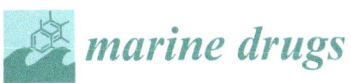

Article

Kinetic and Stoichiometric Modeling-Based Analysis of Docosahexaenoic Acid (DHA) Production Potential by *Crypthecodinium cohnii* from Glycerol, Glucose and Ethanol

Kristaps Berzins [1], Reinis Muiznieks [1], Matiss R. Baumanis [1], Inese Strazdina [1], Karlis Shvirksts [1], Santa Prikule [1], Vytautas Galvanauskas [2,3], Daniel Pleissner [4,5], Agris Pentjuss [1], Mara Grube [1], Uldis Kalnenieks [1] and Egils Stalidzans [1,2,*]

[1] Institute of Microbiology and Biotechnology, University of Latvia, Jelgavas Street 1, LV-1004 Riga, Latvia; kristaps.berzins@lu.lv (K.B.); reinis.muiznieks@lu.lv (R.M.); matiss.baumanis@gmail.com (M.R.B.); inese.strazdina@lu.lv (I.S.); karlis.svirksts@lu.lv (K.S.); santaprikule@gmail.com (S.P.); agris.pentjuss@gmail.com (A.P.); mara.grube@lu.lv (M.G.); uldis.kalnenieks@lu.lv (U.K.)
[2] Biotehniskais Centrs AS, Dzerbenes Street 27, LV-1006 Riga, Latvia; vytautas.galvanauskas@ktu.lt
[3] Department of Automation, Kaunas University of Technology, LT-51367 Kaunas, Lithuania
[4] Sustainable Chemistry (Resource Eficiency), Institute of Sustainable and Environmental Chemistry, Leuphana University of Lüneburg, Universitätsallee 1, C13.203, 21335 Luneburg, Germany; daniel.pleissner@leuphana.de
[5] Institute for Food and Environmental Research (ILU), Papendorfer Weg 3, 14806 Bad Belzig, Germany
* Correspondence: egils.stalidzans@lu.lv; Tel.: +371-29575510

Abstract: Docosahexaenoic acid (DHA) is one of the most important long-chain polyunsaturated fatty acids (LC-PUFAs), with numerous health benefits. *Crypthecodinium cohnii*, a marine heterotrophic dinoflagellate, is successfully used for the industrial production of DHA because it can accumulate DHA at high concentrations within the cells. Glycerol is an interesting renewable substrate for DHA production since it is a by-product of biodiesel production and other industries, and is globally generated in large quantities. The DHA production potential from glycerol, ethanol and glucose is compared by combining fermentation experiments with the pathway-scale kinetic modeling and constraint-based stoichiometric modeling of *C. cohnii* metabolism. Glycerol has the slowest biomass growth rate among the tested substrates. This is partially compensated by the highest PUFAs fraction, where DHA is dominant. Mathematical modeling reveals that glycerol has the best experimentally observed carbon transformation rate into biomass, reaching the closest values to the theoretical upper limit. In addition to our observations, the published experimental evidence indicates that crude glycerol is readily consumed by *C. cohnii*, making glycerol an attractive substrate for DHA production.

Keywords: Krebs cycle; central metabolism; kinetic model; constraint-based model; FTIR spectroscopy

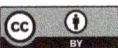

1. Introduction

Knowledge-based bioeconomy implies the conversion of cheap renewable resources into biotechnological products with added value.

Docosahexaenoic acid (DHA) is one of the most important long-chain polyunsaturated fatty acids (LC-PUFAs), with numerous health benefits such as reducing the risk of cardiovascular diseases, cancer, and rheumatoid arthritis; alleviating depression symptoms and post-natal depression; and contributing to immune-modulatory effects [1]. DHA also has an important role in the healthy development of the fetal brain and retina, and thus is commonly used in infant-related food products. The global EPA/DHA market was estimated at USD 2.49 billion in 2019, with a projected annual growth rate of 7% until 2027 [2]. Currently, cold-water marine fish oil is a source of 96% of DHA, but it is not able to meet the increasing demand of DHA for human consumption [3] due to the depletion of wild fish stocks and pollution of the marine environment (with lipophilic environmental pollutants, dioxins, heavy metals, etc.). Moreover, fish and other animals lack certain fatty acid desaturases that are required for the de novo synthesis of LC-PUFAs. Plants, although a commercially important source of oils and fats, do not synthesize LC-PUFAs.

Efforts to explore alternative sources of DHA have been made in the last decade, including the generation of transgenic oilseed plants [4] and large-scale production of DHA-producing microalgae and protists [5]. As microbes synthesize all of their cell lipid fatty acids de novo, the profile of these lipids is relatively simple, more predictable, and can be very rich in specific fatty acids, including LC-PUFAs. Among the protists, *Crypthecodinium cohnii*, a marine heterotrophic dinoflagellate, is successfully used for the industrial production of DHA because it can accumulate DHA at high concentrations within the cells [6]. In contrast to photosynthetic microalgae, heterotrophs, such as *C. cohnii*, do not require light; hence, a high biomass density can be reached in conventional bioreactors.

The established carbon substrates for the growth of *C. cohnii* are glucose, ethanol, and acetate. Ethanol and acetate are found to be superior to glucose for the production of DHA, likely because of their short conversion pathway to acetyl-CoA, the key precursor of fatty acid synthesis [7]. No or marginal growth on sucrose, glycerol, fructose, maltose, rhamnose, arabinose, lactose, and galacturonic acid has been reported previously [6,8,9]. However, several recent papers [10–12] demonstrated *C. cohnii* growth and abundant DHA synthesis in glycerol. Glycerol is an interesting renewable substrate since it is a by-product of biodiesel production and other industries, and is generated globally in large quantities. The contradictory information in the literature about the consumption of glycerol by *C. cohnii*, and DHA production from glycerol, calls for a closer look at this substrate. Notably, glycerol consumption requires just two additional reactions (glycerol kinase and glycerol-3-phosphate dehydrogenase) until it enters the metabolic "highway" of glycolysis.

The systems biology approach is used to gain a mechanistic understanding of the functioning of metabolic pathways and the theoretical limitations of different biotechnologically used but insufficiently explored organisms by combining laboratory experiments and mathematical modeling [13–16]. The implementation of the systems biology approach in education and production can lead to improvements in industrial biotechnology facilitated by interdisciplinary synergy [15,17]. The applications of different modeling approaches shed light on different aspects of the process of interest [18], enabling the implementation of different types of case-specific constraints [19].

In the present work, the authors focused on the experimental work and mathematical modeling of *C. cohnii*-central metabolic fluxes with three substrates: (i) glucose, as the most widely used carbon substrate for laboratory cultivation of this dinoflagellate [6]; (ii) ethanol, reported to be the best substrate for accumulation of DHA [20]; and (iii) glycerol, as an important renewable substrate, yet with somewhat contradictory evidence on its consumption and DHA production in *C. cohnii* [9,11,12]. The enzymatic capacity of metabolic pathways towards Acetyl-CoA (DHA precursor) is analyzed by a kinetic model. The availability of metabolic resources at the central metabolism scale is assessed by a stoichiometric model.

2. Results

2.1. Comparison of Growth, Substrate Consumption, and Accumulation of PUFAs with Glucose, Ethanol and Glycerol

Batch cultivation results with a single carbon substrate, or their combinations with glycerol, are shown in Figures 1 and 2, respectively. The growth on glycerol was compared to the growth on glucose and ethanol within a range of substrate concentrations. As seen in Figure 1, at all concentrations, the tested growth and substrate consumption with glycerol were roughly comparable to those with ethanol but proceeded significantly slower than with glucose. In contrast, Taborda et al. [12] and Safdar et al. [10] reported the growth and uptake rates for glycerol as comparable or even surpassing those with glucose. Apparently, growth parameters might vary depending on the strain, inoculum size and other cultivation parameters. Glycerol can be applied in a wide range of concentrations without any significant variations in its uptake kinetics or growth inhibition. Ethanol, in contrast, is demonstrated to inhibit growth at concentrations above 5 g/L [20]. Clearly, our data confirm that glycerol could serve as the sole carbon substrate for *C. cohnii* cultivation. At the same time, it could potentially be used as a co-substrate for mixotrophic cultivations. Under mixotrophic growth conditions (Figure 2), the uptake of glycerol and glucose occurred simultaneously, although at the initial stage of cultivation, glycerol slightly slowed down glucose consumption (compared with the growth on glucose as the sole carbon source, shown in Figure 1). Additionally, ethanol could be taken up simultaneously with glycerol (Figure 2).

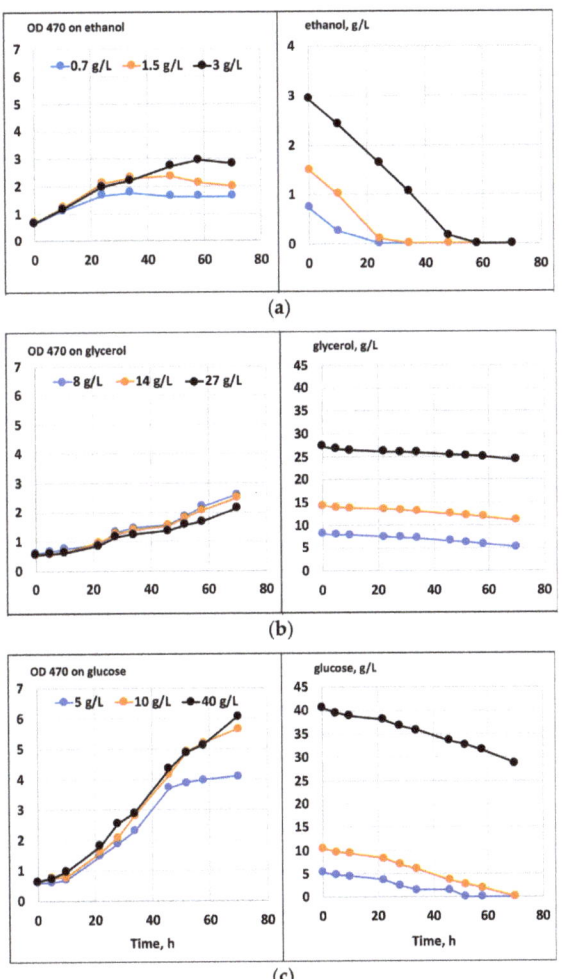

Figure 1. Growth and substrate consumption of *C. cohnii* on media with ethanol (**a**), glycerol (**b**), or glucose (**c**).

The early-stage accumulation of PUFAs in the *C. cohnii* biomass, cultivated on each of the three carbon sources, was monitored by FTIR spectroscopy, following the approach used in Didrihsone et al. [21]. FTIR was chosen as a rapid analytical method, requiring a small sample size and no complex pretreatment steps. The validity of infrared spectroscopy to estimate the content of saturated, monounsaturated and polyunsaturated fatty acids has been reported previously [22–24]. Yoshida and Yoshida [25] evaluated the FTIR spectra of synthetic and dietary triglyceride oils with various PUFAs, including DHA. The second-derivative spectra for the alkene (-HC=CH-) C-H stretching vibrational mode of several synthetic triglycerides and dietary PUFA oils showed that the peak position corresponded to the peak position in raw spectra, and the position was changed from 3005 to 3013 cm^{-1} when the extent of unsaturation was increased from mono-ene to hexa-ene. Particularly in spectra of DHA oils, the alkene peak position was at 3013.4 cm^{-1}. Here, the second-derivative spectra revealed a small peak at 3014 cm^{-1} as a simple, separate spectral feature, and accordingly, could be ascribed to the =CH- stretching of cis-alkene in PUFAs of the *C. cohnii* cells (Figure 3). The vast evidence accumulated so far on the fatty acid composition of *C. cohnii* cells indicates that DHA is the dominant PUFA in this species [26–30]. Apart from DHA (C22:6), there is a small amount of C22:5, while the rest of its fatty acid fraction is composed of C18:1, and of C12-C18 saturated fatty acids. Notably, DHA is the only representative of hexa-enes at measurable quantities; therefore, the spectral feature at 3014 cm^{-1} can be specifically related to *C. cohnii* DHA.

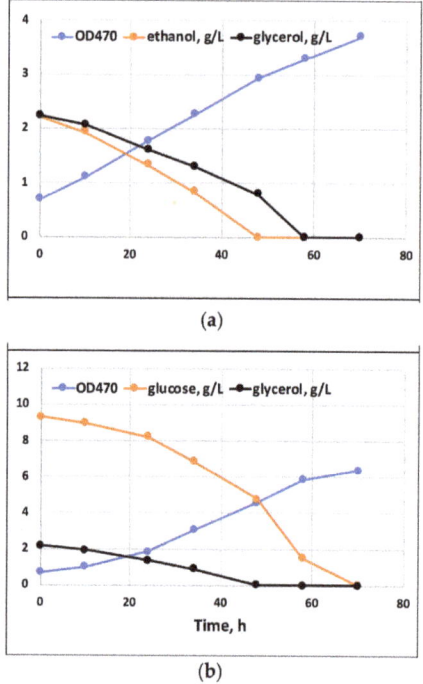

Figure 2. Mixotrophic growth of *C. cohnii* on glycerol with ethanol (**a**) or with glucose (**b**).

The strongest absorbance at 3014 cm^{-1} was found in the glycerol-grown cells. Notably, the accumulation of PUFAs with glycerol was already well-pronounced after 28 h of cultivation. At this early time point, hardly any absorbance was seen in the glucose-grown cells, despite the fact that glucose enabled faster growth. The absorbance of the ethanol-grown cells was more similar to that of the glycerol culture; nevertheless, after 70 h of cultivation, the glycerol-grown cells had accumulated significantly more PUFAs (Figure 3). Previously, we performed a chromatographic analysis of the fatty acid composition of *C. cohnii* CCMP 316 biomass grown in fed-batch mode with ethanol [30]. Following the same methodology, we also analyzed the DHA content of the same strain, grown in batch mode on 40 g L^{-1} glucose under conditions similar to those of the present study (unpublished data). The DHA content in these cultivations was in the range of 3.0–3.5% of the biomass dry weight. Here, this value would correspond to the black lines at the top panel of Figure 3, providing a rough absolute scale for the change of DHA content, seen in the spectra.

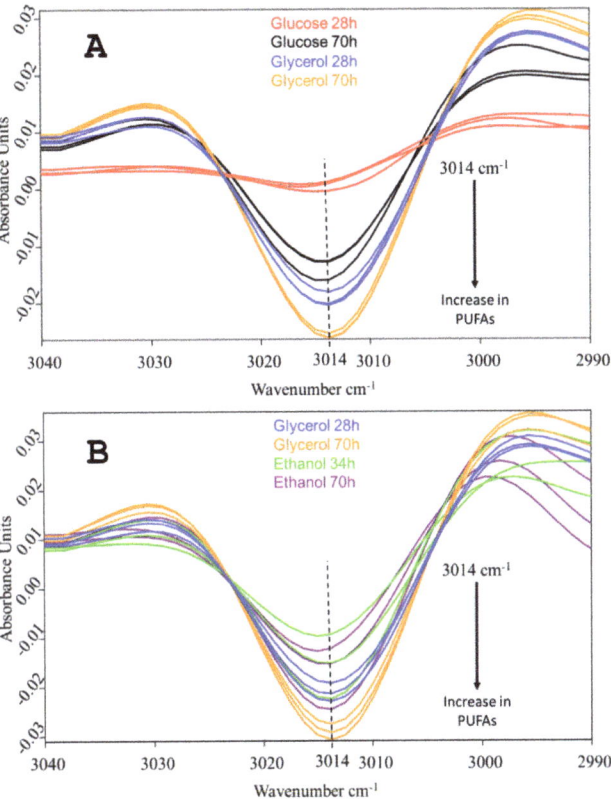

Figure 3. Vector-normalized, second-derivative FTIR spectra of *C. cohnii* biomass, showing relative amounts of accumulated PUFAs when grown with glycerol vs. glucose (**a**) or with glycerol vs. ethanol (**b**). Spectra obtained from cultivations with three concentrations of each carbon source are presented: with 5 g/L, 10 g/L and 40 g/L of glucose; 8 g/L, 14 g/L and 27 g/L of glycerol; and 0.7 g/L, 1.5 g/L and 3 g/L of ethanol.

2.2. Pathway-Scale Kinetic Model of Substrate Uptake

2.2.1. Structure of the Model

A kinetic ordinary differential equation (ODE)-based model of *C. cohnii*, including metabolic reactions that connect glucose, ethanol and glycerol uptake and the Krebs cycle with the production of Acetyl-CoA, the precursor of DHA, was developed. The model is organized into three compartments (extracellular, cytosol and mitochondria). The model contains 35 reactions and 36 metabolites (Figure 4).

The model structure was developed based on research by Zhang's group on transcriptomics [31] and the ^{13}C metabolic flux analysis [32] of DHA production in the case of glucose consumption. This kinetic model structure is similar to the structure proposed in Cui et al. [32]; however, the pentose phosphate pathway and glutamate dehydrogenase reactions were removed to make the kinetic model simpler and because the fluxes through these reactions were relatively small. The model does not include energy and redox cofactor moieties. The kinetic equations and some parameters of the reactions were obtained from the following databases: *Brenda* [33], *SABIO-RK* [34] and *UniProt* [35].

The tricarboxylic acid cycle reaction parameters were adapted from [36]. The equilibrium constant of reactions was assessed using *Equilibrator* [37] and the NIST database (https://randr.nist.gov/enzyme/, accessed on 3 January 2022). The unit used for the reaction fluxes in the model is mmol·L^{-1}·min^{-1}.

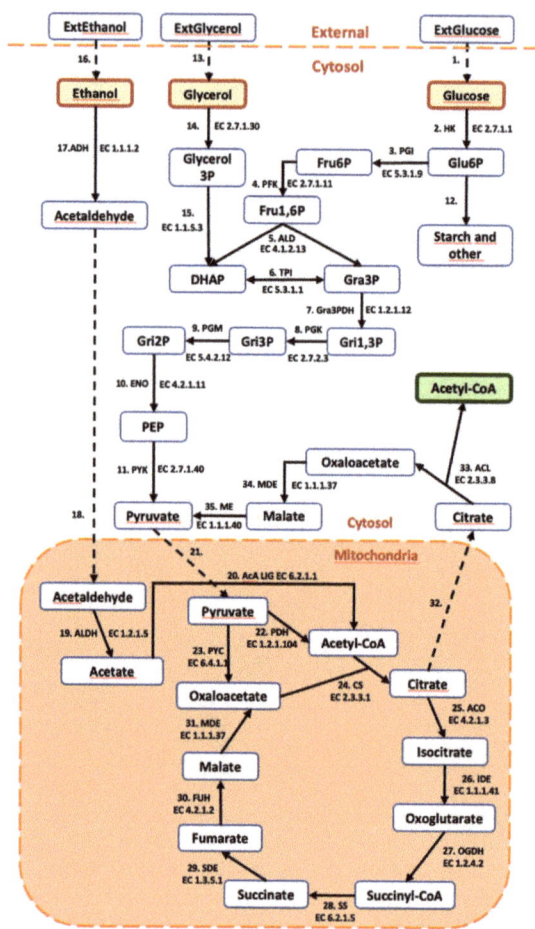

Figure 4. Metabolic network scope of the kinetic model. Dashed lines show transport reactions. Abbreviated metabolites—ExtGlucose: external glucose; ExtGlycerol: external glycerol; ExtEthanol: external ethanol; Glu6P: glucose 6-phosphate; Fru6p: fructose 6-phosphate; Fru1,6P: fructose 1,6-bisphosphate; DHAP: dihydroxyacetone phosphate; Gra3P: glyceraldehyde-3-phopshate; Gri1,3P: glycerate-1,3-biphosphate; Gri3P: glycerate-2-phosphate; Gri2P: Glycerate-2-phosphate; PEP: phosphoenolpyruvate; Acetyl-CoA: acetyl coenzyme-A. (Enzymes: HK: hexokinase; PGI: Phosphoglucose isomerase; PFK: Phosphofuctokinase; ALD: Fructosebiphosphate aldolase; TPI: Triosephosphate isomerase; Gra3PDH: Glyceraldehyde phosphate dehydrogenase; PGK: 3-phosphoglycerate kinase; PGM: Phosphoglycerolmutase; ENO: Phosphopyruvate hydratase; PYK: Pyruvate kinase; PDH: pyruvate dehydrogenase; PYC: pyruvate carboxylase; CS: citrate synthase; ACO: aconitate hydratase; IDE: isocitrate dehydrogenase; OGDH: 2-oxoglutarate dehydrogenase; SS: succinyl-CoA synthetase; SDE: succinate dehydrogenase; FUH: fumarate hydratase; MDE: malate dehydrogenase; ACL: ATP-dependent citrate lyase; ME: malic enzyme; ADH: alcohol dehydrogenase; ALDH: acetaldehyde dehydrogenase; AcA LIG: acetate CoA ligase).

2.2.2. Parameter Estimation Results

Three experimental parameter sets have been developed for the kinetic model to account for different substrate uptakes: glucose, glycerol and ethanol. The most detailed published dataset available corresponds to the consumption of glucose based on ^{13}C metabolic flux analysis [32] with a glucose consumption rate of 3.58 mmoL·min^{-1}·L^{-1} and reaction rates, including the Krebs cycle and Acetyl-CoA production. For modeling purposes, a single, concentration-independent substrate uptake rate for glycerol and ethanol was derived from the cultivation experiments described in Section 2.1.

During the parameter estimation, it became clear that a single set of model parameters could not describe all three examined substrates. The same parameter set of kinetic models could be used for glucose and glycerol experiments. This could be expected because of the common pathway of glucose and glycerol from Gra3P to pyruvate, which then enters the mitochondria, serving as the precursor for both mitochondrial oxaloacetate (reaction PYC) and mitochondrial Acetyl-CoA (reaction PDH). It turned out that, in the case of ethanol that enters the Krebs cycle via Acetyl-CoA, the PDH reaction rate had to be close to zero to facilitate all of the mitochondrial pyruvate flux towards mitochondrial oxaloacetate.

As a result, we developed two structurally identical kinetic models that were able to simulate the experimentally observed data. Both models were deposited in the BioModels [38] database in SBML (level 2 version 4) and COPASI formats: (1) glucose and glycerol consumption model (Biomodels ID: MODEL2112280001) with a Vmax of PDH being 907 mmoL·min^{-1}·L^{-1} (Supplementary Files S1 and S2) ethanol consumption model (Biomodels ID: MODEL2112290001) with a low Vmax of PDH 1e-6 mmol·min^{-1}·L^{-1} (Supplementary File S2). The parameters of the models are summarized in Supplementary File S3.

2.2.3. Simulation Results

The simulations of the glucose/glycerol model confirm the experimentally determined production flux of cellular Acetyl-CoA at 3.87 mmoL·min^{-1}·L^{-1} when consuming glucose at 3.58 mmoL·min^{-1}·L^{-1} (Table 1). The same model predicts the cellular Acetyl-CoA production flux at 1.44 mmoL·min^{-1}·L^{-1} when consuming glycerol at 2.42 mmoL·min^{-1}·L^{-1}. The ethanol model predicts a cellular Acetyl-CoA production flux of 4.76 mmol·min^{-1}·L^{-1} when consuming ethanol at 7.76 mmoL·min^{-1}·L^{-1}. This means that the percentage of substrate that undergoes carbon transformation into two carbon atoms of Acetyl-CoA is 36, 40 and 61% for glucose, glycerol and ethanol, respectively. The most efficient substrate in terms of carbon uptake (C1 moles) at the experimentally observed uptake rate is glucose (21.46 mmoL·min^{-1}·L^{-1}) followed by ethanol (15.52 mmoL·min^{-1}·L^{-1}) and glycerol (7.27 mmoL·min^{-1}·L^{-1}).

Table 1. Some simulated flux rates for different substrates.

Experimental Data	Substrate Concentration mmoL·L^{-1}	Substrate Uptake mmoL·min^{-1}·L^{-1}	Single Carbon (C1) Uptake mmoL·min^{-1}·L^{-1}	Krebs Cycle Flux mmoL·min^{-1}·L^{-1}	ACL EC 2.3.3.8 Flux mmoL·min^{-1}·L^{-1}	Specific Growth Rate μ h^{-1}
Cui et.al. 2018 [32]	Glucose, up to 50	3.58	21.46	2.43	3.87	0.051
This study	Glycerol, up to 130	2.42	7.27	0.90	1.44	0.023
This study	Ethanol, up to 32	7.76	15.52	3.00	4.76	0.046

2.3. Medium-Scale Stoichiometric Model of DHA Production

2.3.1. Validation of the Model

A medium-scale stoichiometric, central, carbon metabolism model of *C. cohnii* has been developed. The model is organized in three compartments (extracellular, cytosol and mitochondria) and has 398 reactions and 468 metabolites. Out of these 398 reactions, 35 are transport reactions (metabolite uptake, shuttle transport, metabolite output). The model simulates the uptake of the substrates, as well as H_2O, O_2, H^+ and ammonia, which is available to the *C. cohnii* for uptake in a bioreactor. The model is available in COBRA format and MS Excel format (Supplementary File S4) and is available in the BioModels database in SBML format (Bomodels ID: MODEL2112300001).

The biomass equation was created by using biomass composition data from Cui et al. [32], determining the amount of each metabolite needed to form 1 gram of biomass [39]. To determine the ratio between the nucleotides that make up the RNA and DNA, *C. cohnii* transcriptome [31] and *Symbiodinium minutum* genome [40] data were used. The unit used for the reaction fluxes in the model is mmol·gDW^{-1}·h^{-1}.

The stoichiometric model was validated using published experimental results, as well as experiments performed during this study (Table 2), reaching the specific growth rate when consuming the substrate at the experimentally observed uptake rate.

Table 2. Validation data.

Reference	Consumption mmoL·gDW^{-1}·h^{-1}	Specific Growth Rate μ h^{-1}
Cui et.al. 2018 [32]	Glucose 0.65	0.051
Cui et.al. 2018 with ETA [32]	Glucose 0.61	0.047
This study	Glucose 0.59	0.044
Taborda et al. 2021 [12]	Glucose 0.37	0.017
This study	Glycerol 0.44	0.023
Taborda et al. 2021 [12]	Glycerol 0.43	0.019
This study	Ethanol 1.41	0.046
Taborda et al. 2021 [12]	Acetate 0.60	0.025

The maximal biomass productivity with the given substrate uptake, according to validation data (Table 2), was determined by maximizing biomass production in the stoichiometric model to demonstrate that, in most cases, the μ_{max} of the model is close or higher than the experimentally observed μ (Figure 5), indicating that model predictions are close to the experimentally determined values or above them. Higher model predictions suggest that the growth in the experiment did not reach the maximal rate for unspecified reasons.

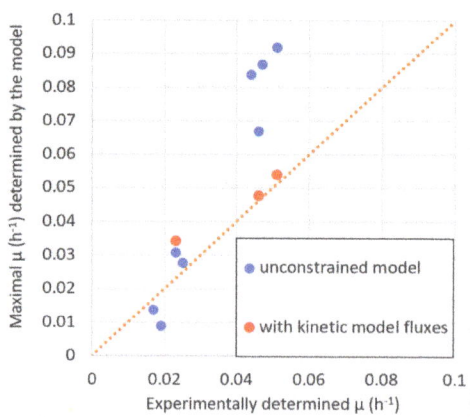

Figure 5. The stoichiometric model predicted the maximal specific growth rate μ_{max} comparison with experimentally determined μ at experimentally determined values of substrate consumption (Table 2).

2.3.2. Validation of Steady-State Fluxes of the Kinetic Model

The structure of the stoichiometric model includes all reactions of the pathway-scale kinetic model. This enables the feasibility testing of steady-state, pathway-scale kinetic model fluxes within the framework of the medium-scale stoichiometric model, namely, the biomass production at the experimentally determined substrate consumption and intracellular reaction rates of Acetyl-CoA production. This model has been validated by three steady-state flux datasets (Supplementary File S5) of simulations mentioned in Table 1.

The stoichiometric model could simulate the kinetic model steady-state fluxes of glucose consumption, largely due to the fact that the fluxes were based on ^{13}C flux experimental data that covered all relevant branches (Supplementary File S5, Sheet "Glucose").

In the case of glycerol, the kinetic model did not take into account the flux to the pentose phosphate pathway. Therefore, larger flux values for the reactions PGI, PFK and FBA were allowed in the stoichiometric model, and the small kinetic model values in glucose and ethanol uptake were set to zero (Supplementary File S5, Sheet "Glycerol").

The kinetic model steady-state flux set for ethanol consumption also had to be corrected to enable the operation of the pentose phosphate pathway in a similar way, as in the case of glycerol (Supplementary File S5, Sheet "Ethanol"). The transport rates of other substrates were set to zero.

Steady states were reached with the accepted variability of some reactions up to 4% for glucose, 10% for glycerol and 3% for ethanol. This variability was introduced to compensate for potential measurement errors and to meet the full balance pre-condition of constraint-based stoichiometric modeling.

2.4. Model-Based Determination of DHA Production Potential

The effectivity of carbon conversion into biomass can be analyzed in several ways. We looked at the biomass production rate and the efficiency of substrate carbon transformation into biomass (Table 3). The experimentally observed biomass production rate μ is the highest in the case of glucose and the lowest in the case of glycerol. However, glycerol shows the highest efficiency of substrate transformation into biomass (57.4 mmoLC1·gDW^{-1}), while glucose is the least efficient (76.5 mmoL mmoLC1·gDW^{-1}). The optimization of the stoichiometric model, without taking into account the fluxes simulated by the kinetic model, reveals that any substrate of interest can be transformed into biomass with a ratio of about 42 mmoLC1·gDW^{-1}. This means that the experimentally observed transformation rate of glycerol is the closest to the theoretical value using 35% more carbon than predicted by the model in an optimal case. In the case of glucose and ethanol, that is 80% and 45%, respectively.

The DHA production potential was determined by the stoichiometric model without taking into account the kinetic model fluxes for different biomass production intensities (Figure 6). The calculations were carried out by the stoichiometric model at experimentally observed substrate uptake rates of glucose, glycerol and ethanol. The maximal specific growth rate (μ_{max}) was determined by maximizing biomass function, assuming that all substrates will be targeted at biomass production with DHA as a part of the biomass. Knowing that the DHA fraction in the experimentally produced biomass was variable (Figure 3), we introduced a DHA production reaction to simulate DHA overproduction, which increases in cases when 80% or 40% of the maximal biomass produced. Taking into account equal substrate transformation ratios into biomass, calculated numbers are equal for all substrates.

The stoichiometric model simulations indicate that DHA production potential increases when biomass production decreases. In the case of the maximal biomass production, the percentage of substrate carbon that forms DHA grows from 27% at the maximal biomass production rate up to 70% in the case of 40% of maximal biomass production rate. The percentage of DHA in total fatty acids (TFA) increases from 39% to 81%, respectively. These calculations are based on the assumption that all metabolic resources that do not form biomass are directed by the available metabolic reactions towards the production of DHA.

Table 3. The efficiency of substrate transformation into biomass for experimentally observed and optimized data.

Experimental Data	Substrate Uptake mmoL·gDW^{-1}·h^{-1}	Carbon (C1) Uptake mmoL·gDW^{-1}·h^{-1}	Experimental		Optimized by Stoichiometric Modeling	
			μ h^{-1}	Carbon C1 per gDW Biomass mmoL·gDW^{-1}	μ_{max} h^{-1}	Carbon C1 per gDW Biomass mmoL·gDW^{-1}
Cui et.al. 2018 [32]	Glucose 0.65 (=3.58 mmol·min^{-1}·L^{-1})	3.9	0.051	76.5	0.092	42.4
This study	Glycerol 0.44 (=2.42 mmol·min^{-1}·L^{-1})	1.32	0.023	57.4	0.031	42.6
This study	Ethanol 1.41 (=7.76 mmol·min^{-1}·L^{-1})	2.82	0.046	61.3	0.067	42.1

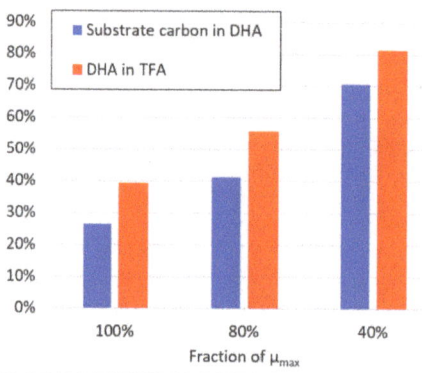

Figure 6. Estimation of DHA production potential by the constraint-based stoichiometric model at different biomass production intensities: 100% (=μ_{max}), 80% and 40%.

3. Discussion

3.1. Combining Kinetic and Stoichiometric Models

In the present study, we created kinetic and stoichiometric models of *C. cohnii*-central metabolism that are validated by ^{13}C fluxomic data [32]. The knowledge of the involvement of central metabolism reactions in the transformation of substrates to DHA is extended by the interaction of pathway-scale kinetic and constraint-based stoichiometric models to a larger scale, thus enabling a narrower scope of feasible metabolic scenarios.

Kinetic models usually cover a pathway-scale number of reactions [41]. Kinetic models contain a mathematical description of the kinetics of reaction mechanisms such as the Michaelis–Menten reaction, mass action and others. This type of model provides an opportunity to quantitatively simulate the values of metabolite concentrations and reaction fluxes. In kinetic modeling, it is optimistically assumed that the necessary energy, redox cofactor and some other metabolites are supplied by the remaining metabolism in some way [19].

In contrast to kinetic models, stoichiometric models require fewer details for individual reactions and, as a consequence, can be applied at the genome-scale [42,43]. The stoichiometric approach can be used for the analysis of feasible steady states, provided that there is information about the reaction stoichiometry. The advantage of stoichiometric models is their ability to find out whether all of the involved metabolites have precursors supplied for their production [19]. In the present work, we combined both modeling approaches [44].

The combination of both models enabled the feasibility of internal fluxes, which were calculated by the kinetic models of ethanol and glycerol, to be tested; they have never been measured experimentally. The test resulted in a rejection of some steady-state fluxes that were suggested by the kinetic model in the case of glycerol and ethanol, showing the usefulness of the iterative application of both model types. Steady-state fluxes that were kinetically feasible in the ODE-based model became unfeasible in the constraint-based stoichiometric model, where all biomass compounds had to be produced in a specific proportion. Thus, the stoichiometric model demonstrated that some fluxes simulated by the kinetic model disabled the production of all necessary metabolites in parallel with the production of biomass at the experimentally observed specific growth rate, suggesting the necessity for additional experiments to determine feasible flux distributions.

3.2. Analysis of Substrate-Specific Functioning of Central Metabolism by Experimental and Modeling Analysis

Our aim here was to employ the model simulation of central metabolism for a better understanding of the conversion of several substrates into the target product: DHA. In particular, we were interested in glycerol as a potential renewable for the synthesis of PUFAs, still poorly studied as a substrate for growth and DHA production in *C. cohnii*. We used both model types to establish (1) if the enzymatic capacity ensured the sufficient supply kinetics of Acetyl-CoA, the key central metabolite needed for DHA production, and (2) if there was the required number of metabolic precursors available for the building blocks of DHA. So far, this kind of approach has not been applied in the analysis of *C. cohnii* or any other dinoflagellates.

Both kinetic and stoichiometric models were used to simulate the observed kinetics for the uptake of glucose, ethanol and glycerol, with a particular focus on the early stages of culture growth. Kinetic and stoichiometric models were able to simulate the experimental observations (Table 2).

At the level of the pathway-scale kinetic model, it was found that the functioning of the model with ethanol as the substrate was only possible if the PDH reaction did not operate (V_{max} of PDH is close to zero). The necessity to block the reaction in the case of ethanol is determined by the fact that, in contrast to the glucose and glycerol pathways, the ethanol catabolic pathway produces mitochondrial Acetyl-CoA, and all pyruvate pools should be redirected for the regeneration of mitochondrial oxaloacetate to provide the acceptor for the CS reaction. There are several possible mechanisms for the heavy reduction in PDH flux: (1) the allosteric inhibition of PDH by Acetyl-CoA [45]; (2) the covalent modification by phosphorylation with ATP [46], and (3) the regulation of PDH expression at the transcriptional level. PDH allosteric inhibition by Acetyl-CoA seems most likely since it is supported by the kinetic model, showing higher concentrations of mitochondrial Acetyl-CoA in the case of ethanol consumption (2.1×10^{-3} mmoL·L^{-1}) than when consuming glucose (4.5×10^{-4} mmoL·L^{-1}) or glycerol (1.8×10^{-3} mmoL·L^{-1}).

We found that with glycerol, the cells grew slower than with glucose yet tended to accumulate more PUFAs, than with both other substrates (Figure 3). This is supported by the experimental observations that the carbon from glycerol is more efficiently transformed into biomass (Table 3). Potentially, another reason why glycerol is advantageous for DHA accumulation might be related to the storage of DHA in the cells. Most of the DHA in *C. cohnii* is incorporated in triacylglycerols [9]. Therefore, as DHA is being produced, part of the available glycerol could be directly utilized for triacylglycerol synthesis, removing the free DHA, and thus stimulating its synthesis. When growing on glucose or ethanol, the supply of glycerol for triacylglycerol synthesis requires additional metabolic reactions and might represent a bottleneck.

Crude glycerol, derived from biodiesel production, contains inhibitory substances, and its utilization for food-grade DHA production poses problems, as previously analyzed by Sijtsma et al. [9]. However, an unexpected observation was recently reported by Taborda et al. [12]. These authors found that crude glycerol was superior to pure glycerol with respect to DHA yields and productivity and was comparable to glucose. This might have far-reaching practical applications, yet still requires a more detailed study.

The fact that the stoichiometric model could find ways to produce DHA equally well from carbon supplied by any of the analyzed substrates indicates that some details of metabolism (inhibition due to substrate concentration or enzyme capacity limitations and other factors), which are not included in the stoichiometric model, would make the substrate conversion rate closer to the experimentally observed conversion rates. Unfortunately, a genome-scale, constraint-based stoichiometric model cannot be developed at this moment as no genome sequence of *C. cohnii* has been published.

The assumption that all free metabolic resources are targeted towards DHA production is introduced for the estimation of the production potential of DHA. Metabolic engineering [47] is needed to find out what fraction of the potential determined by the model is reachable in praxis.

The combination of ODE-based, pathway-scale kinetic modeling and constraint-based stoichiometric modeling with ^{13}C data enables a more detailed insight into the flux distribution within the organism. The combined application of different types of models enables the rejection of many unfeasible hypotheses that may arise due to the limited predictivity of each separate modeling type. Both models and their combinations can be used to explore a wider range of problems in metabolism and its optimization.

4. Materials and Methods

To explore the potential of DHA production from glycerol, glucose and ethanol, the authors combined literature data, their own experimental results, the pathway-scale kinetic model and medium-scale stoichiometric model (Figure 7). The ^{13}C data on the DHA production from glucose [32] were used to parametrize the Krebs cycle of kinetic and stoichiometric models. After that, the substrate consumption rates with corresponding biomass production rates were used to find out the potential amount of DHA that could be produced from the particular substrate. Pathway-scale kinetic models contributed here with detailed kinetic rate equations for substrate-specific transport and metabolic reactions assessing the sufficiency of the enzymatic capacity of reactions and transports. The medium-scale stoichiometric model takes into account the main duties of central metabolism to produce biomass with balanced reactions, leading to a full accounting of all elements of reactions to establish the availability of all molecules that apply balanced reactions. The DNA production potential is estimated by the stoichiometric model by fixing biomass production at a reasonable level and maximizing DHA production from the selected substrate.

4.1. Experimental Materials and Methods

Culture maintenance and cultivations were performed on a medium with sea salts and yeast extract, as described previously [30]. In brief, *Crypthecodinium cohnii* CCMP 316 was obtained from the National Center for Marine Algae and Microbiota, USA. It was cultivated on a complex medium containing 2 g L^{-1} yeast extract, 25 g L^{-1} sea salt (Sigma-Aldrich) and various concentrations of glycerol, glucose and/or ethanol, as specified in the Results section. Cultivations were carried out aerobically at 25 °C in 0.5 L or 1 L Erlenmeyer shaken flasks with 200 mL of culture on a rotary shaker at 140–180 r.p.m. The concentrations of glucose, ethanol and glycerol in culture media were monitored by HPLC, as described previously [30,48].

FTIR spectra of algal biomass were recorded using Vertex 70 coupled with the microplate reader HTS-XT (Bruker, Germany). Spectra were recorded in the frequency range of 3800–600 cm^{-1}, with a spectral resolution of 4 cm^{-1}, and 64 scans were coadded. Only spectra with absorbance within the absorption limits between 0.25 and 0.80 (where the concentration of a component is proportional to the intensity of the absorption band) were used for data analysis. The FTIR spectra were vector normalized and deconvoluted (second derivative) for more precise evaluation of weak-intensity spectral bands and to resolve the overlapping components, if any [49]. Data were processed using OPUS 7.5 software (Bruker Optics GmbH, Ettlingen, Germany). The baseline of each spectrum was corrected by the rubber band method.

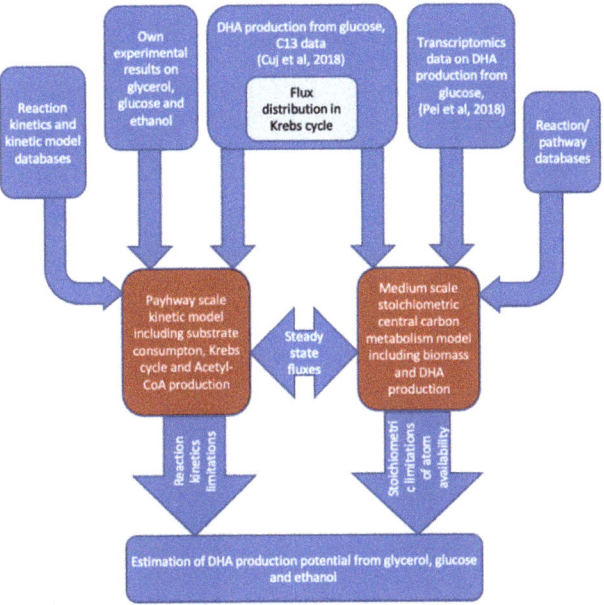

Figure 7. Information flow-to and -from pathway-scale kinetic model and central carbon metabolism scale constraint-based stoichiometric model.

4.2. Development of a Pathway-Scale Kinetic Model

The model was developed in *COPASI* (COmplex PAthway SImulator) simulation software [50,51] version 4.34 (Build 251). The estimation for kinetic equation parameters that were not found in literature or databases was conducted using built-in parameter estimation functionality using global stochastic optimization methods. The model-specific parameter estimation performance of global stochastic optimization methods implemented in *COPASI* was tested using *ConvAn* software [52]. During parameter estimation, multiple parallel optimization runs were applied, using *COPASI* wrapper *SpaceScanner* [53] to select the most efficient global stochastic optimization algorithms, reducing misinterpretation risks of optimization results [54]. The total concentration of used amino acids in the reactions included in the model was limited to avoid unnecessarily high enzyme concentrations that would not be evolutionarily favorable.

Model parameters were either obtained from the literature or inferred from experimental data. An additional parameter V_m was added to the reactions used from [36] to change the V_{max} of these reactions without changing the V_f to V_r ratios. Kinetic equations of all enzymatic reactions had overexpression coefficients k that could be used for optimizing enzyme concentrations to increase Acetyl-CoA or other molecule production. Currently, all coefficients $k = 1$ so that the model corresponds to wild-type concentrations of enzymes.

Species concentration constraints were applied in the parameter estimation task in *COPASI*. From Park et al. [55], it was implemented as a constraint that the metabolite concentrations in this model should not exceed 12 mmol/L, except for cellular ethanol, which was allowed to reach 32 mmoL/L.

The metabolic flux unit in the kinetic model is $mmoL \cdot min^{-1} \cdot L^{-1}$ since it is frequently used in kinetic models, while in the stoichiometric model, the metabolic flux unit is $mmoL \cdot gDW^{-1} \cdot h^{-1}$. To transition from dry-weight-related measurements to absolute weight, it was assumed that dry weight made up 33% of the absolute weight and the cell density was $1 \ g \cdot mL^{-1}$. Mitochondrial volume was made to be 1% of the cytosol volume [56].

To determine the parameters that were dependent on enzyme concentrations, three sets of experimental data were used. The first set included reaction fluxes adapted from Cui et al. ^{13}C metabolic flux analysis for growth on glucose. The second and third sets included experimentally measured glycerol and ethanol consumption rates (Section 2.1) determined during this study. The experimental data of glucose consumption were not used in parameter estimation due to the high similarity with ^{13}C experimental data. The *Parameter estimation* task was used in *COPASI*; the data sets were added as different experiments.

4.3. Development of the Constraint-Based Medium-Scale Stoichiometric Model

A constraint-based, medium-scale stoichiometric model [57] of central carbon metabolism, biomass production and pathways to DHA was developed, extending the scope of the kinetic model. Reactions were included in the model based on the results of transcriptomics [31] and on the reactions from the genome annotation of the *Symbiodinium minutum* genome, which is a phylogenetically close relative of *C. cohnii*. The specific growth rate was calculated by an exponential approximation of the growth curve. It is assumed that DHA production is constant during the growth period.

The model was built and optimized using COBRA Toolbox v3.0 [58] and RAVEN 2.0 [59] functionality. The model was visualized by Paint4Net [60], Escher [61] and IMFLer [62] software.

The model was validated using the experimental data generated during this study and those found in the literature.

5. Conclusions

Kinetic and stoichiometric modeling-based analysis demonstrates the attractiveness of glycerol as a substrate for DHA (main fraction of PUFA [30]) production by *C. cohnii*, along with established substrates, such as ethanol and glucose. This is proven experimentally and analyzed mathematically by mechanistic models of *C. cohnii* metabolism. The promising results on the applicability of crude glycerol [12] increase the attractivity of glycerol even further.

The iterative application of the pathway-scale kinetic model and constraint-based stoichiometric model combines the accuracy of the kinetic model of the main product-forming pathways with the large-scale stoichiometric model's ability to determine if the pathways addressed by the kinetic model could be supplied with all of the necessary molecular components. Simultaneously, biomass could be produced by the metabolic network of the organism of interest. This approach is important for improving the understanding of metabolic network functionality and increasing the predictability and efficiency of metabolic engineering efforts.

Our experiments, in combination with modeling, supported the potential of glycerol as another renewable substrate of *C. cohnii* for the production of DHA. Despite a lower consumption rate and lower specific growth rate, the PUFA content and efficiency of carbon transformation into biomass are better with glycerol than with glucose. Therefore, the sustainability parameters [63] of DHA production from glycerol are expected to be better than in the case of glucose and ethanol.

Supplementary Materials: The following are available online at https://www.mdpi.com/article/10.3390/md20020115/s1, File S1: Kinetic model for Acetyl-CoA production from glucose and glycerol by *C. cohnii*, File S2: Kinetic model for Acetyl-CoA production from ethanol by *C. cohnii*, File S3: Parameters of kinetic models for Acetyl-CoA production from glucose, glycerol and ethanol by *C. cohnii*, File S4: Constraint-based stoichiometric model of central metabolism of *C. cohnii*, File S5: Flux distribution of kinetic models for Acetyl-CoA production from glucose, glycerol and ethanol (columns A–C and F). The supplementary information includes also flux values adapted for stoichiometric model simulations (columns D and E). Reactions marked by yellow are reactions, which are set to zero in stoichiometric model. Reactions marked by green are set to default upper and lower bounds (1000 and −1000 respectivelly).

Author Contributions: Conceptualization, E.S., D.P., A.P., V.G., K.B. and U.K.; methodology, E.S. and U.K.; software, R.M., S.P. and K.B.; validation, R.M., M.R.B. and K.B.; formal analysis, K.S., E.S. and U.K.; investigation, I.S., S.P., R.M., M.R.B., K.S., M.G. and K.B.; resources, I.S., M.G. and U.K.; data curation, S.P., K.B. and M.G.; writing—original draft preparation, R.M., K.B., M.G., E.S. and U.K.; writing—review and editing, R.M., M.R.B., E.S., D.P., A.P., V.G. and U.K.; visualization, R.M. and E.S.; supervision, E.S. and U.K.; project administration, E.S.; funding acquisition, A.P., E.S. and U.K. All authors have read and agreed to the published version of the manuscript.

Funding: This work was funded by the Latvian ERDF project 1.1.1.1/18/A/022. R.M., M.R.B. and A.P. were supported by University of Latvia under project "Climate change and its impacts on sustainability of natural resources" (Nr. Y5-AZ20-ZF-N-270).

Institutional Review Board Statement: Not applicable.

Data Availability Statement: Data is contained within the article or supplementary material.

Conflicts of Interest: The authors declare no conflict of interest.

References

1. Adarme-Vega, T.C.; Thomas-Hall, S.R.; Schenk, P.M. Towards Sustainable Sources for Omega-3 Fatty Acids Production. *Curr. Opin. Biotechnol.* **2014**, *26*, 14–18. [CrossRef] [PubMed]
2. Oliver, L.; Dietrich, T.; Marañón, I.; Villarán, M.C.; Barrio, R.J. Producing Omega-3 Polyunsaturated Fatty Acids: A Review of Sustainable Sources and Future Trends for the EPA and DHA Market. *Resources* **2020**, *9*, 148. [CrossRef]
3. Ji, X.-J.; Ren, L.-J.; Huang, H. Omega-3 Biotechnology: A Green and Sustainable Process for Omega-3 Fatty Acids Production. *Front. Bioeng. Biotechnol.* **2015**, *3*, 1301–1315. [CrossRef] [PubMed]
4. Graham, I.A.; Larson, T.; Napier, J.A. Rational Metabolic Engineering of Transgenic Plants for Biosynthesis of Omega-3 Polyunsaturates. *Curr. Opin. Biotechnol.* **2007**, *18*, 142–147. [CrossRef]
5. Santos-Sánchez, N.F.; Valadez-Blanco, R.; Hernández-Carlos, B.; Torres-Ariño, A.; Guadarrama-Mendoza, P.C.; Salas-Coronado, R. Lipids Rich in ω-3 Polyunsaturated Fatty Acids from Microalgae. *Appl. Microbiol. Biotechnol.* **2016**, *100*, 8667–8684. [CrossRef] [PubMed]
6. Mendes, A.; Reis, A.; Vasconcelos, R.; Guerra, P.; Lopes Da Silva, T. Crypthecodinium Cohnii with Emphasis on DHA Production: A Review. *J. Appl. Phycol.* **2009**, *21*, 199–214. [CrossRef]
7. Sijtsma, L.; de Swaaf, M.E. Biotechnological Production and Applications of the ω-3 Polyunsaturated Fatty Acid Docosahexaenoic Acid. *Appl. Microbiol. Biotechnol.* **2004**, *64*, 146–153. [CrossRef] [PubMed]
8. de Swaaf, M.E.; de Rijk, T.C.; Eggink, G.; Sijtsma, L. Optimisation of Docosahexaenoic Acid Production in Batch Cultivations by Crypthecodinium Cohnii. *Prog. Ind. Microbiol.* **1999**, *35*, 185–192. [CrossRef]
9. Sijtsma, L.; Anderson, A.J.; Ratledge, C. Alternative Carbon Sources for Heterotrophic Production of Docosahexaenoic Acid by the Marine Alga Crypthecodinium Cohnii. In *Single Cell Oils*; Elsevier: Amsterdam, The Netherlands, 2010; pp. 131–149.
10. Safdar, W.; Zan, X.; Song, Y. Synergistic Effects of PH, Temperature and Agitation on Growth Kinetics and Docosahexaenoic Acid Production of C. Cohnii Cultured on Different Carbon Sources. *Int. J. Res. Agric. Sci.* **2017**, *4*, 94–101.
11. Moniz, P.; Silva, C.; Oliveira, A.C.; Reis, A.; Lopes da Silva, T. Raw Glycerol Based Medium for Dha and Lipids Production, Using the Marine Heterotrophic Microalga Crypthecodinium Cohnii. *Processes* **2021**, *9*, 2005. [CrossRef]
12. Taborda, T.; Moniz, P.; Reis, A.; da Silva, T.L. Evaluating Low-Cost Substrates for Crypthecodinium Cohnii Lipids and DHA Production, by Flow Cytometry. *J. Appl. Phycol.* **2021**, *33*, 263–274. [CrossRef]
13. Pentjuss, A.; Kalnenieks, U. Assessment of Zymomonas Mobilis Biotechnological Potential in Ethanol Production by Flux Variability Analysis. *Biosyst. Inf. Technol.* **2014**, *3*, 1–5. [CrossRef]
14. Pentjuss, A.; Stalidzans, E.; Liepins, J.; Kokina, A.; Martynova, J.; Zikmanis, P.; Mozga, I.; Scherbaka, R.; Hartman, H.; Poolman, M.G.; et al. Model-Based Biotechnological Potential Analysis of Kluyveromyces Marxianus Central Metabolism. *J. Ind. Microbiol. Biotechnol.* **2017**, *44*, 1177–1190. [CrossRef] [PubMed]
15. Otero, J.M.; Nielsen, J. Industrial Systems Biology. *Biotechnol. Bioeng.* **2010**, *105*, 439–460. [CrossRef] [PubMed]
16. Palsson, B.O. Metabolic Systems Biology. *FEBS Lett.* **2009**, *583*, 3900–3904. [CrossRef] [PubMed]
17. Cvijovic, M.; Höfer, T.; Aćimović, J.; Alberghina, L.; Almaas, E.; Besozzi, D.; Blomberg, A.; Bretschneider, T.; Cascante, M.; Collin, O.; et al. Strategies for Structuring Interdisciplinary Education in Systems Biology: An European Perspective. *NPJ Syst. Biol. Appl.* **2016**, *2*, 16011. [CrossRef] [PubMed]
18. Stelling, J. Mathematical Models in Microbial Systems Biology. *Curr. Opin. Microbiol.* **2004**, *7*, 513–518. [CrossRef]
19. Stalidzans, E.; Seiman, A.; Peebo, K.; Komasilovs, V.; Pentjuss, A. Model-Based Metabolism Design: Constraints for Kinetic and Stoichiometric Models. *Biochem. Soc. Trans.* **2018**, *46*, 261–267. [CrossRef]
20. de Swaaf, M.E.; Pronk, J.T.; Sijtsma, L. Fed-Batch Cultivation of the Docosahexaenoic-Acid-Producing Marine Alga Crypthecodinium Cohnii on Ethanol. *Appl. Microbiol. Biotechnol.* **2003**, *61*, 40–43. [CrossRef]

21. Didrihsone, E.; Dubencovs, K.; Grube, M.; Shvirksts, K.; Suleiko, A.; Suleiko, A.; Vanags, J. Cryptecodinium Cohnii Growth and Omega Fatty Acid Production in Mediums Supplemented with Extract from Recycled Bio-Mass. *Mar. Drugs* **2022**, *20*, 68. [CrossRef] [PubMed]
22. Ripoche, A.; Guillard, A.S. Determination of Fatty Acid Composition of Pork Fat by Fourier Transform Infrared Spectroscopy. *Meat Sci.* **2001**, *58*, 299–304. [CrossRef]
23. Ami, D.; Posteri, R.; Mereghetti, P.; Porro, D.; Doglia, S.M.; Branduardi, P. Fourier Transform Infrared Spectroscopy as a Method to Study Lipid Accumulation in Oleaginous Yeasts. *Biotechnol. Biofuels* **2014**, *7*, 12. [CrossRef] [PubMed]
24. Ferreira, R.; Lourenço, S.; Lopes, A.; Andrade, C.; Câmara, J.S.; Castilho, P.; Perestrelo, R. Evaluation of Fatty Acids Profile as a Useful Tool towards Valorization of By-Products of Agri-Food Industry. *Foods* **2021**, *10*, 2867. [CrossRef]
25. Yoshida, S.; Yoshida, H. Noninvasive Analyses of Polyunsaturated Fatty Acids in Human Oral Mucosa in Vivo by Fourier-Transform Infrared Spectroscopy. *Biopolymers* **2004**, *74*, 403–412. [CrossRef] [PubMed]
26. Mendes, A.; Guerra, P.; Madeira, V.; Ruano, F.; Lopes da Silva, T.; Reis, A. Study of Docosahexaenoic Acid Production by the Heterotrophic Microalga Cryptecodinium Cohnii CCMP 316 Using Carob Pulp as a Promising Carbon Source. *World J. Microbiol. Biotechnol.* **2007**, *23*, 1209–1215. [CrossRef]
27. Chalima, A.; Taxeidis, G.; Topakas, E. Optimization of the Production of Docosahexaenoic Fatty Acid by the Heterotrophic Microalga Cryptecodinium Cohnii Utilizing a Dark Fermentation Effluent. *Renew. Energy* **2020**, *152*, 102–109. [CrossRef]
28. Diao, J.; Li, X.; Pei, G.; Liu, L.; Chen, L. Comparative Metabolomic Analysis of Cryptecodinium Cohnii in Response to Different Dissolved Oxygen Levels during Docosahexaenoic Acid Fermentation. *Biochem. Biophys. Res. Commun.* **2018**, *499*, 941–947. [CrossRef]
29. Lopes da Silva, T.; Reis, A. The Use of Multi-Parameter Flow Cytometry to Study the Impact of n-Dodecane Additions to Marine Dinoflagellate Microalga Cryptecodinium Cohnii Batch Fermentations and DHA Production. *J. Ind. Microbiol. Biotechnol.* **2008**, *35*, 875–887. [CrossRef] [PubMed]
30. Strazdina, I.; Klavins, L.; Galinina, N.; Shvirksts, K.; Grube, M.; Stalidzans, E.; Kalnenieks, U. Syntrophy of Cryptecodinium Cohnii and Immobilized Zymomonas Mobilis for Docosahexaenoic Acid Production from Sucrose-Containing Substrates. *J. Biotechnol.* **2021**, *338*, 63–70. [CrossRef]
31. Pei, G.; Li, X.; Liu, L.; Liu, J.; Wang, F.; Chen, L.; Zhang, W. De Novo Transcriptomic and Metabolomic Analysis of Docosahexaenoic Acid (DHA)-Producing Cryptecodinium Cohnii during Fed-Batch Fermentation. *Algal Res.* **2017**, *26*, 380–391. [CrossRef]
32. Cui, J.; Diao, J.; Sun, T.; Shi, M.; Liu, L.; Wang, F.; Chen, L.; Zhang, W. 13C Metabolic Flux Analysis of Enhanced Lipid Accumulation Modulated by Ethanolamine in Cryptecodinium Cohnii. *Front. Microbiol.* **2018**, *9*, 956. [CrossRef] [PubMed]
33. Chang, A.; Jeske, L.; Ulbrich, S.; Hofmann, J.; Koblitz, J.; Schomburg, I.; Neumann-Schaal, M.; Jahn, D.; Schomburg, D. BRENDA, the ELIXIR Core Data Resource in 2021: New Developments and Updates. *Nucleic Acids Res.* **2021**, *49*, D498–D508. [CrossRef] [PubMed]
34. Wittig, U.; Kania, R.; Golebiewski, M.; Rey, M.; Shi, L.; Jong, L.; Algaa, E.; Weidemann, A.; Sauer-Danzwith, H.; Mir, S.; et al. SABIO-RK–Database for Biochemical Reaction Kinetics. *Nucleic Acids Res.* **2012**, *40*, D790–D796. [CrossRef] [PubMed]
35. Bateman, A.; Martin, M.J.; O'Donovan, C.; Magrane, M.; Alpi, E.; Antunes, R.; Bely, B.; Bingley, M.; Bonilla, C.; Britto, R.; et al. UniProt: The Universal Protein Knowledgebase. *Nucleic Acids Res.* **2017**, *45*, D158–D169. [CrossRef]
36. Singh, V.K.; Ghosh, I. Kinetic Modeling of Tricarboxylic Acid Cycle and Glyoxylate Bypass in Mycobacterium Tuberculosis, and Its Application to Assessment of Drug Targets. *Theor. Biol. Med. Model.* **2006**, *3*, 27. [CrossRef]
37. Flamholz, A.; Noor, E.; Bar-Even, A.; Milo, R. Equilibrator—The Biochemical Thermodynamics Calculator. *Nucleic Acids Res.* **2012**, *40*, D770–D775. [CrossRef]
38. Malik-Sheriff, R.S.; Glont, M.; Nguyen, T.V.N.; Tiwari, K.; Roberts, M.G.; Xavier, A.; Vu, M.T.; Men, J.; Maire, M.; Kananathan, S.; et al. BioModels-15 Years of Sharing Computational Models in Life Science. *Nucleic Acids Res.* **2020**, *48*, D407–D415. [CrossRef]
39. Feist, A.M.; Palsson, B.O. The Biomass Objective Function. *Curr. Opin. Microbiol.* **2010**, *13*, 344–349. [CrossRef]
40. Shoguchi, E.; Shinzato, C.; Kawashima, T.; Gyoja, F.; Mungpakdee, S.; Koyanagi, R.; Takeuchi, T.; Hisata, K.; Tanaka, M.; Fujiwara, M.; et al. Draft Assembly of the Symbiodinium Minutum Nuclear Genome Reveals Dinoflagellate Gene Structure. *Curr. Biol.* **2013**, *23*, 1399–1408. [CrossRef]
41. Almquist, J.; Cvijovic, M.; Hatzimanikatis, V.; Nielsen, J.; Jirstrand, M. Kinetic Models in Industrial Biotechnology—Improving Cell Factory Performance. *Metab. Eng.* **2014**, *24*, 38–60. [CrossRef]
42. Price, N.D.; Papin, J.A.; Schilling, C.H.; Palsson, B.O. Genome-Scale Microbial in Silico Models: The Constraints-Based Approach. *Trends Biotechnol.* **2003**, *21*, 162–169. [CrossRef]
43. Thiele, I.; Palsson, B.O. A Protocol for Generating a High-Quality Genome-Scale Metabolic Reconstruction. *Nat. Protoc.* **2010**, *5*, 93–121. [CrossRef]
44. Kalnenieks, U.; Pentjuss, A.; Rutkis, R.; Stalidzans, E.; Fell, D.A. Modeling of Zymomonas Mobilis Central Metabolism for Novel Metabolic Engineering Strategies. *Front. Microbiol.* **2014**, *5*, 42. [CrossRef]
45. Schrenk, D.F.; Bisswanger, H. Measurements of Electron Spin Resonance with the Pyruvate Dehydrogenase Complex from Escherichia Coli. *Eur. J. Biochem.* **1984**, *143*, 561–566. [CrossRef] [PubMed]
46. Pelley, J.W. Glycolysis and Pyruvate Oxidation. In *Elsevier's Integrated Biochemistry*; Elsevier: Amsterdam, The Netherlands, 2007; pp. 47–53.

47. Nielsen, J. Metabolic Engineering: Techniques for Analysis of Targets for Genetic Manipulations. *Biotechnol. Bioeng.* **1998**, *58*, 125–132. [CrossRef]
48. Strazdina, I.; Balodite, E.; Lasa, Z.; Rutkis, R.; Galinina, N.; Kalnenieks, U. Aerobic Catabolism and Respiratory Lactate Bypass in Ndh-Negative Zymomonas Mobilis. *Metab. Eng. Commun.* **2018**, *7*, e00081. [CrossRef]
49. Susi, H.; Byler, D.M. Resolution-Enhanced Fourier Transform Infrared Spectroscopy of Enzymes. *Methods Enzymol.* **1986**, *130*, 290–311. [CrossRef] [PubMed]
50. Hoops, S.; Sahle, S.; Gauges, R.; Lee, C.; Pahle, J.; Simus, N.; Singhal, M.; Xu, L.; Mendes, P.; Kummer, U. COPASI—A complex pathway simulator. *Bioinformatics* **2006**, *22*, 3067–3074. [CrossRef]
51. Mendes, P.; Hoops, S.; Sahle, S.; Gauges, R.; Dada, J.O.; Kummer, U. Computational Modeling of Biochemical Networks Using COPASI. In *Methods in Molecular Biology, Systems Biology*; Maly, I.V., Ed.; Humana Press: Totowa, NJ, USA, 2009; Volume 500, pp. 17–59. ISBN 978-1-934115-64-0.
52. Kostromins, A.; Mozga, I.; Stalidzans, E. ConvAn: A Convergence Analyzing Tool for Optimization of Biochemical Networks. *Biosystems* **2012**, *108*, 73–77. [CrossRef]
53. Elsts, A.; Pentjuss, A.; Stalidzans, E. SpaceScanner: COPASI Wrapper for Automated Management of Global Stochastic Optimization Experiments. *Bioinformatics* **2017**, *33*, 2966–2967. [CrossRef]
54. Stalidzans, E.; Landmane, K.; Sulins, J.; Sahle, S. Misinterpretation Risks of Global Stochastic Optimisation of Kinetic Models Revealed by Multiple Optimisation Runs. *Math. Biosci.* **2019**, *307*, 25–32. [CrossRef] [PubMed]
55. Park, J.O.; Rubin, S.A.; Xu, Y.-F.; Amador-Noguez, D.; Fan, J.; Shlomi, T.; Rabinowitz, J.D. Metabolite Concentrations, Fluxes and Free Energies Imply Efficient Enzyme Usage. *Nat. Chem. Biol.* **2016**, *12*, 482–489. [CrossRef] [PubMed]
56. Uchida, M.; Sun, Y.; McDermott, G.; Knoechel, C.; le Gros, M.A.; Parkinson, D.; Drubin, D.G.; Larabell, C.A. Quantitative Analysis of Yeast Internal Architecture Using Soft X-ray Tomography. *Yeast* **2011**, *28*, 227–236. [CrossRef] [PubMed]
57. Bordbar, A.; Monk, J.M.; King, Z.A.; Palsson, B.O. Constraint-Based Models Predict Metabolic and Associated Cellular Functions. *Nat. Rev. Genet.* **2014**, *15*, 107–120. [CrossRef] [PubMed]
58. Heirendt, L.; Arreckx, S.; Pfau, T.; Mendoza, S.N.; Richelle, A.; Heinken, A.; Haraldsdóttir, H.S.; Wachowiak, J.; Keating, S.M.; Vlasov, V.; et al. Creation and Analysis of Biochemical Constraint-Based Models Using the COBRA Toolbox v.3.0. *Nat. Protoc.* **2019**, *14*, 639–702. [CrossRef]
59. Wang, H.; Marcišauskas, S.; Sánchez, B.J.; Domenzain, I.; Hermansson, D.; Agren, R.; Nielsen, J.; Kerkhoven, E.J. RAVEN 2.0: A Versatile Toolbox for Metabolic Network Reconstruction and a Case Study on Streptomyces Coelicolor. *PLoS Comput. Biol.* **2018**, *14*, e1006541. [CrossRef]
60. Kostromins, A.; Stalidzans, E. Paint4Net: COBRA Toolbox Extension for Visualization of Stoichiometric Models of Metabolism. *Biosystems* **2012**, *109*, 233–239. [CrossRef] [PubMed]
61. King, Z.A.; Dräger, A.; Ebrahim, A.; Sonnenschein, N.; Lewis, N.E.; Palsson, B.O. Escher: A Web Application for Building, Sharing, and Embedding Data-Rich Visualizations of Biological Pathways. *PLoS Comput. Biol.* **2015**, *11*, e1004321. [CrossRef]
62. Petrovs, R.; Stalidzans, E.; Pentjuss, A. IMFLer: A Web Application for Interactive Metabolic Flux Analysis and Visualization. *J. Comput. Biol.* **2021**, *28*, 1021–1032. [CrossRef]
63. Stalidzans, E.; Dace, E. Sustainable Metabolic Engineering for Sustainability Optimisation of Industrial Biotechnology. *Comput. Struct. Biotechnol. J.* **2021**, *19*, 4770–4776. [CrossRef] [PubMed]

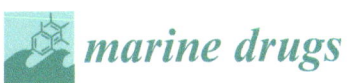

Article

Crypthecodinium cohnii Growth and Omega Fatty Acid Production in Mediums Supplemented with Extract from Recycled Biomass

Elina Didrihsone [1,*], Konstantins Dubencovs [1,2,3], Mara Grube [4], Karlis Shvirksts [4], Anastasija Suleiko [1], Arturs Suleiko [1,2] and Juris Vanags [1,2,3]

1. Latvian State Institute of Wood Chemistry, LV1006 Riga, Latvia; gmtd@inbox.lv (K.D.); anastasija.gurcinska@gmail.com (A.S.); arturs.suleiko@bioreactors.net (A.S.); btc@edi.lv (J.V.)
2. A/S Biotehniskais Centrs, LV1006 Riga, Latvia
3. Institute of General Chemical Engineering, Faculty of Materials Science and Applied Chemistry, Riga Technical University, LV1048 Riga, Latvia
4. Institute of Microbiology and Biotechnology, University of Latvia, LV1004 Riga, Latvia; mara.grube@lu.lv (M.G.); karlis.svirksts@lu.lv (K.S.)
* Correspondence: elina.didrihsone@kki.lv

Abstract: *Crypthecodinium cohnii* is a marine heterotrophic dinoflagellate that can accumulate high amounts of omega-3 polyunsaturated fatty acids (PUFAs), and thus has the potential to replace conventional PUFAs production with eco-friendlier technology. So far, *C. cohnii* cultivation has been mainly carried out with the use of yeast extract (YE) as a nitrogen source. In the present study, alternative carbon and nitrogen sources were studied: the extraction ethanol (EE), remaining after lipid extraction, as a carbon source, and dinoflagellate extract (DE) from recycled algae biomass *C. cohnii* as a source of carbon, nitrogen, and vitamins. In mediums with glucose and DE, the highest specific biomass growth rate reached a maximum of 1.012 h^{-1}, while the biomass yield from substrate reached 0.601 $g \cdot g^{-1}$. EE as the carbon source, in comparison to pure ethanol, showed good results in terms of stimulating the biomass growth rate (an 18.5% increase in specific biomass growth rate was observed). DE supplement to the EE-based mediums promoted both the biomass growth (the specific growth rate reached 0.701 h^{-1}) and yield from the substrate (0.234 $g \cdot g^{-1}$). The FTIR spectroscopy data showed that mediums supplemented with EE or DE promoted the accumulation of PUFAs/docosahexaenoic acid (DHA), when compared to mediums containing glucose and commercial YE.

Keywords: *Crypthecodinium cohnii*; omega-3 fatty acid; biomass recycling; dinoflagellate extract; FTIR spectroscopy

1. Introduction

One of the most commercially important representatives of the omega-3 fatty acids' (FAs) group is docosahexaenoic acid (DHA), which is a long-chain, highly polyunsaturated omega-3 (n-3) fatty acid (LC-PUFA). DHA is considered one of the most significant and beneficial fatty acids for the health of infants and adults. Numerous research papers have reported that DHA supports the human cardiovascular and nervous systems, prevents the occurrence of inflammatory diseases, alleviates depression, and treats psoriasis and rheumatoid arthritis. Furthermore, DHA plays a key role in the healthy development of the fetal brain and retina, thus it is commonly included in infant-oriented food products and supplements [1,2].

Currently, the main source of DHA is fish oil. However, when compared to microbial DHA, fish-derived PUFAs lack the flexibility of its biosynthetic counterpart, as availability of raw materials (e.g., fish oil for its production) strongly depends on fish resources (e.g., seasonality and geographical location). The fish oil purification process is also quite difficult, and the resulting product remains unsuitable for all dietary requirements (e.g., vegetarians and vegans) [3–5]. Furthermore, fish oil has a specific odour and taste, which is unpleasant for a noticeable part of people, especially infants. Therefore, omega-3 FA obtainment from fish is suboptimal and poses a negative effect on the environment. Moreover, conventional DHA production currently cannot meet the increasing demand for omega-3 FA for human consumption [5].

A wide misconception is that fish produce DHA themselves through specific metabolic pathways, which are semi-unique to aquatic life forms. Marine organisms, especially different families of fish, in their natural habitats accumulate omega-3 FAs in their organisms through feeding on zooplankton, which in turn consumes the primary omega-3 FAs producers, namely microalgae [2]. However, in fish farms, the use of eicosapentaenoic acid (EPA) and DHA as feed supplements has become a conventional practice. The demand for products containing omega-3 FA has significantly increased during the past decades. However, due to insufficient fish resources, the global market currently is in crisis. As of now, the global fish oil production reaches approximately 1 million metric tonnes per year, of which ~70% is generally used for aquafeeds [6].

Considering all of the above mentioned, direct methods for FAs acquisition from unicellular microorganisms, which have the ability to synthesize DHA on their own, becomes preferable, even though the cost of edible microbial oil is estimated to reach 3000–5000 USD per kg [7], which is considerably higher than conventional fish oil, estimated to exceed 2000 USD per metric ton [6]. Besides, the concentration of DHA in single cell oil (SCO), for example, from *Crypthecodinium cohnii*, can reach much higher concentrations when compared to fish oil (54% and 12% by mass, respectively) [8,9].

Cultivated microalgae-derived oil does not contain heavy metals and cholesterol, and has a neutral taste, which can be easily enhanced depending on the consumer requirements [2]. The average lipid content in microalgae biomass is from 20 to 50% by mass. However, under stress conditions, it can reach even higher levels (up to 85%) [10]. Microalgae species such as *C. cohnii*, *Nannochloropsis gaditana*, *Isochrysis galbana* and *Phaeodactylum tricornutum* were proven to be suitable for production of PUFAs on a commercial scale [10]. Multiple commercial scale applications were already previously studied and successfully put into commission (e.g., microalgae cultivation in tubular and flat panel bioreactors [10] and transgenic oilseed plants [11]), which indicates the severity of the DHA shortage that the world is experiencing right now.

A marine dinoflagellate *C. cohnii* can accumulate PUFAs in significant amounts (up to 25% of DHA or 35% of FAs of dry weight [2,8])and therefore it has been used previously for industrial production of omega-3 fatty acids [12]. However, in *C. cohnii* cultivation processes, yeast extract (YE) is conventionally used as the nitrogen source, which noticeably affects the cost of the target products [3]. Therefore, the identification of a cheap and renewable substrate for a highly efficient DHA production by *C. cohnii* is necessary. In the literature, suitable carbon sources have been widely studied (e.g., glucose, acetate, glycerol, oleic acid, acetic acid, ethanol, rapeseed meal hydrolysate, crude waste molasses, cheese whey, corn steep liquor, tagatose, carob syrup, date syrup, and galacturonic acid) [3,4,13–16]. The results (see Table 1) show that the highest biomass concentrations were achieved using acetic acid and ethanol in fed-batch fermentations (109 g·L^{-1} and 83 g·L^{-1}, respectively [17,18]) and in batch fermentations with glucose and acetate (27.7 g·L^{-1} and 7.03 g·L^{-1}, respectively [4,19]). The highest DHA concentrations 19 g·L^{-1} and 11.7 g·L^{-1} were achieved using acetic acid and ethanol, respectively, as carbon sources in fed-batch fermentations [17,18]. In batch fermentations, the highest DHA titres have been achieved with glucose (1.6 g·L^{-1} and 1.4 g·L^{-1}) [19,20]. However, the effect of nitrogen sources on the cultivation efficiency has not been studied as extensively as carbon sources. Suitable nitrogen sources for marine protists are tryptone, yeast extract, peptone, soy peptone, urea, monosodium glutamate, nitrate, ammonia, and ammonium chloride [3,13]. It also should be noted that some marine protists (e.g., *Schizochytrium* species) can utilize a wider range of nitrogen sources than others (e.g., *Crypthecodinium* species) [13]. Although nitrogen source variation in *C. cohnii* cultivations has been employed, e.g., urea, yeast extract, meat extract, glutamic acid, ammonium sulphate, ammonium bicarbonate, sodium nitrite, and ammonium nitrate [15,21,22], yet mostly the effect of the nitrogen source on the *C. cohnii* growth has not been the focus of the past studies. The highest DHA titres in microalgae cells—0.99 g·L^{-1}, has been observed when sodium nitrate was utilized [22]. The highest total lipid content, 28.48%, 18.67%, and 18.14% of dry cell weight (DCW), has been observed utilizing threonine, yeast extract, and sodium nitrate, respectively [21–23]. Moreover, to the authors' knowledge, there have been no attempts to use a recycled waste product as a nitrogen source as it will be outlined in the present study.

Table 1. *C. cohnii* growth parameters, DHA, and lipid production with different carbon and nitrogen sources.

Carbon Source	Nitrogen Source	Fermentation Mode	μ_{max}, h^{-1}	Biomass, g·L^{-1}	$Y_{x/s}$, g·g^{-1}	DHA, g·L^{-1}	Lipid,% of DCW	Ref.
Acetate	Ammonium sulphate *	Batch	-	~7.7	-	-	-	[21]
	Yeast extract *		-	~6.0	-	-	18.67 **	
			0.025	7.03	-	0.03118 ± 0.00160	12.43 ± 0.62	[4]
Acetic acid	Ammonium sulphate *	Fed-batch	-	-	-	0.1016	-	[21]
	Yeast extract *		-	-	-	0.1629	-	
			0.053	109	0.13	19	55.69 **	[17]
Ethanol	Yeast extract	Fed-batch	0.05	83	0.31	11.7	42.17 **	[18]
Galacturonic acid	Yeast extract	Batch	-	3.07 ± 0.04	-	0.05273 ± 0.00015	46.58 **	[16]
Glucose	Sodium nitrate *	Batch	-	23.7 ± 0.61	0.38	0.99	18.14 **	[22]
	Threonine *		-	25.3	0.95 ± 0.09	-	28.46 **	[23]
	Yeast extract, tryptone		0.067	2.046	0.499	0.159	-	[24]
			0.017	2.66	-	0.01634 ± 0.00168	14.70 ± 0.07	[4]
	Yeast extract		-	6.4	-	1.4	-	[20]
			-	27.7	-	1.6	13.36	[19]
Glycerol (crude)	Yeast extract	Batch	0.018	5.05	-	0.02696 ± 0.00107	14.70 ± 0.73	[4]
Glycerol (pure)	Yeast extract	Batch	0.019	6.33	-	0.01307 ± 0.00072	11.04 ± 0.50	
Molasses	Yeast extract	Batch	0.013	3.91	-	0.01956 ± 0.00100	11.12 ± 0.56	
Molasses (crude waste)	Rapeseed meal hydrolysate	Batch	-	3.43	-	0.00872	-	[25]
Organosolv pulps	Yeast extract	Batch	-	5.2	-	0.8	-	[20]

Where μ_{max} is the specific biomass growth rate and $Y_{x/s}$ is the biomass yield from a substrate (carbon source); * The focus of the study is an effect of nitrogen source on *C. cohnii* growth parameters; ** Recalculated values of the results available in the literature.

An alternative way of cultivation could be to use the extraction ethanol (EE), remaining after lipid extraction, as a source of carbon, and extracts from recycled dinoflagellate biomass as a source of carbon, nitrogen, and vitamins. A substitute of conventional nitrogen sources, dinoflagellate extract (DE), is obtained from de-oiled microalgae biomass (i.e., after lipid extraction, by hydrolysis, neutralization with calcium carbonate, sedimentation, separation, evaporation of liquid phase, and drying). The described process can also be called biomass recycling.

The aim of the present study was to evaluate the growth and metabolic response of *C. cohnii* to different carbon and nitrogen sources in growth media including conventional commercially available YE, and two novel extracts (EE, Des). This approach provides more efficient use of the lipid extraction by-products/waste products and circular DHA production process (Scheme 1), and therefore could be beneficial to the bio-economy.

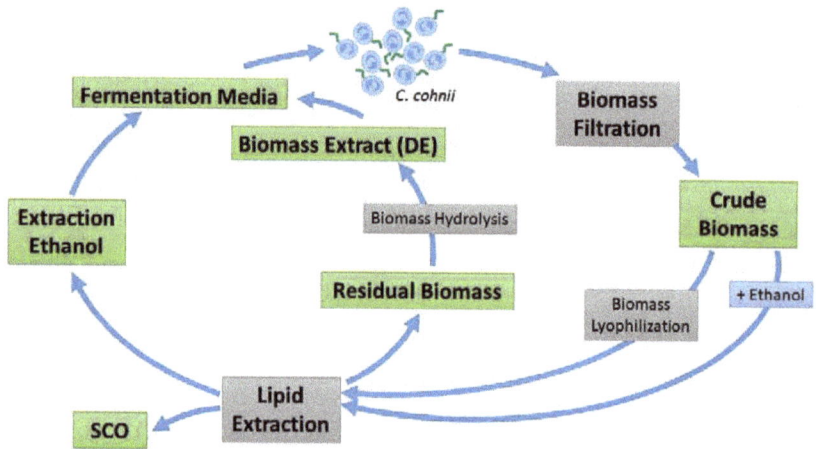

Scheme 1. Dinoflagellate extract (DE) and single cell oil (SCO) acquisition process.

2. Results

To access the possibility of replacing YE with cheaper alternative sources of nitrogen and nutrients for the cultivation of *C. cohnii* and DHA production, we used extracts obtained from de-oiled dinoflagellate biomass, as well as ethanol, which was used as part of one of the oil extraction methods. Two main methods were used to extract oil from the dinoflagellate biomass (see Scheme 2). In the first case, the oil was extracted from lyophilized biomass using hexane. Thus, obtaining a SCO, which after esterification can be separated into FAs. A waste product of this process is de-oiled microalgae biomass, which is hydrolysed to obtain dinoflagellate extract (DE) (see Scheme 2A). In the second case, the oil extraction is carried out through saponification of fats in wet biomass with KOH in the presence of ethanol. Thus, obtaining the hydroalcoholic phase, containing soaps, and de-oiled microalgae biomass. Ethanol, which is used in this process, extracts multiple components from the biomass and can serve as a source of carbon and organic nitrogen, vitamins, nutrients, and salts for subsequent cultivations (see Scheme 2B).

The first method requires additional biomass processing before the oil extraction (e.g., freezing and drying (lyophilization)). On the contrary, the second method requires an additional extraction step. The obtained DEs by the first and second method were called DE_A and DE_B, respectively. Experiments on the effect of the DE on the growth of *C. cohnii* were carried out in mediums with glucose as the main carbon source. EE was used as an alternative source of carbon.

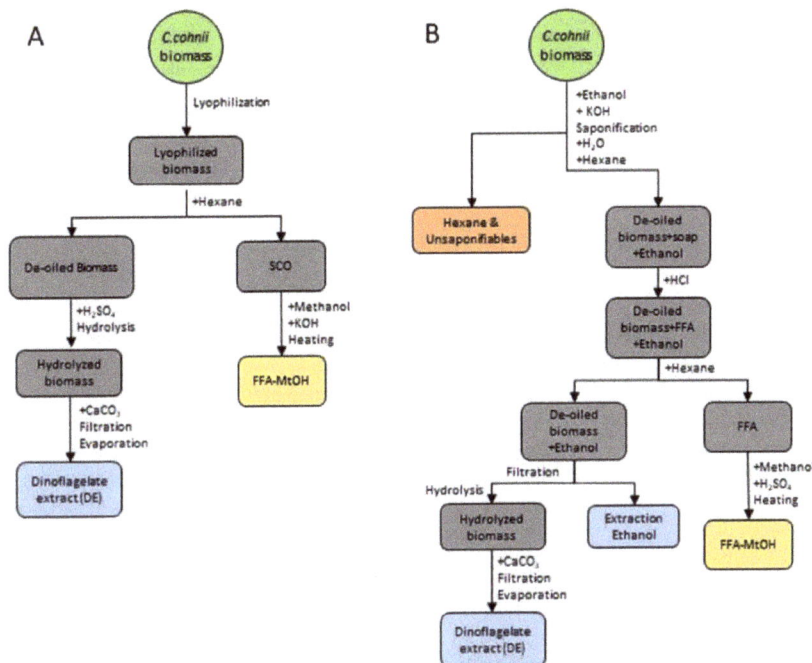

Scheme 2. Dinoflagellate extract, extraction ethanol, and free fatty acid (FFA) methyl ester acquisition from (**A**) lyophilized biomass and (**B**) wet biomass.

2.1. Experiments with Glucose as the Carbon Source

Multiple cultivation experiments were carried out using a complex medium containing glucose, sea salt, and YE and/or DE to study the effect of DE on the growth rate, biomass, and lipids including DHA by *C. cohnii*. The media composition used in the experiments with glucose as the main carbon source are summarized in Table 2. The mediums under study contained either only YE, only DE, or YE and DE (25/75 w/w). Selection of the initial glucose concentration (10 g·L^{-1}) is justified by the fact that the mentioned amount of substrate is enough for the biomass to fully consume 1 g·L^{-1} of YE. Furthermore, de Swaaf et al. [17], Jiang et al. [26], and Diao et al. [27], as part of previously reported studies, have shown that the maximum biomass growth rate is achieved if the glucose concentration is maintained in the range of 5–25 g·L^{-1}. Additionally, de Swaaf et al. has demonstrated, that biomass growth inhibition begins at glucose concentrations of 20–25 g·L^{-1}. The specific biomass growth rates and yields in different mediums are shown in Table 2. The maximum specific biomass growth rate and yield from glucose were observed in the medium containing exclusively DE$_A$, and were equal to 1.012 and 0.601 g·g^{-1}, respectively. The lowest specific growth rate (0.655 h^{-1}) was observed with the medium, which contained only DE$_B$. A similar growth rate (0.615 h^{-1}) was observed with the reference medium with no added extracts.

The addition of 25% YE to 75% DE$_B$ into the cultivation medium (DE$_{B75}$) increased the specific biomass growth rate by 37% (up to 0.901 h^{-1}), while the yield of biomass remained mostly unchanged (0.398 g·g^{-1}). However, the addition of 25% of YE to DE$_A$ (medium DE$_{A75}$) lowered the specific biomass growth rate to 0.9 h^{-1}, in comparison to the mediums containing only DE extracts.

Table 2. The medium compositions and the growth parameters of *C. cohnii* with glucose as carbon source.

Medium	Component, g·L^{-1}					μ_{max}, h^{-1}	$Y_{x/s}$, g·g^{-1}
	Sea Salts	Glucose	YE	DE$_A$	DE$_B$		
YE	12.5	10.0	1.0	-	-	0.930	0.446
DE$_A$	12.5	10.0	-	1.0	-	1.012	0.601
DE$_B$	12.5	10.0	-	-	1.0	0.655	0.398
DE$_{A75}$	12.5	10.0	0.25	0.75	-	0.900	0.403
DE$_{B75}$	12.5	10.0	0.25	-	0.75	0.901	0.371
Glucose	12.5	10.0	-	-	-	0.615	0.397

Where μ_{max} is the specific biomass growth rate and $Y_{x/s}$ is the biomass yield from a substrate.

Figure 1 shows the biomass growth (A) and glucose consumption (B) curves in mediums given in Table 2. It can be seen that all mediums containing YE ensured complete assimilation of glucose in 7–14 days, while in mediums containing DE, only half of the initially supplemented substrate was assimilated until the 14th experiment day.

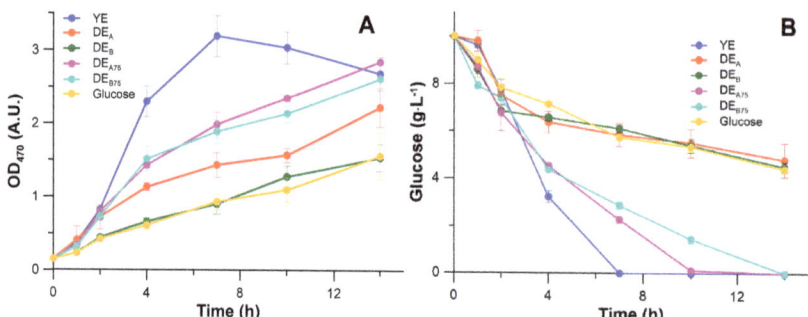

Figure 1. Cultivation of *C. cohnii* with glucose as a carbon source—(**A**) optical density (OD) change over time and (**B**) glucose concentration change over time.

Almost all growth curves, except the DE$_A$ medium, reached the lag phase during the first day of cultivation. The medium containing only YE showed the highest average specific growth rate for the first three days until all glucose was consumed. After that, the growth passed into the stationary phase and cyst formation began. In other mediums, the maximum specific growth rate was observed only on the first cultivation day, after which the biomass growth remained constant.

2.2. Experiments with Ethanol as the Carbon Source

The EE, collected after the lipid extraction from *C. cohnii* biomass, was used as the main carbon source in complex mediums containing YE and DE as sources of nitrogen and nutrients. The media compositions, the specific biomass growth rates, and biomass yields are summarized in Table 3.

The highest specific growth rate and biomass yield were obtained in mediums containing YE and reached 0.757 h^{-1} and 0.282 g·g^{-1}, respectively. In mediums with DE, the growth rates were slightly lower than using YE and reached 0.701 h^{-1} for DE$_A$ and 0.651 h^{-1} for DE$_B$. The biomass yield on the 14th day of cultivation in mediums containing DE$_A$ and DE$_B$, reached 0.234 and 0.221 g·g^{-1}, respectively.

Table 3. The medium compositions and the growth parameters of *C. cohnii* with extraction ethanol (EE) as carbon source.

Medium	Component, g·L^{-1}						μ_{max}, h^{-1}	$Y_{x/s}$, g·g^{-1}
	Sea Salts	EE	Ethanol	YE	DE$_A$	DE$_B$		
EE_YE	12.5	5.9	-	1.0	-	-	0.757	0.282
EE_DE$_A$	12.5	5.9	-	-	1.0	-	0.701	0.234
EE_DE$_B$	12.5	5.9	-	-	-	1.0	0.651	0.221
EE_DE$_{A75}$	12.5	5.9	-	0.25	0.75	-	0.658	0.238
EE_DE$_{B75}$	12.5	5.9	-	0.25	-	0.75	0.606	0.218
EE	12.5	5.9	-	-	-	-	0.470	0.124
Ethanol	12.5	-	4.7	-	-	-	0.383	0.122

Where μ_{max} is the specific biomass growth rate and $Y_{x/s}$ is the biomass yield from a substrate.

From Figure 2 it can be observed that in the case of YE and DE$_A$, the specific biomass growth rate reached the maximum and remained constant until the 4th cultivation day until the substrate was not entirely consumed. In turn, the biomass growth rate in mediums containing only DE$_B$ was relatively high only on the first day of cultivation, after which it gradually decreased. It should be noted that during cultivation in mediums containing YE, similarly as in the glucose experiment, the lag phase was observed during the first day of cultivation.

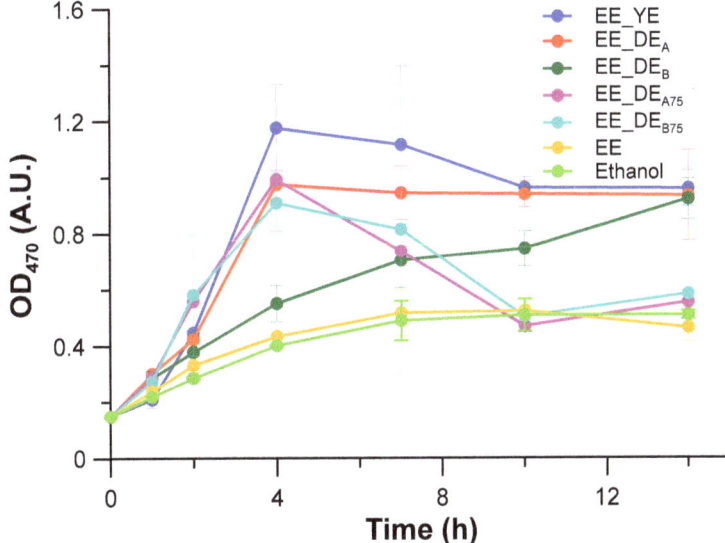

Figure 2. The optical density (OD) change over time of *C. cohnii* in mediums with extraction ethanol (EE) as a carbon source.

Experiments on pure and extraction ethanol (EE) were conducted to evaluate their effect on the biomass growth rate and yield. The specific growth rate in the case of EE was 0.470 h^{-1}, which is for 20% more than in pure ethanol (0.383 h^{-1}) and 50% more than in mediums containing YE or DE. The maximum biomass yield in both cases was very similar (0.124 g·g^{-1} for EE and 0.122 g·g^{-1} for pure ethanol), but with EE it was reached on the seventh day, and with pure ethanol on the 10th cultivation day.

2.3. Evaluation of Lipid/FA and PUFA Accumulation in C. cohnii Biomass by FTIR

FTIR is a rapid method, particularly used for monitoring the relative content of each macromolecular component under varying growth conditions [28–31]. FTIR spectroscopy of *C. cohnii* biomass was used to evaluate the growth medium-induced production of lipids/FA and PUFAs. Fish oil supplements naturally contain about 30% of EPA and DHA in the form of triacylglycerols (TAGs), a tri-ester [32,33]. The FTIR spectrum of fish oil (Figure 3) reveals three high-intensity absorption bands at 2925, 2854 cm^{-1} (CH$_3$ and CH$_2$ vibrations, respectively), and 1745 cm^{-1} (C=O vibrations of lipid esters) that are indicative of lipids, FAs or triglycerides and therefore are indicative of total lipids. The spectrum also revealed a smaller peak at 3011 cm^{-1} (olefinic group = CH), which is typical for unsaturated fatty acids (PUFAs/DHA) [34–39].

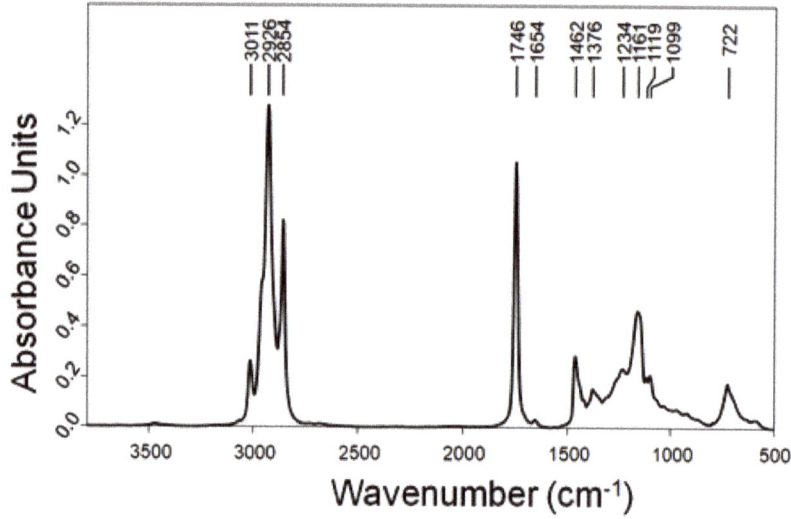

Figure 3. FTIR spectrum of fish oil food supplement (LYSI HF, Iceland). 10 mL contains: FA (2155 mg) incl. EPA (690 mg) and DHA (920 mg), and vitamins: E (9,2 mg), A (460 µg), and D (20 µg).

The characteristic absorption bands of the major cell components in the FTIR spectra are at 1080 cm^{-1} of carbohydrates; 1250 cm^{-1} of nucleic acids; 1650 and 1545 cm^{-1} of proteins (Amide I and Amide II, stretching vibrations of C=O bond of amide and bending vibrations of the N-H bond, respectively); triplet bands in 2800–3000 cm^{-1} and 1744 cm^{-1} of lipids/FA (C-H stretching in CH$_3$ and CH$_2$ and C=O of esters/ester carbonyl, respectively) and ~3014 cm^{-1} of PUFAs/DHA (olefinic HC=CH stretching mode) [28,40]. The position and intensities of particular absorption bands allow to monitor or evaluate the macromolecular composition of cells as well as the accumulation of lipids/FAs and PUFAs [40–43]. PUFAs in the FTIR spectrum show a peak in the range of 3005–3013 cm^{-1}, particularly the specific peak of DHA oils is at ~3013,4 cm^{-1} [44].

Samples for FTIR were collected only on day 14, due to the amount of accumulated biomass in the experimental setup. For data analysis of *C. cohnii* cells, only spectra with absorption limits between 0.25 and 0.80 were used, and therefore, in accordance with the Lambert-Bouger-Beer law, the concentration of a component is proportional to the intensity of the absorption band. The spectra were vector normalized and therefore the intensity of the vibration band was proportional to the amount of band vibrations, i.e., the intensity is proportional to concentration. Therefore, the latter allows to cross-compare the cell biomass composition, accumulation, and number of macromolecular components (e.g., proteins, carbohydrates, FAs, PUFAs, DHA, etc). This is an especially valuable FTIR spectroscopy approach for quick and informative evaluation of large sample sets to select the best growth conditions for the production/accumulation of the targeted metabolites. Further quantitative and qualitative analyses of the most relevant samples can be carried out more precisely by FTIR spectroscopy, chromatography, mass spectroscopy, etc. Therefore, even though FTIR is a semi-quantitative method and does not provide precise values, it remarkably saves resources and time for evaluation of different biotechnological processes.

FTIR spectra of *C. cohnii* grown in mediums with YE, DE_A, DE_{A75}, DE_{B75}, or glucose (Figure 4) showed that the macromolecular composition of cells is different depending on the growth medium composition. The spectrum profile of the *C. cohnii* cells grown in medium containing YE was noticeably different from others of this experimental set. Spectra of the cells grown with YE showed similar amounts of total carbohydrates but higher content of proteins and lower content of total lipids than in cells grown in mediums with DE_A, DE_{A75} DE_{B75}, or glucose. The vector normalized spectra of cells grown without YE showed similar content of the total carbohydrates and proteins, but the content of lipids/FA and PUFAs/DHA varied. The highest number of total lipids/FAs (2925, 2854, and 1745 cm^{-1}) was detected in cells grown in mediums with glucose but lower with DE_{A75} and DE_{B75}. However, a higher amount of PUFAs/DHA (3014 cm^{-1}) was detected in cells grown in medium with DE_{A75}.

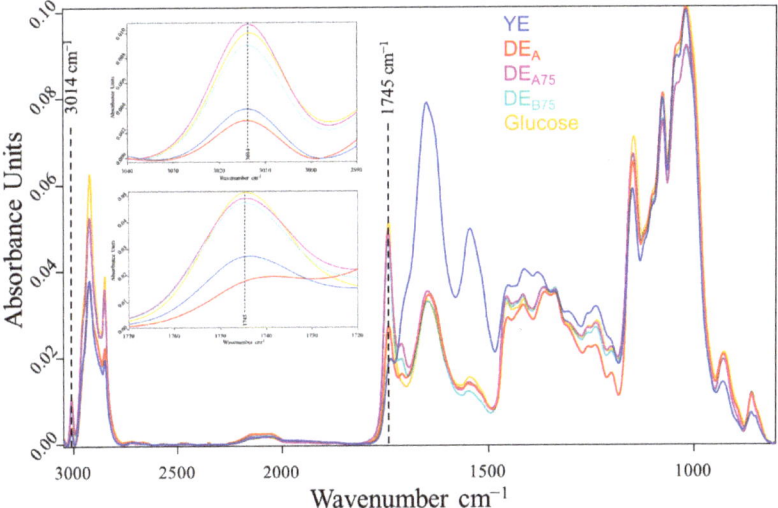

Figure 4. Vector normalized FTIR spectra of *C. cohnii* biomass after 14 days of growth in mediums, with YE, DE_A, DE_{A75}, DE_{B75}, or glucose.

FTIR spectra of *C. cohnii* cultivated in mediums with EE-YE, EE-DE_A, EE-DE_B, EE-DE_{A75}, EE-DE_{B75}, EE, or pure ethanol are shown in Figure 5. FTIR spectra showed different cell macromolecular compositions, which can be grouped into two clusters. The first group EE-YE, EE-DE_{A75}, and EE-DE_{B75} produce relatively high amounts of proteins, low amounts of total carbohydrates, and lesser amounts of total lipids than cells grown with EE-DE_A, EE-DE_B, EE, or pure ethanol. The FTIR spectra of the second group (i.e., cells grown in EE-DE_A, EE-DE_B, EE, or pure ethanol showed more total lipids/FA and PUFAs/DHA compared to those of the first group). The highest content of FAs and PUFAs/DHA was detected in *C. cohnii* grown in mediums with EE/EE-DE_A and EE-DE_B.

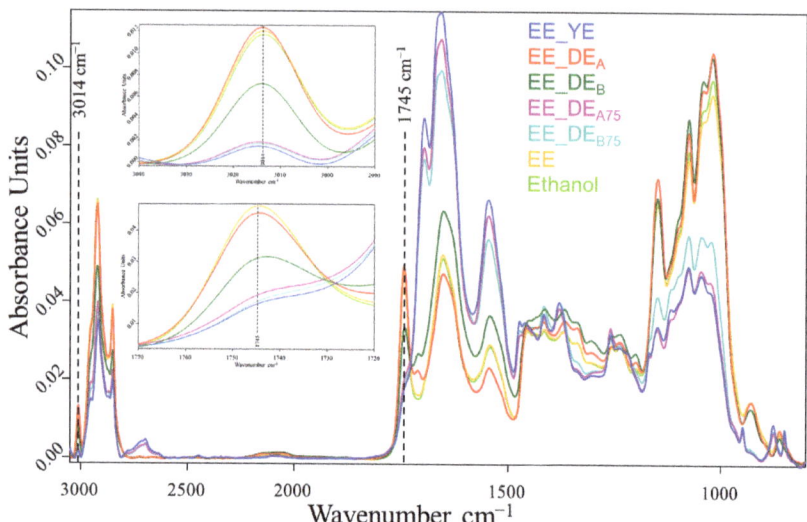

Figure 5. Vector normalized FTIR spectra of *C. cohnii* biomass after 14 days of growth in seven different mediums with ethanol.

3. Discussion

The main components of the culture medium for *C. cohnii* are the substrate (glucose, glycerol, ethanol, acetic acid), yeast extract, and sea salt (artificial or natural). The biomass yield from each component of the cultivation medium was determined during bioreactor cultivations and reached 0.7 g·g^{-1} for glucose, 5.3 g·g^{-1} for yeast extract, and 0.87 g·g^{-1} for sea salt (results not shown). Despite the fact that, compared to other components, a small amount (in terms of mass) of yeast extract is used, its price is the highest (8–10 USD/kg) and makes up more than half of the cultivation medium cost. Considering that the costs of raw materials for the production of SCO is about half of all production expenses, the reduction of the necessary amounts of cultivation medium components poses a significant effect on the overall process economy.

The obtained results of this study show that DE_A stimulated a similar biomass growth rate when compared to YE, while the biomass yield was significantly higher if glucose was used as a carbon source. The absence of a lag phase during cultivation in mediums containing only DE_A, both with glucose or ethanol, unlike mediums with YE, indicates that the mineral and vitamin composition of DE_A is more preferable for proliferation of *C. cohnii* cells. However, a decrease of the biomass growth rate in mediums with DE_A should be noted. The increase in biomass titres after cultivation for four days (media with DE_A) and seven days (media with DE_{A75}) becomes constant and equal to that obtained in the control medium (with glucose). Therefore, despite the high initial biomass growth rates, the efficiency of DE_A is approximately two times lower when compared to that of YE. The latter can be compensated by increasing the initial concentrations of DE_A or the addition of small amounts of YE to the cultivation medium, which in itself depends on the economic feasibility of the process.

The use of DE_B as a nitrogen source, in the case of both glucose and ethanol, had a minimal effect on the growth rate and biomass yield. Obviously, many thermal and chemical biomass processing steps, which are necessary to obtain DE_B, completely or to a larger extent degrade the initial vitamins present in *C. cohnii* biomass.

EE, although it did not significantly affect the biomass growth rate, showed the same biomass yield when compared to the control sample (pure ethanol), which indicates the feasibility of using it as a carbon source for *C. cohnii* cultivation.

Cross comparison of the FTIR spectral data showed that the growth medium components clearly affect the biochemical composition of *C. cohnii* cells. When grown in mediums with YE, EE-YE, EE-DE$_{A75}$, or EE-DE$_{B75}$, *C. cohnii* cells contained more proteins (compared to the cells grown in any other studied mediums) but the absorption band at 1745 cm^{-1} (ester C=O bonds of lipids/FA) was not detected, thus indicating that the cells did not overproduce lipids/FA. In the context of searching for the growth conditions promoting the accumulation of PUFAs/DHA the most promising results were acquired when *C. cohnii* was cultivated in the mediums with DE$_{A75}$ and glucose (Figure 4), EE-DE$_A$, EE-DE$_B$, EE, or ethanol (Figure 5). However, further quantitative analyses of the main cell macromolecular components (carbohydrates, proteins, and lipids) are needed to identify the most efficient growth media that promotes the overproduction of PUFAs/DHA by *C. cohnii*.

To summarize the above mentioned, DE$_A$ and EE can both be successfully used as alternative sources of nitrogen, nutrients, and carbon to reduce the costs of conventional SCO and DHA production processes.

Moreover, the production of DE$_A$ can be optimized through the use of hydrochloric acid and sodium hydroxide. The hydrolysate obtained in this way, after neutralization with acid, can be directly used to create a suitable dinoflagellate cultivation medium. Furthermore, the use of the above-mentioned hydrolysate will make it possible to exclude such energy-demanding steps of the production process as evaporation and simultaneously significantly reduce the amount of sea salt, which otherwise should be added in the cultivation medium in large quantities.

4. Materials and Methods

4.1. Cultivation Conditions

Crypthecodinium cohnii CCMP 316 was obtained from the Provasoli-Guillard National Center for Marine Algae and Microbiota (NCMA) (USA). The culture inoculum was grown in a custom-made setup (see Scheme 3) consisting of 250 mL bottles with a working volume of 150 mL. The growth medium containing glucose 5 g·L^{-1}, yeast extract 2 g·L^{-1} and sea salts 25 g·L^{-1}, with aeration 30 mL/min, rotation speed 130 rpm (provided by an orbital shaker PSU-20i, Biosan, Riga, Latvia) was maintained at 25 °C. The cultivation medium compositions for experiments are shown in Table 4, as well as in Tables 2 and 3. The initial optical density (OD$_{470}$) of experiments was set to 0.15.

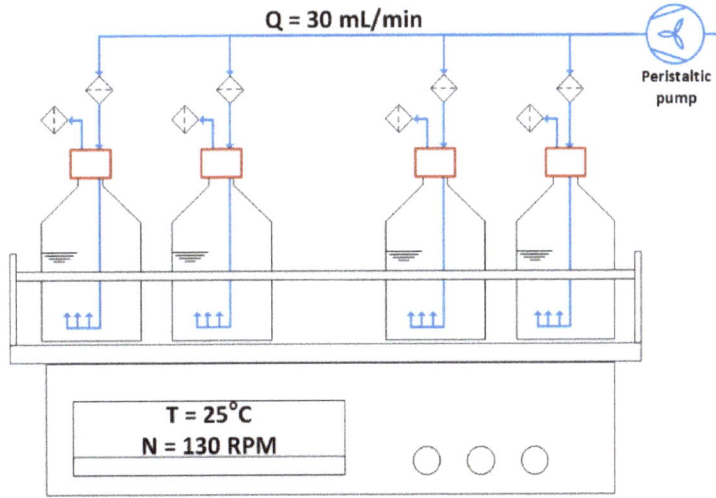

Scheme 3. *C. cohnii* cultivation experiment setup.

Table 4. The medium compositions for *C. cohnii* cultivations.

Medium	Component, g·L^{-1}						
	Sea Salts	Glucose	EE	Ethanol	YE	DE$_A$	DE$_B$
YE	12.5	10.0	-	-	1.0	-	-
DE$_A$	12.5	10.0	-	-	-	1.0	-
DE$_B$	12.5	10.0	-	-	-	-	1.0
DE$_{A75}$	12.5	10.0	-	-	0.25	0.75	-
DE$_{B75}$	12.5	10.0	-	-	0.25	-	0.75
Glucose	12.5	10.0	-	-	-	-	-
EE_YE	12.5	-	5.9	-	1.0	-	-
EE_DE$_A$	12.5	-	5.9	-	-	1.0	-
EE_DE$_B$	12.5	-	5.9	-	-	-	1.0
EE_DE$_{A75}$	12.5	-	5.9	-	0.25	0.75	-
EE_DE$_{B75}$	12.5	-	5.9	-	0.25	-	0.75
EE	12.5	-	5.9	-	-	-	-
Ethanol	12.5	-	-	4.7	-	-	-

4.2. Dinoflagellate Extract and Extraction Ethanol Obtainment

Dinoflagellate extracts (DEs) were obtained by recycling de-oiled *C. cohnii* biomass from the cultivation process in a laboratory scale bioreactor EDF-5.4_1 (JSC Biotehniskais centrs, Riga, Latvia) by a method adapted from Gao et al. [45]. The de-oiled biomass was hydrolysed with H_2SO_4 at 121 °C for 20 min. The hydrolysed solution was neutralized with an appropriate amount of $CaCO_3$. The solid fraction was separated from the hydrolysate by filtration. Most of the liquid hydrolysate was evaporated by heating at 120 °C, 600 rpm. The remaining moisture was evaporated by drying the sample in an oven at 80 °C overnight. The obtained dry extract pellets were grinned into a fine powder, hereinafter referred to as DE. De-oiled biomass for DE$_A$ obtainment was produced by a method adapted from Halim et al. [46]. Lipids were extracted from lyophilized biomass with the use of Soxhlet extraction with hexane as the solvent, containing 0.01% butylated hydroxytoluene (BHT). De-oiled biomass for DE$_B$ obtainment was produced by a method adapted from Mendes et al. [47]. Lipids were extracted with hexane (BHT concentration in hexane 0.01%) from the wet biomass, followed by incubation overnight at 20 °C with ethanol and KOH, simultaneously the extraction ethanol (EE) was obtained and separated. The acidification with HCl and additional hexane extractions were performed, the resulting suspension was used for DE obtainment as described above.

4.3. Optical Density and Glucose Concentration Measurements

C. cohnii growth was monitored via optical density (OD) measurements at a wavelength of 470 nm with a spectrophotometer Jenway 6300 (Cole-Parmer, Saint Neots, UK). The glucose concentration was measured enzymatically with an AccuChek ACTIVE blood sugar analyzer (Roche, Basel, Switzerland). Samples for OD and glucose measurements were taken on days 1, 2, 4, 7, 10, and 14. The experiments were performed in at-least triplicate and the experimental data was expressed as mean ± standard deviation (SD).

4.4. Determination of Biomass Dry Cell Weight

The biomass dry cell weight (DCW) in relation to the absorbance at a wavelength of 470 nm was determined gravimetrically as described in [48]. During the present study, the correlation coefficients value was determined as 1.415 g (DCW)·L^{-1}·A.U.$^{-1}$.

4.5. Fourier Transform Infrared Spectroscopy

Fourier transform infrared (FTIR) spectra of biomass were recorded using Vertex 70 coupled with the HTS XT microplate reader (Bruker Optik GmbH, Ettlingen, Germany) Sample aliquots were pipetted on a 384 well microplate dried and recorded in the frequency range of 4000–600 cm^{-1}. Omega fatty acids were identified by absorption bands at ~1743 cm^{-1} and ~3012 cm^{-1}. Due to the experimental setup and amount of accumulated biomass during the cultivation processes, samples for FTIR were collected only on day 14.

For data analyses only spectra with absorption limits between 0.25 and 0.80 were used, and therefore, in accordance with the Lambert-Bouger-Beer law, the concentration of a component is proportional to the intensity of the absorption band. Spectra were vector normalized, and therefore the intensity of the vibration band was proportional to the amount of band vibrations (i.e., the intensity is proportional to concentration).

5. Conclusions

FTIR spectra of *C. cohnii* cells clearly showed the medium-induced metabolic responses, including variations of the produced total lipids/FA, PUFAs, and DHA. Further studies of the concentrations and composition of PUFAs produced under various cultivation conditions together with the cell growth data would allow us to identify the most efficient cultivation medium composition. Nevertheless, current observations point out to the positive effect (both in terms of process economy and process efficiency) of supplementing the standard *C. cohnii* cultivation medium with recycled components (e.g., dinoflagellate extracts and extraction ethanol).

Author Contributions: Conceptualization, K.D. and E.D.; methodology, E.D., M.G. and A.S. (Anastasija Suleiko); formal analysis, K.D.; investigation, E.D., M.G., K.S. and A.S. (Anastasija Suleiko); resources, J.V.; writing—original draft preparation, E.D.; writing—review and editing, K.D., A.S. (Arturs Suleiko), A.S. (Anastasija Suleiko), M.G., J.V. and E.D.; visualization, A.S. (Arturs Suleiko), K.D. and K.S.; supervision, K.D. All authors have read and agreed to the published version of the manuscript.

Funding: This research was funded by European Regional Development Fund, grant number 1.1.1.1/18/A/022.

Institutional Review Board Statement: Not applicable.

Conflicts of Interest: The authors declare no conflict of interest.

References

1. Adarme-Vega, T.C.; Thomas-Hall, S.R.; Schenk, P.M. Towards sustainable sources for omega-3 fatty acids production. *Curr. Opin. Biotechnol.* **2014**, *26*, 14–18. [CrossRef] [PubMed]
2. Stramarkou, M.; Oikonomopoulou, V.; Chalima, A.; Boukouvalas, C.; Topakas, E.; Krokida, M. Optimization of green extractions for the recovery of docosahexaenoic acid (DHA) from Crypthecodinium cohnii. *Algal Res.* **2021**, *58*, 102374. [CrossRef]
3. da Silva, T.L.; Moniz, P.; Silva, C.; Reis, A. The dark side of microalgae biotechnology: A heterotrophic biorefinery platform directed to ω-3 rich lipid production. *Microorganisms* **2019**, *7*, 670. [CrossRef] [PubMed]
4. Taborda, T.; Moniz, P.; Reis, A.; da Silva, T.L. Evaluating low-cost substrates for Crypthecodinium cohnii lipids and DHA production, by flow cytometry. *J. Appl. Phycol.* **2021**, *33*, 263–274. [CrossRef]
5. Ji, X.-J.; Ren, L.-J.; Huang, H. Omega-3 Biotechnology: A Green and Sustainable Process for Omega-3 Fatty Acids Production. *Front. Bioeng. Biotechnol.* **2015**, *3*, 190–209. [CrossRef]
6. Sharma, J.; Sarmah, P.; Bishnoi, N.R. Market Perspective of EPA and DHA Production from Microalgae. In *Nutraceutical Fatty Acids from Oleaginous Microalgae*; Scrivener Publishing LLC: Beverly, MA, USA, 2020; pp. 281–297. [CrossRef]
7. Braunwald, T.; French, W.T.; Claupein, W.; Graeff-Hönninger, S. Economic assessment of microbial biodiesel production using heterotrophic yeasts. *Int. J. Green Energy* **2016**, *13*, 274–282. [CrossRef]
8. Jovanovic, S.; Dietrich, D.; Becker, J.; Kohlstedt, M.; Wittmann, C. Microbial production of polyunsaturated fatty acids—high-value ingredients for aquafeed, superfoods, and pharmaceuticals. *Curr. Opin. Biotechnol.* **2021**, *69*, 199–211. [CrossRef]
9. Petrie, J.R.; Shrestha, P.; Zhou, X.R.; Mansour, M.P.; Liu, Q.; Belide, S.; Nichols, P.D.; Singh, S.P. Metabolic Engineering Plant Seeds with Fish Oil-Like Levels of DHA. *PLoS ONE* **2012**, *7*, 2–8. [CrossRef] [PubMed]
10. Santos-Sánchez, N.F.; Valadez-Blanco, R.; Hernández-Carlos, B.; Torres-Ariño, A.; Guadarrama-Mendoza, P.C.; Salas-Coronado, R. Lipids rich in ω-3 polyunsaturated fatty acids from microalgae. *Appl. Microbiol. Biotechnol.* **2016**, *100*, 8667–8684. [CrossRef]

11. Graham, I.A.; Larson, T.; Napier, J.A. Rational metabolic engineering of transgenic plants for biosynthesis of omega-3 polyunsaturates. *Curr. Opin. Biotechnol.* **2007**, *18*, 142–147. [CrossRef]
12. Mendes, A.; Reis, A.; Vasconcelos, R.; Guerra, P.; Lopes Da Silva, T. Crypthecodinium cohnii with emphasis on DHA production: A review. *J. Appl. Phycol.* **2009**, *21*, 199–214. [CrossRef]
13. Xiao, R.; Li, X.; Zheng, Y. Comprehensive Study of Cultivation Conditions and Methods on Lipid Accumulation of a Marine Protist, Thraustochytrium striatum. *Protist* **2018**, *169*, 451–465. [CrossRef]
14. Lv, M.; Wang, F.; Zeng, L.; Bi, Y.; Cui, J.; Liu, L.; Bi, Y.; Chen, L.; Zhang, W. Identification and metabolomic analysis of a starch-deficient Crypthecodinium cohnii mutant reveals multiple mechanisms relevant to enhanced growth and lipid accumulation. *Algal Res.* **2020**, *50*, 102001. [CrossRef]
15. Rumiani, L.A.; Jalili, H.; Amrane, A. Enhanced docosahexaenoic acid production by Crypthecodinium cohnii under combined stress in two-stage cultivation with date syrup based medium. *Algal Res.* **2018**, *34*, 75–81. [CrossRef]
16. Paz, A.; Karnaouri, A.; Templis, C.C.; Papayannakos, N.; Topakas, E. Valorization of exhausted olive pomace for the production of omega-3 fatty acids by Crypthecodinium cohnii. *Waste Manag.* **2020**, *118*, 435–444. [CrossRef]
17. De Swaaf, M.E.; Sijtsma, L.; Pronk, J.T. High-cell-density fed-batch cultivation of the docosahexaenoic acid producing marine alga Crypthecodinium cohnii. *Biotechnol. Bioeng.* **2003**, *81*, 666–672. [CrossRef]
18. De Swaaf, M.E.; Pronk, J.T.; Sijtsma, L. Fed-batch cultivation of the docosahexaenoic-acid-producing marine alga Crypthecodinium cohnii on ethanol. *Appl. Microbiol. Biotechnol.* **2003**, *61*, 40–43. [CrossRef]
19. de Swaaf, M.E.; de Rijk, T.C.; Eggink, G.; Sijtsma, L. Optimisation of docosahexaenoic acid production in batch cultivations by Crypthecodinium cohnii. *Prog. Ind. Microbiol.* **1999**, *35*, 185–192. [CrossRef]
20. Karnaouri, A.; Asimakopoulou, G.; Kalogiannis, K.G.; Lappas, A.A.; Topakas, E. Efficient production of nutraceuticals and lactic acid from lignocellulosic biomass by combining organosolv fractionation with enzymatic/fermentative routes. *Bioresour. Technol.* **2021**, *341*, 125846. [CrossRef] [PubMed]
21. Chalima, A.; Taxeidis, G.; Topakas, E. Optimization of the production of docosahexaenoic fatty acid by the heterotrophic microalga Crypthecodinium cohnii utilizing a dark fermentation effluent. *Renew. Energy* **2020**, *152*, 102–109. [CrossRef]
22. Safdar, W.; Shamoon, M.; Zan, X.; Haider, J.; Sharif, H.R.; Shoaib, M.; Song, Y. Growth kinetics, fatty acid composition and metabolic activity changes of Crypthecodinium cohnii under different nitrogen source and concentration. *AMB Express* **2017**, *7*, 85. [CrossRef]
23. Safdar, W.; Zan, X.; Shamoon, M.; Sharif, H.R.; Mukama, O.; Tang, X.; Song, Y. Effects of twenty standard amino acids on biochemical constituents, docosahexaenoic acid production and metabolic activity changes of Crypthecodinium cohnii. *Bioresour. Technol.* **2017**, *238*, 738–743. [CrossRef] [PubMed]
24. Jiang, Y.; Chen, F.; Liang, S.Z. Production potential of docosahexaenoic acid by the heterotrophic marine dinoflagellate Crypthecodinium cohnii. *Process Biochem.* **1999**, *34*, 633–637. [CrossRef]
25. Gong, Y.; Liu, J.; Jiang, M.; Liang, Z.; Jin, H.; Hu, X.; Wan, X.; Hu, C. Improvement of omega-3 docosahexaenoic acid production by marine dinoflagellate Crypthecodinium cohnii using rapeseed meal hydrolysate and waste molasses as feedstock. *PLoS ONE* **2015**, *10*, e0125368. [CrossRef]
26. Jiang, Y.; Chen, F. Effects of medium glucose concentration and pH on docosahexaenoic acid content of heterotrophic Crypthecodinium cohnii. *Process Biochem.* **2000**, *35*, 1205–1209. [CrossRef]
27. Diao, J.; Song, X.; Zhang, X.; Chen, L.; Zhang, W. Genetic Engineering of Crypthecodinium cohnii to increase growth and lipid accumulation. *Front. Microbiol.* **2018**, *9*, 492. [CrossRef] [PubMed]
28. Grube, M.; Bekers, M.; Upite, D.; Kaminska, E. IR-spectroscopic studies of Zymomonas mobilis and levan precipitate. *Vib. Spectrosc.* **2002**, *28*, 277–285. [CrossRef]
29. Fuchino, K.; Kalnenieks, U.; Rutkis, R.; Grube, M.; Bruheim, P. Metabolic profiling of glucose-fed metabolically active resting Zymomonas mobilis strains. *Metabolites* **2020**, *10*, 81. [CrossRef]
30. Grube, M.; Kalnenieks, U.; Muter, O. Metabolic response of bacteria to elevated concentrations of glyphosate-based herbicide. *Ecotoxicol. Environ. Saf.* **2019**, *173*, 373–380. [CrossRef]
31. Grube, M.; Shvirksts, K.; Krafft, C.; Kokorevicha, S.; Zandberga, E.; Abols, A.; Line, A.; Kalnenieks, U. Miniature diamond-anvil cells for FTIR-microspectroscopy of small quantities of biosamples. *Analyst* **2018**, *143*, 3595–3599. [CrossRef]
32. Killeen, D.P.; Marshall, S.N.; Burgess, E.J.; Gordon, K.C.; Perry, N.B. Raman Spectroscopy of Fish Oil Capsules: Polyunsaturated Fatty Acid Quantitation Plus Detection of Ethyl Esters and Oxidation. *J. Agric. Food Chem.* **2017**, *65*, 3551–3558. [CrossRef]
33. Karunathilaka, S.R.; Choi, S.H.; Mossoba, M.M.; Yakes, B.J.; Brückner, L.; Ellsworth, Z.; Srigley, C.T. Rapid classification and quantification of marine oil omega-3 supplements using ATR-FTIR, FT-NIR and chemometrics. *J. Food Compos. Anal.* **2019**, *77*, 9–19. [CrossRef]
34. Guillén, M.D.; Cabo, N. Characterization of edible oils and lard by fourier transform infrared spectroscopy. Relationships between composition and frequency of concrete bands in the fingerprint region. *JAOCS J. Am. Oil Chem. Soc.* **1997**, *74*, 1281–1286. [CrossRef]
35. Dean, A.P.; Sigee, D.C.; Estrada, B.; Pittman, J.K. Using FTIR spectroscopy for rapid determination of lipid accumulation in response to nitrogen limitation in freshwater microalgae. *Bioresour. Technol.* **2010**, *101*, 4499–4507. [CrossRef]

36. Vongsvivut, J.; Heraud, P.; Zhang, W.; Kralovec, J.A.; McNaughton, D.; Barrow, C.J. Quantitative determination of fatty acid compositions in micro-encapsulated fish-oil supplements using Fourier transform infrared (FTIR) spectroscopy. *Food Chem.* **2012**, *135*, 603–609. [CrossRef] [PubMed]
37. Ferreira, R.; Lourenço, S.; Lopes, A.; Andrade, C.; Câmara, J.S.; Castilho, P.; Perestrelo, R. Evaluation of fatty acids profile as a useful tool towards valorization of by-products of agri-food industry. *Foods* **2021**, *10*, 2867. [CrossRef] [PubMed]
38. Ripoche, A.; Guillard, A.S. Determination of fatty acid composition of pork fat by Fourier transform infrared spectroscopy. *Meat Sci.* **2001**, *58*, 299–304. [CrossRef]
39. Meng, W.; Jiang, Y.; Rothschild, D.; Lipke, M.; Hall, G.; Wang, L. Modeling the structure and infrared spectra of omega-3 fatty acid esters. *J. Chem. Phys.* **2020**, *153*. [CrossRef] [PubMed]
40. Ami, D.; Posteri, R.; Mereghetti, P.; Porro, D.; Doglia, S.M.; Branduardi, P. Fourier transform infrared spectroscopy as a method to study lipid accumulation in oleaginous yeasts. *Biotechnol. Biofuels* **2014**, *7*, 12. [CrossRef]
41. Berzins, K.; Muiznieks, R.; Baumanis, M.R.; Strazdina, I.; Shvirksts, K.; Prikule, S.; Galvanauskas, V.; Pleissner, D.; Pentjuss, A.; Grube, M.; et al. Kinetic and stoichiometric modeling based analysis of docosahexaenoic acid (DHA) production potential by C.cohnii from glycerol, glucose and ethanol. *Mar. Drugs* **2022**. Under review.
42. Shapaval, V.; Afseth, N.K.; Vogt, G.; Kohler, A. Fourier transform infrared spectroscopy for the prediction of fatty acid profiles in Mucor fungi grown in media with different carbon sources. *Microb. Cell Fact.* **2014**, *13*, 1–11. [CrossRef]
43. Vongsvivut, J.; Heraud, P.; Gupta, A.; Puri, M.; McNaughton, D.; Barrow, C.J. FTIR microspectroscopy for rapid screening and monitoring of polyunsaturated fatty acid production in commercially valuable marine yeasts and protists. *Analyst* **2013**, *138*, 6016–6031. [CrossRef]
44. Yoshida, S.; Yoshida, H. Noninvasive analyses of polyunsaturated fatty acids in human oral mucosa in vivo by fourier-transform infrared spectroscopy. *Biopolymers* **2004**, *74*, 403–412. [CrossRef] [PubMed]
45. Gao, M.-T.; Shimamura, T.; Ishida, N.; Takahashi, H. Investigation of utilization of the algal biomass residue after oil extraction to lower the total production cost of biodiesel. *J. Biosci. Bioeng.* **2012**, *114*, 330–333. [CrossRef] [PubMed]
46. Halim, R.; Danquah, M.K.; Webley, P.A. Extraction of oil from microalgae for biodiesel production: A review. *Biotechnol. Adv.* **2012**, *30*, 709–732. [CrossRef] [PubMed]
47. Mendes, A.; Da Silva, T.L.; Reis, A. DHA concentration and purification from the marine heterotrophic microalga Crypthecodinium cohnii CCMP 316 by winterization and urea complexation. *Food Technol. Biotechnol.* **2007**, *45*, 38–44.
48. Dubencovs, K.; Liepins, J.; Suleiko, A.; Suleiko, A.; Vangravs, R.; Kassaliete, J.; Scerbaka, R.; Grigs, O. Optimization of synthetic media composition for Kluyveromyces marxianus fed-batch cultivation. *Fermentation* **2021**, *7*, 62. [CrossRef]

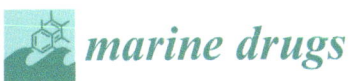

Article

A $^{13}CO_2$ Enrichment Experiment to Study the Synthesis Pathways of Polyunsaturated Fatty Acids of the Haptophyte *Tisochrysis lutea*

Marine Remize [1,2,*], Frédéric Planchon [1], Matthieu Garnier [3], Ai Ning Loh [4], Fabienne Le Grand [1], Antoine Bideau [1], Christophe Lambert [1], Rudolph Corvaisier [1], Aswani Volety [5] and Philippe Soudant [1,*]

[1] UMR 6539 LEMAR, CNRS, IRD, Ifremer, University of Brest, 29280 Plouzane, France; Frederic.Planchon@univ-brest.fr (F.P.); fabienne.legrand@univ-brest.fr (F.L.G.); Antoine.Bideau@univ-brest.fr (A.B.); christophe.lambert@univ-brest.fr (C.L.); rudolph.corvaisier@univ-brest.fr (R.C.)
[2] GREENSEA, Promenade du Sergeant Navarro, 34140 Meze, France
[3] PBA, Ifremer, Rue de l'Ile d'Yeu, BP 21105, CEDEX 03, 44311 Nantes, France; Matthieu.Garnier@ifremer.fr
[4] Center for Marine Science, Department of Earth and Ocean Sciences, University of North Carolina Wilmington, 5600 Marvin K. Moss Ln, Wilmington, NC 28403, USA; lohan@uncw.edu
[5] 50 Campus Drive, Elon University, Elon, NC 27244, USA; avolety@elon.edu
* Correspondence: marineremize@greensea.fr (M.R.); philippe.soudant@univ-brest.fr (P.S.)

Abstract: The production of polyunsaturated fatty acids (PUFA) in *Tisochrysis lutea* was studied using the gradual incorporation of a ^{13}C-enriched isotopic marker, $^{13}CO_2$, for 24 h during the exponential growth of the algae. The ^{13}C enrichment of eleven fatty acids was followed to understand the synthetic pathways the most likely to form the essential polyunsaturated fatty acids 20:5n-3 (EPA) and 22:6n-3 (DHA) in *T. lutea*. The fatty acids 16:0, 18:1n-9 + 18:3n-3, 18:2n-6, and 22:5n-6 were the most enriched in ^{13}C. On the contrary, 18:4n-3 and 18:5n-3 were the least enriched in ^{13}C after long chain polyunsaturated fatty acids such as 20:5n-3 or 22:5n-3. The algae appeared to use different routes in parallel to form its polyunsaturated fatty acids. The use of the PKS pathway was hypothesized for polyunsaturated fatty acids with n-6 configuration (such as 22:5n-6) but might also exist for n-3 PUFA (especially 20:5n-3). With regard to the conventional n-3 PUFA pathway, Δ6 desaturation of 18:3n-3 appeared to be the most limiting step for *T. lutea*, "stopping" at the synthesis of 18:4n-3 and 18:5n-3. These two fatty acids were hypothesized to not undergo any further reaction of elongation and desaturation after being formed and were therefore considered "end-products". To circumvent this limiting synthetic route, *Tisochrysis lutea* seemed to have developed an alternative route via Δ8 desaturation to produce longer chain fatty acids such as 20:5n-3 and 22:5n-3. 22:6n-3 presented a lower enrichment and appeared to be produced by a combination of different pathways: the conventional n-3 PUFA pathway by desaturation of 22:5n-3, the alternative route of ω-3 desaturase using 22:5n-6 as precursor, and possibly the PKS pathway. In this study, PKS synthesis looked particularly effective for producing long chain polyunsaturated fatty acids. The rate of enrichment of these compounds hypothetically synthesized by PKS is remarkably fast, making undetectable the ^{13}C incorporation into their precursors. Finally, we identified a protein cluster gathering PKS sequences of proteins that are hypothesized allowing n-3 PUFA synthesis.

Keywords: long-chain PUFA synthesis; desaturases; elongases; PKS pathway; 20:5n-3 (EPA); 22:6n-3 (DHA); *Tisochrysis lutea*; ^{13}C artificial enrichment

1. Introduction

Long chain polyunsaturated fatty acids (LC-PUFA) such as 20:5n-3 (EPA) and 22:6n-3 (DHA) are important compounds for most marine metazoans for their growth, reproduction, and development. They are not able to synthetize them in sufficient quantities and thus have to acquire them from their diet. On the basis of the food web, protists are the

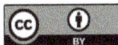

main producers of these fatty acids and present a key role in marine ecosystem functioning. 20:5n-3 and 22:6n-3 are also particularly important in human nutrition. They are known to have beneficial effects on cardiovascular diseases or diabetes. However, due to high demand for human nutrition and aquaculture of carnivore species, a shortage of these two compounds found in fish oil is predicted to occur by 2050 [1]. Despite their economic and ecologic interests, biological and ecological processes responsible for their synthesis are still under investigation. It is, then, of first concern to understand how 20:5n-3 and 22:6n-3 are produced at the basis of the food webs, and how global changes could affect their availability at higher trophic levels.

In phytoplankton and microzooplankton, fatty acids are synthetized via different metabolic pathways [2–4]. The most "conventional" pathway is the fatty acid synthase (FAS) pathway, followed by the elongation and front-end desaturation steps of the n-3 and n-6 pathways. Starting with the initial formation of acetyl-CoA and then malonyl-CoA in aerobic conditions, these pathways produce more complex fatty acids by progressive addition of two atoms of carbon (elongation steps) or desaturations of precursors such as 16:0 or 18:0 [5–7]. These two pathways can be connected by the so-called ω-3 desaturase (or methyl end desaturase) pathway. Within the n-3 and n-6 pathways, an alternative route of Δ8 desaturation can also bypass the Δ6 desaturation step and has already been identified in Haptophyte [8]. These routes allowed the synthesis of 20:5n-3 as well as 22:6n-3 (Figure 1).

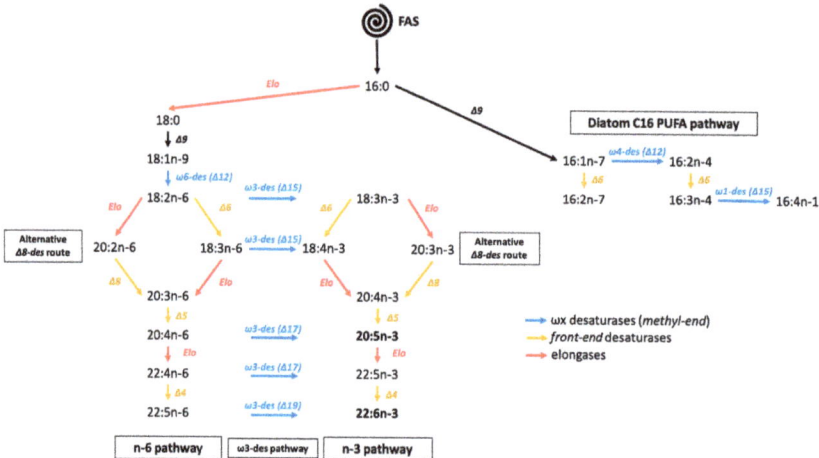

Figure 1. Microalgae fatty acid synthesis pathways. Desaturases are noted with "ΔX" (yellow arrows) and "ωY-des (ΔX)" (blue arrows), where X refers to the location of carbon holding the newly formed double bond from the front end (or carboxyl end) and Y its position from the methyl end. Elo: elongase, FAS: fatty acid synthase.

An alternative O_2 independent pathway, called the polyketide synthase (PKS) pathway, is responsible of long chain PUFA synthesis such as 20:5n-3 and 22:6n-3 [3,9,10]. It has been found in bacteria and protists such as thraustochytrids, dinophytes, and haptophytes [11–15]. The PKS pathway relies on the same four basic enzymatic reactions (condensation, reduction, dehydration, and reduction) as the FAS pathway. Opposed to the conventional pathway, the PKS pathway is less energy consuming, because it requires fewer reduction and dehydration steps than "conventional" pathways [3]. The metabolites used to form the carbon chain are simultaneously desaturated and elongated, creating long-chain PUFA [3,16,17].

Even if some microalgae species share all or part of O_2-dependent n-3 and n-6 pathways and O_2-independent PKS pathways, PUFA composition of primary producers varies greatly according to species. Diatoms synthetize more 20:5n-3 as well as C16 PUFA, while dinophytes or haptophytes contain more 22:6n-3 or C_{18} PUFA. Other groups such as cyanobacteria or some chlorophytes classes are unable to build 20:5n-3 or 22:6n-3 or only in very low proportions (<1%) [18–21].

To improve knowledge of the synthesis routes and production of 20:5n-3 and 22:6n-3, studies have focused on identifying genes coding for the different elongase and desaturase [10,22–25]. Moreover, in recent years, the use of ^{13}C substrate allowed monitoring the incorporation of labelled substrates into targeted organic macromolecules. Different metabolic intermediates or end products such as fatty acids [26–29] are monitored and quantified. This has already been applied to *E. coli* [30], yeast [29], and microalgae [31–35]. The development of technics such as gas chromatography coupled to mass spectrometry (GC-c-IRMS) consists of a noticeable improvement in the direct resolution of isotopic composition of organic macromolecules the so-called compounds specific isotope analysis (CSIA) including fatty acids [36–39].

The present study aims at investigating the synthesis pathways of essential PUFA 20:5n-3 and 22:6n-3 using stable isotope (^{13}C) labelling experiment of the haptophyte *Tisochrysis lutea*. *T. lutea* is intensively used in aquaculture (hatchery) and industry [40]. The incorporation of ^{13}C was monitored in 11 FA during 24 h at a high temporal resolution (each 0.5 to 2 h). Progressive accretion of the ^{13}C-labelled CO_2 into FA (from precursors to PUFA of interest) allowed us to constrain FAS, elongase/desaturase, and PKS involvement in 20:5n-3 and 22:6n-3 production by *Tisochrysis lutea*. In parallel to the monitoring of ^{13}C incorporation into FA, growth, physiological status, and other cellular parameters (morphology, viability, esterase activity, and lipid content) were monitored by flow cytometry analysis.

2. Results

2.1. Algae Physiology and Biochemistry during the 24 h Experiment

Cell abundance for *Tisochrysis lutea* during the 24 h of experiment increased sharply from t_0 to t_{24}. The experiment allowed cell concentration to double for the three balloons (Figure 2A). Despite the attention given to homogenization at the time of subculture from inoculum, the second enriched balloon had a cell concentration twice higher than Tl1 and TlT. This difference remained constant during the entire experiment. Cell abundance varied from 4.3×10^6 cells·mL^{-1} to 9.5×10^6 cells·mL^{-1} for the most concentrated balloon Tl2 and from, on average, 2.6×10^6 cells·mL^{-1} to 6.4×10^6 cells·mL^{-1} for the two others (Figure 2A). Despite the concentration differences, the general slopes for the three balloons were very similar (0.22 cells·mL^{-1}·h^{-1} for Tl2 and 0.15 cells·mL^{-1}·h^{-1} for Tl1 + TlT) (Figure 2A). Bacteria were also found in higher abundance Tl2 (Figure 2B), almost five times higher than in Tl1 and TlT. However, bacteria increased only by a factor of 1.2 for Tl2 between t_0 and t_{24} versus a factor 3.5 in average for Tl1 and TlT. Bacteria concentration was around 6.6 times higher than algae concentration for Tl1 and TlT on average over the 24 h of the experiment. For Tl2, bacteria concentration was 16 times higher than algae concentration at the beginning of the experiment, but this ratio decreased progressively until t_{24} (8.7 times higher) (Figure 2B).

FSC and SSC were, respectively, considered a proxy of cell size and cell complexity, and FL3 was considered a proxy of chlorophyll content. SSC and red fluorescence (FL3) did not significantly vary during the entire experiment (Bartlett tests, $p > 0.05$ and ANOVA $p > 0.05$) (Table S1). FSC increased slightly with time for the three balloons (Bartlett test, $p > 0.05$ and ANOVA $p = 0.03$) (Table S1). The percentage of dead microalgae (as measured by SYTOX staining assay) remained below 7% for the 24h of the experiment (Table S1).

Particulate organic carbon concentration increased similarly to the cell abundance for the two labelled balloons from 3.6 to 9.0 mmolC·L^{-1} for Tl1, from 4.5 to 11.6 mmolC·L^{-1} for Tl2, and from 3.4 to 8.2 mmolC·L^{-1} for TlT (Figure 3A). Increase in POC, as a function of experiment duration ($R^2 = 0.81$, $p < 0.0001$), occurred at a relatively constant rate of 0.2 mmolC·L^{-1}·h^{-1} for Tl1, Tl2, and TlT considered together. Total fatty acid (TFA) concentration also increased for the three balloons (between 0.26 mmolC·L^{-1} to 0.60 mmolC·L^{-1} for Tl1, from 0.25 mmolC·L^{-1} to 0.80 mmolC·L^{-1} for Tl2, and from 0.17 mmolC·L^{-1}

to 0.55 mmolC·L^{-1} for TIT) (Figure 3B). The slope was 15 μmolC·L^{-1}·h^{-1} ($R^2 = 0.72$, $p < 0.0001$). POC was significantly correlated to cell concentration ($R^2 = 0.80$ $p < 0.0001$). The slope of the relation between POC and cell abundance is a proxy of carbon content per cell for *T. lutea*, which was, on average for the three balloons, equal to 1.07 fmolC·cell^{-1} (Figure 3C). TFA concentration was linearly and positively correlated with POC concentration ($R^2 = 0.73$, $p < 0.0001$). The slope of the regression between TFA and POC concentration indicates that TFA represent in average 7.7% of bulk POC (Figure 3D).

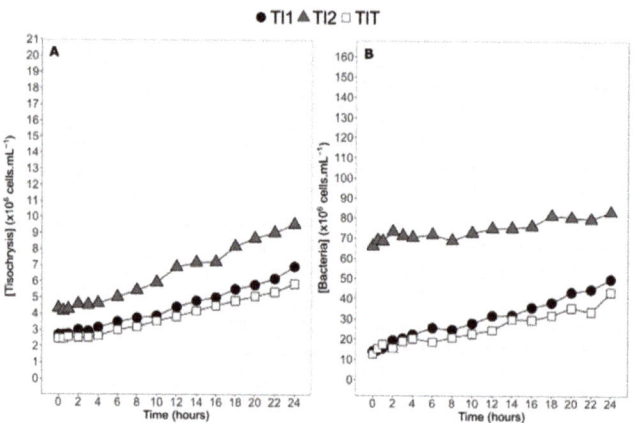

Figure 2. Temporal dynamics of cell concentrations of the two enriched balloons of *Tisochrysis lutea* (TI1 and TI2, filled black circles and filled gray triangles, respectively) and of the control balloon (TIT, empty squares) (**A**) and corresponding bacteria concentrations (**B**) during the 24 h experiment.

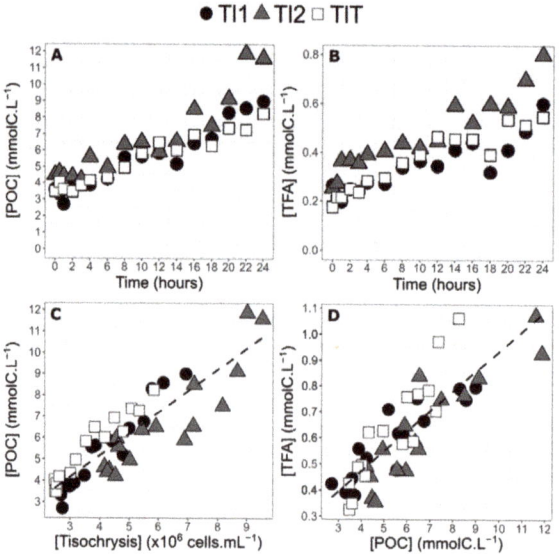

Figure 3. Particulate organic carbon (POC) concentration (**A**) of the two enriched balloons of *Tisochrysis lutea* (TI1 and TI2, filled black circles and filled gray triangles, respectively) and of the control balloon (TIT, empty squares) and total fatty acids (TFA) concentration according to culture age in hours (**B**). POC concentration according to algae concentration (**C**). Relation between total fatty acids and POC concentration (**D**). All regressions (dotted lines) have been calculated with data from the three balloons combined together.

2.2. ^{13}C Atomic Enrichment (AE) of Particulate Organic Carbon and Dissolved Inorganic Carbon

Dissolved inorganic carbon (DIC) progressively enriched in the two balloons with $^{13}CO_2$ (Figure 4A). The enrichment trends were similar for the two balloons after t_4, with an important increase in the DIC atomic enrichment until t_{20} (up to 58.1 and 61.1% for Tl1 and Tl2, respectively). The increase in AE tended to stabilize after t_{20}. Final levels of enrichment were 61.5 and 64.6% for Tl1 and Tl2, respectively (Figure 4A). Atomic enrichment (AE_{POC}) increased sharply after t_4 for the two balloons until the end of the experiment. Enrichment levels at t_{24} were 25.2 and 34.7% for Tl1 and Tl2, respectively (Figure 4B).

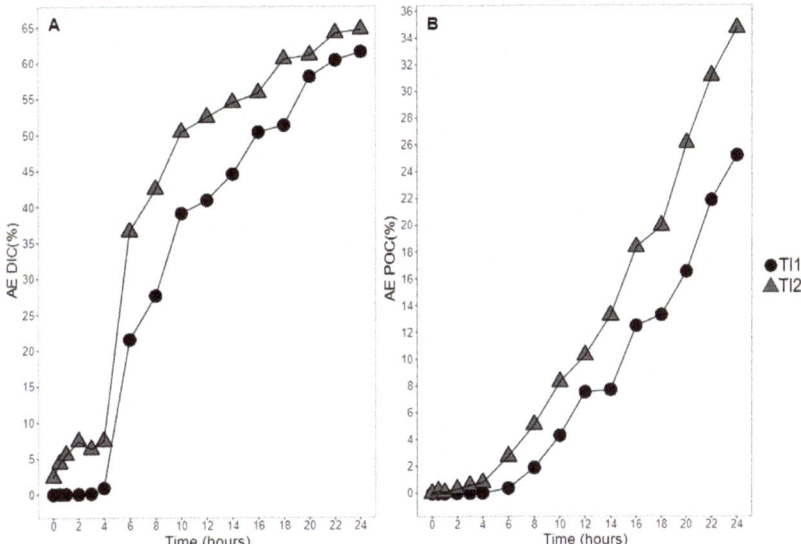

Figure 4. Atomic enrichment of the dissolved inorganic carbon (DIC) (**A**) and particulate organic carbon (POC) (**B**) of the two enriched balloons of *Tisochrysis lutea* (Tl1 and Tl2, filled black circles and filled gray triangles, respectively).

2.3. Fatty Acid Composition in Neutral and Polar Lipids in T. lutea

Neutral lipids and polar lipids represented, respectively, 37% and 63% of TFA on average for the three balloons (Figure 5A). The proportions of individual fatty acid in NL and PL did not vary throughout the experiment. Total bacteria fatty acids (iso15:0, ante15:0, iso16:0, iso17:0, 15:0, 17:0, 21:0, 15:1n-5—Tables S2–S4) remained below 1% for both NL and PL fractions during the 24 h. Branched fatty acids were only present in trace amounts (Tables S2–S4). Concentrations in $\mu g \cdot L^{-1}$ and $\mu molC \cdot L^{-1}$ as well as proportions in% of all identified and quantified FA in neutral and polar lipid fractions according to sampling time are available in the Supplementary Files (Tables S2–S4).

We focus the presentation of the results on the polar lipid fraction, as it is the predominant fraction containing FA (Figure 5B). During the experiment, thirty two fatty acids (FA), as listed in the Material and Methods section, were identified and quantified for *T. lutea*, with 12 being over 1% of the TFA in PL (14:0, 16:0, 18:0, 16:1n-7, 18:1n-9, 18:1n-7, 18:2n-6, 18:3n-3, 18:4n-3, 18:5n-3, 22:5n-6, and 22:6n-3) (Figure 5A). Although under 1% for PL, the 16:3n-6, 20:5n-3, and 22:5n-3 were also presented due to their potential synthesis significance (Figure 5A). PUFA (in average 30%) and SFA (21%) were the main FA categories for polar lipids (PL) during the 24 h. PUFA n-3 represented 25% of the TFA, PUFA n-6 5%.

In PL, 14:0 and 22:6n-3 (respectively, 21% and 18% on average over the 24 h) were the most abundant, followed by 18:1n-9, 18:4n-3, and 16:0 (11–13% of TFA). Finally, 18:3n-3, 18:5n-3, and 22:5n-6 ranged from 3 to 4% of the TFA (Figure 5B). Patterns observed for NL are available in Supplementary Files (Figure S1).

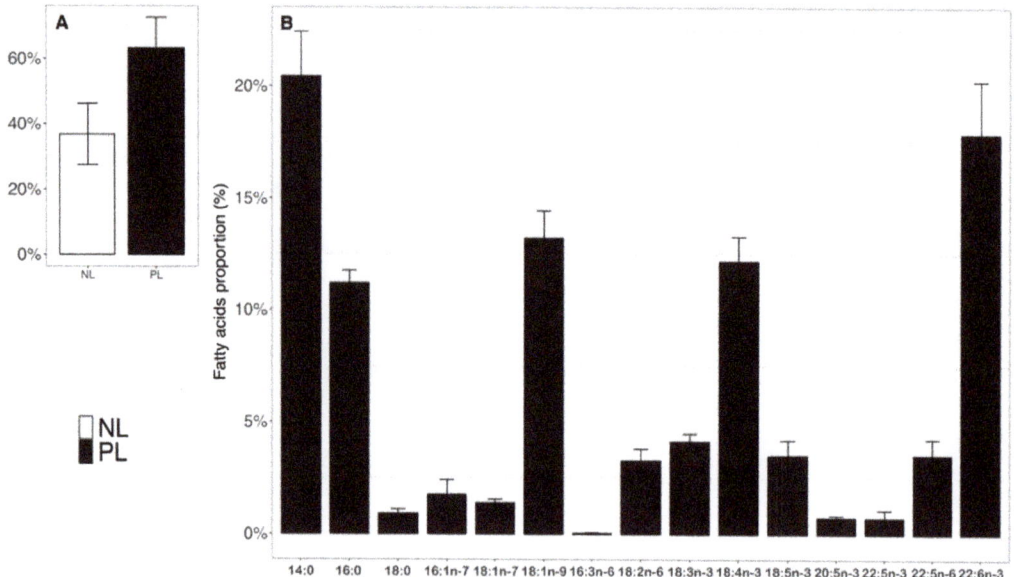

Figure 5. Proportions (%) of NL vs. PL (**A**) and proportions (%) of fifteen fatty acids in the PL fraction in average over the 24 h (**B**).

2.4. Fatty Acid ^{13}C Atomic Enrichment

Figure 6 shows the atomic enrichment (AE) of the eleven fatty acids over time. Despite the different timing and level of enrichment between the two balloons, the temporal dynamic of fatty acids enrichment remained similar. The 18:2n-6 and 18:1n-9 + 18:3n-3 had the highest AE during the entire experiment. 22:5n-6, 16:0, and finally, 20:5n-3 were next. The less enriched fatty acids in the polar lipid fraction were in decreasing order 22:5n-3, 22:6n-3, 18:4n-3, 18:5n-3, and finally, 18:0 (Figure 6). For the NL (Supplementary Files, Figure S2), 20:5n-3, 22:5n-6, 18:1n-9, 16:0, and 18:2n-6 were always the most enriched. The sequence for the other fatty acids remained close to that of polar lipids. It has to be noted that enrichments of 20:5n-3 and, to a lesser extent, of 22:5n-3 were higher in NL than in PL.

Table 1 explored FA synthesis pathways with regard to their most expected direct precursor. Most ratios were below 1, except for the 20:5n-3/18:5n-3 ratio, which was above 1. Similar patterns were observed in NL (Supplementary Files, Table S5).

Table 1. Mean ratio of atomic enrichment (AE) for pairs of FA (FA$_A$ vs. FA$_B$) in the polar lipids (PL) (mean ± SD, n = 9 sampling dates t_8 to t_{24}) for the two enriched balloons (Tl1, Tl2, Tl = *Tisochrysis lutea*).

	Polar Lipids			
	Tl1		Tl2	
Fatty Acid B/Fatty Acid A	Mean *	SD	Mean *	SD
18:5n-3/18:4n-3	0.78	0.10	0.78	0.14
20:5n-3/18:5n-3	2.00	0.92	1.77	0.51
22:5n-3/20:5n-3	0.98	0.20	0.97	0.06
22:6n-3/22:5n-3	0.88	0.03	0.87	0.02
22:6n-3/20:5n-3	0.86	0.17	0.84	0.03
22:6n-3/22:5n-6	0.61	0.05	0.59	0.06

* If the AE of the product (B) exceeds the AE of the reactant (A), ratio > 1, then it is necessary to consider another formation process for B. If the ratio is <1, transformation of A into B is considered possible. If the ratio is close to 1, the fatty acids A and B are at the equilibrium in terms of label incorporated, implying B is then synthesized simultaneously or very rapidly from A.

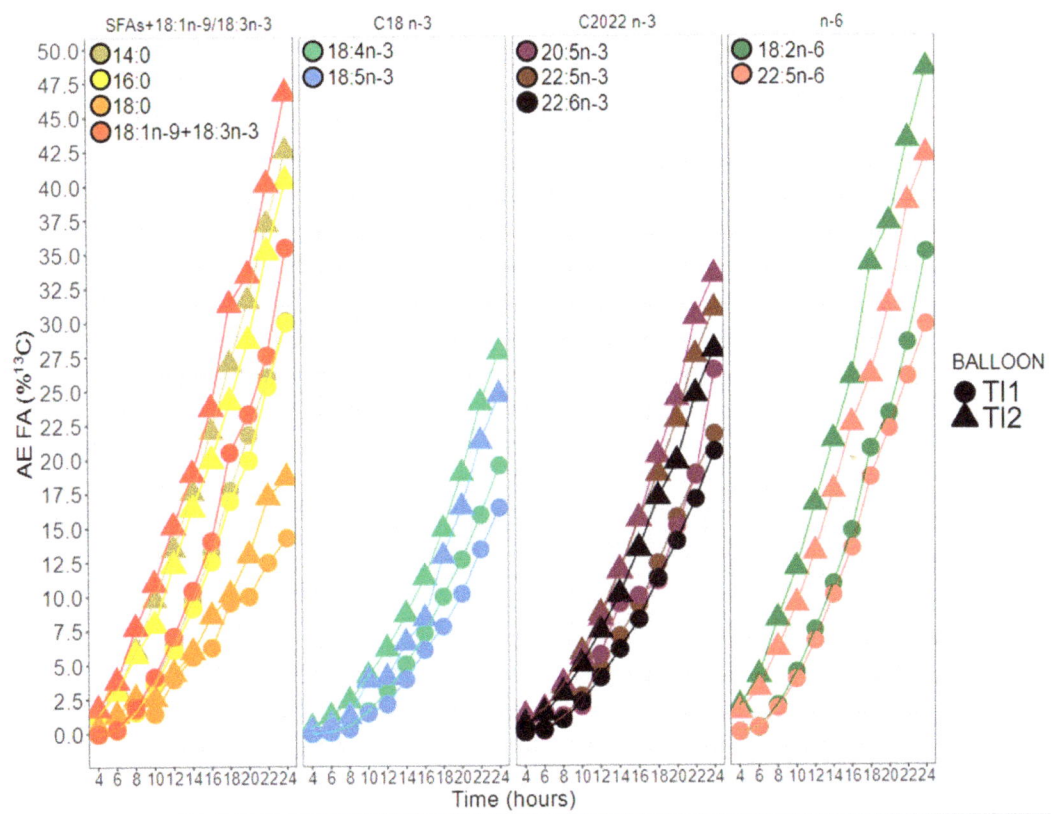

Figure 6. Atomic enrichment of 11 main fatty acids in the polar lipid (PL) fraction during a 24 h ^{13}C labelling experiment of the two enriched balloons of *Tisochrysis lutea* (TI1 and TI2, filled circles and filled triangles, respectively).

2.5. Identification of Candidate Proteins for PKS Synthesis in T. lutea

Thirty sequences of potential candidate proteins involved in *T. lutea* PUFA synthesis have been identified and are presented in Supplementary File (Table S6). Only fourteen presented the four main domains potentially coding for the enzymes used in PKS PUFA synthesis pathways: ketoacyl reductase (KR), polyketide synthase (KS), dehydrase/dehydrogenase (DH), and enoyl reductase (ER). Among these sequences, four sequences (TISO_14962, TISO_14968, TISO_14975, and TISO_14977) were part of the same cluster (group of homologous proteins) and presented multiple KS, KR, ER, and DH domains as well as phosphopantetheine (PP)-binding domains (Figure 7). TISO_14962 also possessed methyltransferases and thioesterase domains (Figure 7). TISO_14977 presented a domain acknowledged to be involved in acetyl-CoA synthesis. Within this cluster, TISO_14973 was also selected, as it contains an atypical domain, specifically recognized as being involved in n-3 PUFA synthesis. Nine other sequences (TISO_04539, TISO_06404, TISO_06537, TISO_08047, TISO_11097 TISO_16495, TISO_27353, TISO_37260, and TISO_37631) were also found, containing the four main domains (up to 18 for KR in TISO_08047). Except TISO_37631, these sequences also have thioesterase, sulfotransferase, or peptide-synthesis-related domains, and thus they might be in charge of the synthesis of more complex lipids.

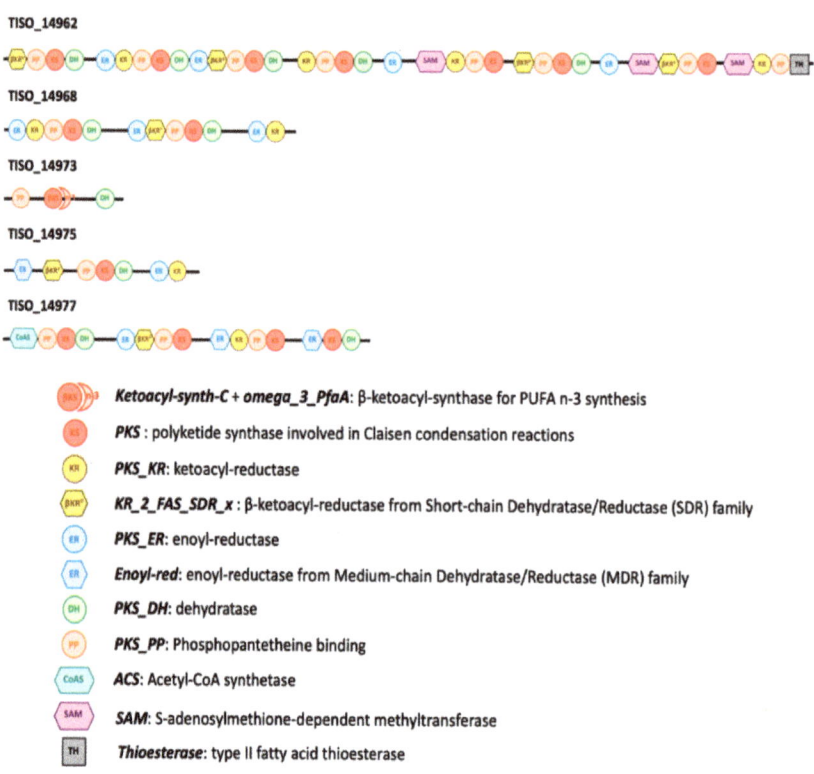

Figure 7. Cluster of candidate proteins suspected involved in PKS PUFA synthesis pathway in *T. lutea*. The name of each protein is annotated with TISO_ (for *Tisochrysis lutea*) and associated number. In the legend, the text written in bold italic correspond to domain names as shown in NCBI conserved domain database, followed by its suspected role.

3. Discussion

This study investigated long-chain PUFA synthesis pathways in the haptophyte *Tisochrysis lutea* using the incorporation of $^{13}CO_2$. Addition of $^{13}CO_2$ did not affect *T. lutea* physiology. Cell viability remained above 93% during the experiment, while cell complexity and chlorophyll content did not vary significantly according to sampling time. Cell size (as attested by FSC) increased slightly during the 24 h experiment. *T. lutea* produced FA to a level of 7% of POC; predominantly in the form of PL (66%).

Major FA of *T. lutea* were similar in proportions to those found in other prymnesiophycea (Haptophytes), i.e., 14:0, 16:0, 18:1n-9, 18:4n-3, and 22:6n-3 [41–45]. As reported before in Huang et al. (2019) [46], *T. lutea* had a low content of neutral lipids during exponential phase, and PUFA were mainly found in the polar fraction. *Tisochrysis lutea* accumulates neutral lipids mainly during stationary phase or under nutritive limitations [45].

The final level of atomic enrichment (AE) into the different FA witnessed active synthesis, as most fatty acids had a higher AE than that of POC (30% on average for the two balloons). 22:5n-6 was the most enriched long chain PUFA (LC-PUFA) in the PL fraction. 22:5n-6 and 18:2n-6 were the only ^{13}C labelled n-6 fatty acids detectable by GC-c-IRMS. None of the known synthesis intermediates (18:3n-6, 20:3n-6, 20:4n-6, and 22:4n-6) between 18:2n-6 and 22:5n-6 [4] had measurable ^{13}C-labelling and were below 1% in the FA profile during our experiment. It is then difficult to hypothesize the pathway used to create 22:5n-6 with this missing information. However, even though the different intermediates were undetectable, 18:2n-6 and 22:5n-6 atomic enrichments being very close cannot exclude them to be related to each other. While studying the existence of an alternative ∆8 desaturase in Haptophyte, Qi et al. (2002) [8] noticed the absence of intermediates of the n-6 ∆8 desaturase pathway (20:2n-6, 20:3n-6 and 20:4n-6)) in *Isochrysis galbana*. It was attributed to relatively high active enzymes that could form the end-product 22:5n-6 with a rapid flow through these n-6 intermediates. Our results agree with this, as ^{13}C enrichment of n-6 intermediates could not be detected by compound specific isotope analysis. To demonstrate the existence of these pathways, it would be interesting to combine functional analysis of desaturases by expression in yeast and GC-c-IRMS monitoring of the intermediates after ^{13}C labelling of their precursors.

However, it is also possible that another pathway not involving "classical" n-6 FA intermediates exist in *T. lutea*. Previous studies showed the existence of PKS genes in various species of the prymnesiophytes including *Isochrysis galbana* [47], closely phylogenetically related to *Tisochrysis lutea*. We identified five candidates; proteins potentially involved in PKS synthesis pathway in *T. lutea*. Even if their function has not been verified, it is possible that at least one of the proteins presented in Figure 7 was responsible for the formation of n-6 PUFA in the haptophyte. Thus, our hypothesis is that an n-6 PKS pathway might also exist in *T. lutea* (Figure 8). Finally, PKS and "classical" n-6 routes might not be completely independent and could interact in the synthesis of 22:5n-6 in *T. lutea*.

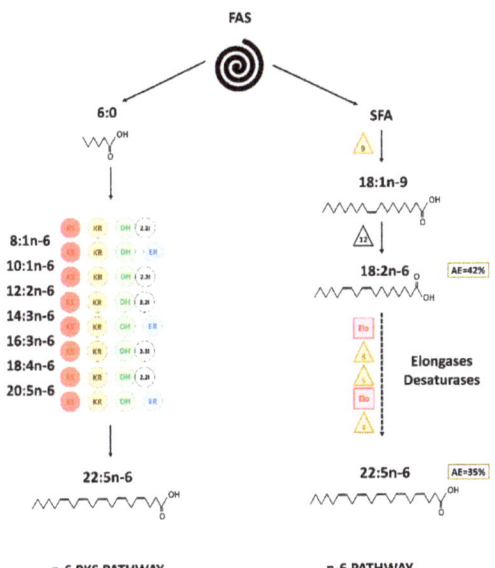

Figure 8. Hypothesized pathways for 22:5n-6 synthesis in *T. lutea* in the PL. Numbers in the boxes correspond to final AE value. The triangles symbolize the desaturases (front-end in yellow and methyl-end in purple), the circles the enzymes involved PKS pathway (KR: 3-ketoacyl synthase, KS: 3-ketoacyl-ACP-reductase, DH: dehydrase, 2.2I: 2-trans, 2-cis isomerase, 2.3I: 2-trans, 2-cis isomerase, ER: enoyl reductase), and the squares the elongases.

Despite being one of the most abundant FA, 18:4n-3 showed a low ^{13}C-enrichment (23%). The synthesis of 18:4n-3 from 18:3n-3 by ∆6 desaturase had already been described by *Isochrysis* sp. [48]. We assume that such activity also exists in *Tisochrysis*, phylogenetically close to *Isochrysis*. However, as 18:3n-3 co-elute with 18:1n-9, it was not possible to measure its AE and to assess whether this could be a limiting step in n-3 pathway (Figure 9). The 18:5n-3 had the lowest enrichment, and the ratio 18:5n-3/18:4n-3 was below the threshold value (R = 0.78), indicating a feasible transformation of 18:4n-3 into 18:5n-3. The existence of ∆3 desaturase that could support the production of 18:5n-3 (18:5∆3,6,9,12,15) from 18:4n-3

(18:4Δ6,9,12,15) had been suggested by Joseph (1975) [49] to explain the presence of this unusual FA in dinophytes. A more recent study by Ahman et al. (2011) [23] showed in *Ostreococcus lucimarinus* that a Δ4 desaturase was surprisingly able to add a double bond in 18:4n-3 at the Δ3 position leading to the formation of 18:5n-3 when the gene was expressed in yeast cell and supplemented by 18:4n-3 as substrate. With our results and the discovery of Ahman et al. (2011) [23], we proposed that a Δ4 desaturase of *T. lutea* might be able to act as a Δ3 desaturase on 18:4n-3 to produce 18:5n-3 (Figure 9). Desaturation of 18:4n-3 into 18:5n-3 had been previously hypothesized by Kotajima et al. (2014) [50] in the prymnesiophyte *Emiliania huxleyi*.

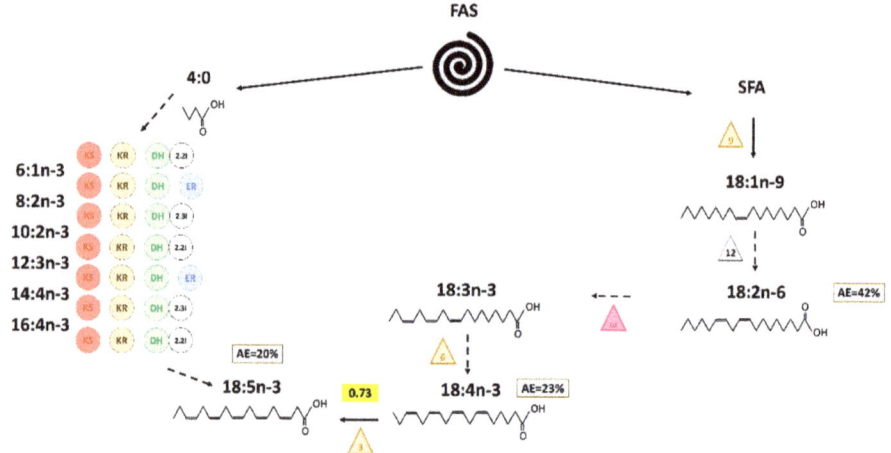

Figure 9. Hypothesized pathways to produce 18:5n-3 in *T. lutea*. Numbers in boxes correspond to final mean AE value, and number in the yellow box the mean value of ratio of the two surrounding fatty acids. The triangles symbolize the desaturases (front-end in yellow and methyl-end in purple), the circles the enzymes involved PKS pathway (KR: 3-ketoacyl synthase, KS: 3-ketoacyl-ACP-reductase, DH: dehydrase, 2.2I: 2-trans, 2-cis isomerase, 2.3I: 2-trans, 2-cis isomerase, ER: enoyl reductase). The directions with dashed arrows cannot be proven with the enrichment dynamics.

The 18:5n-3 was also described as an intermediate of 22:6n-3 synthesis by PKS pathway [4]. However, its low enrichment, as compared to 22:6n-3, appeared not compatible with a hypothetical production through this pathway. Nevertheless, one may speculate that there are two separated PKS pathways, one for the 22:6n-3 and one for the 18:5n-3, as these two PUFA are localized in different cell compartments. The 18:5n-3 is generally associated with chloroplastic glycolipids, while the 22:6n-3 is predominant in the other cellular compartments [51–53].

Surprisingly, 20:5n-3 in PL was more enriched than 18:4n-3, its precursor in the n-3 pathway [4]. As AE of 20:5n-3 is higher than AE of 18:4n-3, it seems very unlikely that 20:5n-3 was produced via the pathway involving 18:4n-3 elongation and 20:4n-3 Δ5 desaturation. The existence of the alternative Δ8 desaturase pathway have been studied before in *Isochrysis galbana* and *Pavlova lutheri* [8,54,55]. However, as for the n-6 PUFA, intermediates (20:3n-3 and 20:4n-3) of the alternative Δ8 pathway were not detected by fatty acid analysis of *Isochrysis galbana* [8]. Similarly, in our study, intermediates (20:3n-3 and 20:4n-3) of this pathway to synthesize 20:5n-3 have not been found in sufficient amount to be measured by CSIA. As proposed by Qi et al. (2002) [8] for *Isochrysis galbana*, the synthesis of 20:5n-3 via 20:3n-3 and 20:4n-3 by *Tisochrysis lutea* might be very rapid, explaining why these two intermediates were only found in trace amounts (0.12% and 0.02% in PL, and 0.05% and 0.33% in NL, respectively).

Due to their lower enrichments, 18:4n-3 and 18:5n-3 seemed unlikely involved in long chain PUFA synthesis such as 20:5n-3 and 22:6n-3. Based on the enrichment dynamics, elongation of 20:5n-3 into 22:5n-3 and further desaturation into 22:6n-3, respectively, by Δ5 elongase and Δ4 desaturase could be possible in *Tisochrysis lutea*. Ratio 22:5n-3/20:5n-3 in PL was within the threshold, indicating a simultaneous enrichment of both 20:5n-3 and 22:5n-3 in *T. lutea*. Such enzymes have been evidenced in haptophytes [54,56,57].

Considering the diversity of PKS gene in haptophytes [47], the possibility of production of 22:6n-3 directly by PKS PUFA synthesis pathway might be possible, as previously shown with thraustochytrids [10,58]. Synthesis of 22:6n-3 by PKS pathway might be at play in parallel with the n-3 pathway. Indeed, we identified a protein cluster gathering the four main domains potentially coding for the enzymes used in PKS PUFA synthesis pathways: ketoacyl reductase (KR), polyketide synthase (KS), dehydrase/dehydrogenase (DH), and enoyl reductase (ER). Protein clusters are groups of similar proteins that most likely shared the same or similar functions [59]. By considering this cluster (candidate proteins TISO_14962, TISO_14968, TISO_14968, TISO_14973, TISO_14975, and TISO_14977, Figure 8), it could be possible that these proteins act together and allow n-3 PUFA synthesis via PKS pathway. Interestingly, protein TISO_14973, while possessing only two of the four domains of interest (KS and DH), presented a specific n-3 domain. This protein might act concomitantly with the other proteins of the same cluster and allow the access to the missing reductase activities (KR and ER). Finally, the ratio 22:5n-6/22:6n-3 was below the threshold value making possible the conversion of 22:5n-6 into 22:6n-3 if we assumed that ω3-desaturase might exist in haptophyte. Synthesis of 22:6n-3 by both n-3 and n-6 pathway might be feasible in *Tisochrysis lutea* (Figure 10). These different ways to produce 22:6n-3 might contribute to betaine lipids synthesis. Indeed, betaine lipids are generally highly unsaturated in C_{20} and C_{22} PUFA, especially in 22:6n-3 in haptophytes [60–63].

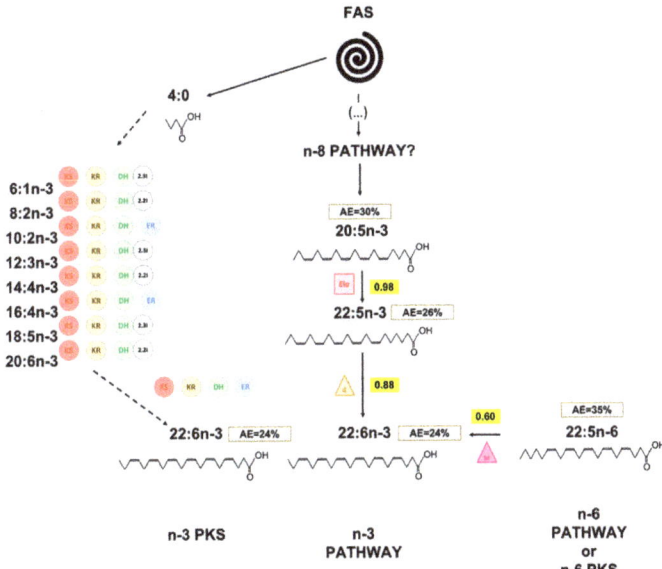

Figure 10. Hypothesized pathways to produce DHA in *T. lutea*. Numbers in boxes correspond to final mean AE value, and number in the yellow box is the mean value of ratio of the two surrounding fatty acids. The triangles symbolize the desaturases (front-end in yellow and methyl-end in purple), the circles the enzymes involved in PKS pathway (KR: 3-ketoacyl synthase, KS: 3-ketoacyl-ACP-reductase, DH: dehydrase, 2.2I/2.3I: 2-trans, 2-cis or 2-trans, 3-cis isomerases, ER: enoyl-reductase), and the squares the elongases.

4. Material and Methods

4.1. Algal Culture and ^{13}C Labelling

This study was conducted following the experimental design described by Remize et al. (2020) [34]. The marine prymnesiophyte *Tisochrysis lutea* (T-iso, CCAP 927/14) was cultured in 2 L batch condition in balloons under continuous light (24 h light cycle, 100 µmoles photons m$^{-2}\cdot$s^{-1}) at 20 °C and with pH regulation at 7.50 ± 0.05 by CO_2 injection. Filtered seawater was previously enriched with Conway medium [64] and inoculated with *T. lutea* preculture in a growing stage (exponential phase, four days old). The experimental setup was composed of two cultures (Tl1 and Tl2) receiving the labelling ^{13}C-CO_2 gas (Sigma-Aldrich, <3%atom ^{18}O, 99.0%atom ^{13}C) and one culture (TlT) receiving petrochemical CO_2 gas. ^{13}C-incorporation in Tl1 and Tl2 began after inoculation (t_0) and was maintained for 24 h (t_{24}).

During the first hours of the experiment, the $^{13}CO_2$ injection tube of balloon Tl1 had been temporarily disconnected from the system. Consequently, balloon Tl2 received earlier the $^{13}CO_2$ and thus started to incorporate ^{13}C before balloon Tl1.

4.2. Samples Collection

Sampling was performed as described in Remize et al. (2020) [34], i.e., at 30 min, 1 h, 2 h, 3 h, 4 h, and then every 2 h. A total of 16 samples was collected during the 24 h monitoring. At each sampling time, a total volume of 30 to 70 mL was collected for (i) flow cytometry analysis of cellular parameters, (ii) bulk isotopic analysis of particulate organic carbon (^{13}C-POC) and dissolved inorganic carbon (^{13}C-DIC) by EA-IRMS, (iii) fatty acid (FA) analysis in neutral lipids (NL) and polar lipids (PL) by GC-FID, and (iv) compound specific isotope analysis (CSIA) of FA (^{13}C-FA) by GC-IRMS, as described in the following paragraphs.

4.3. Flow Cytometry Analysis

Algae growth cellular variables were measured using an Easy-Cyte Plus 6HT flow cytometer (Guava Merck Millipore®, Darmstadt, Germany) equipped with a 488 nm blue laser, detectors of forward (FSC) and side (SSC) light scatters, and three fluorescence detectors: green (525/30 nm), yellow (583/26 nm), and red (680/30 nm). The protocol, the variables studied, and the probes used for this cytometry following are described in Remize et al. (2020) [34]. Briefly, forward scatter (FSC), side scatter (SSC), and red fluorescence (FL3, red emission filter long pass, 670 nm) are used to study, respectively, cell size, complexity, and chlorophyll content. The fluorescent probe (SYTOX, Molecular Probes, Invitrogen, Eugene OR, USA, final concentration of 0.05 µM) was used to assess cell viability on FL1 detector (green fluorescence). The concentration of bacteria was also monitored by using SYBR®Green (Molecular Probes, Invitrogen, Eugene, OR, USA, #S7563) on FL1 detector. Concentrations of algae and bacteria were given cells per mL, and cellular variables were expressed in arbitrary units (a.u).

4.4. POC Concentration and Bulk Carbon Isotopic Composition

For particulate organic carbon (POC) and stable isotopic composition measurements, 30–70 mL of samples were filtered through pre-combusted 0.7 µm nominal pore-size glass fiber filters (Whatman GF/F, Maidstone, UK). The filter was processed, subsampled, and encapsulated as described in Remize et al. (2020) [34]. POC concentrations of all samples were measured using a CE Elantech NC2100 (ThermoScientific, Lakewood, NJ, USA) according to protocol by Remize et al. (2020) [34]. Bulk carbon isotopic composition (^{13}C-POC) was analyzed by continuous flow on an Elemental Analyzer (EA, Flash 2000; Thermo Scientific, Bremen, Germany) coupled to a Delta V+ isotope ratio mass spectrometer (Thermo Scientific). Calibration was performed with international standards and in-house standard described in Table 2.

Table 2. List of international and in-house standards used for EA-IRMS and GB-IRMS analysis.

Description	Nature	Analysis	$\delta^{13}C$ (‰)	SD
IAEA-CH$_6$	Sucrose (C$_{12}$H$_{22}$O$_{11}$)	13C-POC	−10.45	0.03
IAEA-600	Caffeine (C$_8$H$_{10}$N$_4$O$_2$)	13C-POC	−27.77	0.04
Acetanilide	Acetanilide (C$_8$H$_9$NO)	13C-POC	+29.53	0.01
CA21 (in-house std)	Calcium carbonate (CaCO$_3$)	13C-DIC	+1.476	
Na$_2$CO$_3$ (in-house std)	Sodium carbonate	13C-DIC	−6.8805	
NaHCO$_3$ (in-house std)	Sodium bicarbonate	13C-DIC	−5.9325	

4.5. DIC Concentration and Bulk Carbon Isotopic Composition

Samples for dissolved inorganic carbon (DIC) concentration and stable isotopic composition were collected from the filtrate of POC samples and processed as described in Remize et al. (2020) [34]. Analyses were conducted in a gas bench coupled to a Delta Plus mass spectrometer from Thermo Fisher Scientific, Bremen, Germany (GB-IRMS).

4.6. Isotopic Data Processing

We used the atomic proportion of ^{13}C in percent (%atom of ^{13}C) to express the results instead of the δ notation due to ^{13}C-labelling. Conversion between δ notation and %atom ^{13}C notation can be done as follow [65]:

$$\%atom^{13}C = 100 \times \frac{\left(\frac{\delta^{13}C}{1000}+1\right) \times \left(\frac{^{13}C}{^{12}C}\right)_{VPDB}}{1+\left(\frac{\delta^{13}C}{1000}+1\right) \times \left(\frac{^{13}C}{^{12}C}\right)_{VPDB}} \quad (1)$$

where $(^{13}C/^{12}C)_{PDB}$ = 0.0112372, the ratio of ^{13}C to ^{12}C in the international reference VPDB standard.

Atomic enrichment (AE) of POC and DIC is then calculated from atom%^{13}C-POC correction by POC$_{control}$ values (i.e., corrected by 1.08%) and from atom%^{13}C DIC corrected by control values (DIC$_{control}$ = 1.12%), respectively, according to the following equations:

$$AE_{POC} = \%atom^{13}C - POC_{control} \quad (2)$$

$$AE_{DIC} = \%atom^{13}C - DIC_{control} \quad (3)$$

4.7. Fatty Acids Analysis

4.7.1. Fatty Acids Analysis by Gas Chromatography Flame Ionisation Detector (GC-FID)

Lipid extraction, separation of neutral and polar lipid fractions, and transesterification processes are described elsewhere [34]. Fatty acids methyl esters (FAME) samples were analyzed by gas chromatography on a Varian CP8400 gas chromatograph (Agilent, Santa Clara, CA, USA) and separated concomitantly on two columns: one polar (ZB-WAX: 30 mm × 0.25 mm ID × 0.2 µm, Phenomenex, Torrance CA, USA) and the other apolar (ZB-5HT: 30 m × 0.25 mm ID × 0.2 µm, Phenomenex, Torrance CA, USA). The FAME of *T. lutea* were quantified using C23:0 as an internal standard (2.3 µg in each lipid fraction prior transmethylation) and were identified by comparison of their retention times with commercial standards (Supelco 37 component FAME mix, the PUFA No. 1 and No. 3 and the Bacterial Acid Methyl Ester Mix from Sigma-Aldrich, Darmstadt, Germany) and in-house standards mixtures. FA concentrations were reported as µg C·L^{-1} and as % of total fatty acids from each lipid fraction. Thirty two fatty acids (FA) were thus identified and quantified: iso15:0, anteiso15:0, 14:0, 15:0, 16:0, 18:0, 22:0, 24:0, 14:1n-5, 16:1n-9, 16:1n-7, 17:1n-1, 18:1n-9, 18:1n-7, 16:2n-7, 16:2n-4, 16:4n-3, 18:2n-6, 18:3n-6, 18:3n-3, 18:4n-3, 18:5n-3, 20:2n-6, 20:3n-6, 20:4n-6, 20:4n-3, 20:5n-3, 22:2n-6, 22:4n-6, 22:5n-6, 22:5n-3, and 22:6n-3. Individual fatty acid and total fatty acid concentrations (as the sum of both fractions, named thereafter TFA) obtained in µg·L^{-1} by GC-FID were also expressed in µmolC·L^{-1}

($\mu g \cdot L^{-1}$/molecular weight of individual fatty acid × carbon number of individual fatty acid) to ease the comparison with POC concentrations expressed in $\mu molC \cdot L^{-1}$ as well.

4.7.2. Fatty Acid Compound-Specific Isotope Analysis and Processing

Samples for compound-specific isotope analyses (CSIA) of FAME were performed on a Thermo Fisher Scientific GC ISOLINK TRACE ULTRA (Bremen, Germany) using the same apolar column as mentioned above for FAME analysis. Only the fatty acids with the highest concentrations, as measured by GC-FID analyses, were considered for CSIA (namely 14:0, 16:0, 18:0, 18:1n-9, 18:2n-6, 18:3n-3, 18:4n-3, 18:5n-3, 20:5n-3, 22:5n-6, 22:5n-3, and 22:6n-3). The other FA presenting a too low signal amplitude (<800 mV) on the GC-c-IRMS did not allow precise isotope ratio analysis. Additionally, 18:1n-9 and 18:3n-3 co-eluted for GC-c-IRMS on the apolar column, but most of the isotopic signature for neutral lipids (NL) is attributed to 18:1n-9. However, in the polar fraction (PL), 18:1n-9 and 18:3n-3 are in relatively similar proportion and so were considered together. Additionally, ^{13}C enrichment of 18:5n-3 could only be measured in the polar lipid fraction, but its concentration was too low in neutral lipid fraction to measure its isotope composition.

To evidence FA conversion of fatty acid A into fatty acid B in *T. lutea*, we calculated the AE_{FA} ratio (R) of product B over expected precursor A. R was defined with a confidence interval calculated at α = 0.1 (defined arbitrarily) as follows:

$$R = \frac{AE_{FA(B)}}{AE_{FA(A)}} \quad (4)$$

where A is the fatty acid hypothesized to be a precursor to fatty acid B, and $AE_{FA(A)}$ and $AE_{FA(B)}$ are their respective atomic enrichments at each sampling time.

If the AE of the product (B) exceeds the AE of the reactant (A), ratio > 1, then it is necessary to consider another formation process for B, since any molecule formed from A would have the same AE as A or below. If the ratio is <1, transformation of A into B is considered possible. If the ratio is close to 1, the fatty acids A and B are at equilibrium in terms of label incorporated, implying B is then synthesized simultaneously or very rapidly from A.

4.8. Identification within the in Silico Proteome of T. lutea of PKS Enzymes Involved PUFA Synthesis

The in silico proteome generated from last annotated version of the genome of *T. lutea* was used to identify putative proteins involved in n-3 PUFA PKS pathways [66]. We used the PKS previously identified in the haptophyte *Chrysochromulina tobin* as query for a BLASTp analysis, using e-value <10^{-3} as threshold [67]. Analysis of conserved domain was performed using the NCBI CD database V3,18 with e-value <10^{-2} as threshold. The genome location of genes encoding selected proteins was identified to evaluate genes' proximity and occurrence of gene clusters. Proteins and cluster of proteins containing the four domains ketoacyl reductase (KR), dehydrase/dehydrogenase (DH), enoyl reductase (ER), and polyketide synthase (KS) were selected as candidates.

4.9. Statistical Analysis

To assess the potential effect of time and difference between balloons during algae development and of $^{13}CO_2$ incorporation, Bartlett tests and ANOVA were performed on physiological and biochemical parameters, as well as PERMANOVA analysis on FA percentage separately in NL and PL. All statistical analyses were performed using R software.

5. Conclusions

The synthesis of long-chain PUFA in *Tisochrysis lutea* appeared to involve multiple pathways (Figures 8–10). First, the assumption of the use of PKS pathway for 22:5n-6 (DPA-6) was attested regarding the fast enrichment observed for this FA as well as the absence of detectable intermediates more or equally enriched. PKS pathway appeared to be particularly efficient in *T. lutea* and induced a strong incorporation of the ^{13}C-marker. However, the possibility of use of the conventional n-6 PUFA pathway should not be excluded, as 18:2n-6 presented a similar level of enrichment as 22:5n-6. It would only endorse that following desaturation and elongation steps to form 22:5n-6 were particularly dynamic and thus did not allow the accumulation of the ^{13}C-label into n-6 intermediates. Within n-3 PUFA pathway, the Δ6-desaturase route seemed slower than the n-6 pathway in *T. lutea* in producing the two C$_{18}$ polyunsaturated fatty acids 18:4n-3 and 18:5n-3. We assumed 18:4n-3 and 18:5n-3 were unlikely synthesis intermediates of 20:5n-3 and 22:6n-3, as their enrichments were lower than the latter. Although 22:6n-3 was present in higher proportion than 22:5n-6, it was not enriched as fast, possibly because its synthesis may be more complex. Indeed, 22:6n-3 could be synthesized by *Tisochrysis lutea* via a combination multiples pathway: from 22:5n-6 via ω-3 desaturase pathway, from desaturation and elongation of 20:5n-3 and 22:5n-3, and via PKS pathway. Further studies are needed to better constrain the plausible routes taken by this prymnesiophyte to produce long chain PUFA.

Supplementary Materials: The following are available online at https://www.mdpi.com/article/10.3390/md20010022/s1, Table S1: Cellular parameters of *Tisochrysis lutea* (morphology (FSC and SSC), viability (FL1-SYTOX), and chlorophyll content (FL3) using flow cytometry analysis (mean ± SD of the 3 balloons). Values for SYTOX are in%, values for FL3/SSC/FSC in arbitrary unit (a.u), Table S2: Concentrations in µg·L^{-1} of all identified and quantified FA in neutral and polar lipid fractions according to sampling time, Table S3: Concentrations in µmolC·L^{-1} of all identified and quantified FA in neutral and polar lipid fractions according to sampling time, Table S4: Concentrations in% of all identified and quantified FA in neutral and polar lipid fractions according to sampling time. Table S5: Mean ratio of atomic enrichment (AE) for pairs of FA (FAA vs. FAB) in the neutral lipids (NL) (mean ± SD, n = 9 sampling dates t8 to t24) for the two enriched balloons (Tl1, Tl2, Tl = *Tisochrysis lutea*). If the ratio is equal to or close to 1, A and B are assumed at equilibrium, and B is synthesized quickly from A; if the ratio is below 1, the transformation of B from A is possible but slow. Finally, if the ratio is above 1, A is not a main precursor of B, which has to be synthesized by a different pathway. Table S6: List of the potential candidate protein sequences involved in *Tisochrysis lutea* PKS synthesis pathway. The suspected function of each protein has been assumed using the NCBI conserved domain database (CDD) (Marchler-Bauer et al., 2017) by identifying the role of each domain recognized in the sequence. In columns KS/KR/DH/ER are written the number of domain corresponding to these functions in the studied sequences. ACS: acetyl-CoA synthetase, A_NRPS: adenylation domain of the non-ribosomal peptide synthetase (NRPS), Croto: crotonase/enoyl-CoA hydratase, EntF: enterobactin non-ribosomal peptide synthetase or thioesterase domain of Type I PKS, FAAL: fatty acyl-AMP ligase, GrsT: alpha/beta hydrolase, HM: hydroxymethylglutaryl-CoA synthase, MT: methyltransferase, PP: phosphopantetheine-binding (="swinging arm"), Sulf: sulfotransferase, Thio: thioesterase. Figure S1: Proportions (%) of NL vs. PL (A) and proportions (%) of fifteen fatty acids in the NL fraction in average over the 24 h (B). Figure S2: Atomic enrichment of 11 main fatty acids in the polar lipid (NL) fraction during a 24h ^{13}C labelling experiment. Tl: *Tisochrysis lutea*. Reference [68] is cited in the supplementary materials.

Author Contributions: Conceptualization, M.R., F.P. and P.S.; data curation, M.R.; Formal analysis, F.P.; funding acquisition, M.R., A.N.L., A.V. and P.S.; investigation, M.R., F.P., F.L.G., C.L., M.G. and P.S.; methodology, M.R., F.P., A.N.L., F.L.G., A.B., M.G. and P.S.; project administration, M.R. and P.S.; resources, R.C.; software, M.R., F.L.G. and A.B.; supervision, M.R., F.P., A.N.L. and P.S.; validation, M.R. and C.L.; visualization, M.R.; writing—original draft, M.R.; writing—review and editing, M.R., F.P., A.N.L., F.L.G., A.B., C.L., M.G, R.C., A.V. and P.S. All authors have read and agreed to the published version of the manuscript.

Funding: This research was funded by the Université de Bretagne Occidentale (UBO) and the Center for Marine Sciences (CMS) at the University of North Carolina Wilmington (UNCW), the Interdisciplinary School for the Blue Planet (ISblue), and the Walter-Zellidja grant of the Académie Française.

Institutional Review Board Statement: Not applicable.

Informed Consent Statement: Not applicable.

Acknowledgments: We would like to thank Philippe Miner, Nelly Le Goic, Margaux Mathieu-Resuge, Elodie Fleury, Adeline Bidault, Korydwen Terrasson, and Corentin Baudet for their help during sampling and Oanez Lebeau for her support during the isotopic analyses.

Conflicts of Interest: The authors declare no conflict of interest. The funders had no role in the design of the study; in the collection, analyses, or interpretation of data; in the writing of the manuscript, or in the decision to publish the results.

References

1. FAO. *The State of World Fisheries and Aquaculture 2020*; FAO: Quebec, QC, Canada, 2020; ISBN 978-92-5-132692-3.
2. Arao, T.; Yamada, M. Biosynthesis of Polyunsaturated Fatty Acids in the Marine Diatom, Phaeodactylum Tricornutum. *Phytochemistry* **1994**, *35*, 1177–1181. [CrossRef]
3. Metz, J.G.; Roessler, P.; Facciotti, D.; Levering, C.; Dittrich, F.; Lassner, M.; Valentine, R.; Lardizabal, K.; Domergue, F.; Yamada, A.; et al. Production of Polyunsaturated Fatty Acids by Polyketide Synthases in Both Prokaryotes and Eukaryotes. *Science* **2001**, *293*, 290–293. [CrossRef] [PubMed]
4. Bell, M.V.; Tocher, D.R. Biosynthesis of polyunsaturated fatty acids in aquatic ecosystems: General pathways and new directions. In *Lipids in Aquatic Ecosystems*; Kainz, M., Brett, M.T., Arts, M.T., Eds.; Springer: New York, NY, USA, 2009; pp. 211–236. ISBN 978-0-387-88607-7.
5. Gurr, M.I.; Harwood, J.L.; Frayn, K.N. Fatty acids structure and metabolism: Fatty acids biosynthesis. In *Lipid Biochemistry: An Introduction*; Wiley-Blackwell: New York, NY, USA, 2002; pp. 21–59. ISBN 0-632-05409-3.
6. Guschina, I.A.; Harwood, J.L. Lipids and Lipid Metabolism in Eukaryotic Algae. *Prog. Lipid Res.* **2006**, *45*, 160–186. [CrossRef]
7. Harwood, J.L.; Guschina, I.A. The Versatility of Algae and Their Lipid Metabolism. *Biochimie* **2009**, *91*, 679–684. [CrossRef]
8. Qi, B.; Beaudoin, F.; Fraser, T.; Stobart, A.K.; Napier, J.A.; Lazarus, C.M. Identification of a cDNA encoding a novel C18-Δ9 polyunsaturated fatty acid-specific elongating activity from the docosahexaenoic acid (DHA)-producing microalga, Isochrysis galbana. *FEBS Lett.* **2002**, *510*, 159–165. [CrossRef]
9. Hauvermale, A.; Kuner, J.; Rosenzweig, B.; Guerra, D.; Diltz, S.; Metz, J.G. Fatty Acid Production in Schizochytrium Sp.: Involvement of a Polyunsaturated Fatty Acid Synthase and a Type I Fatty Acid Synthase. *Lipids* **2006**, *41*, 739–747. [CrossRef] [PubMed]
10. Ye, C.; Qiao, W.; Yu, X.; Ji, X.; Huang, H.; Collier, J.L.; Liu, L. Reconstruction and Analysis of the Genome-Scale Metabolic Model of Schizochytrium limacinum SR21 for Docosahexaenoic Acid Production. *BMC Genom.* **2015**, *16*, 799. [CrossRef]
11. Ratledge, C. Fatty Acid Biosynthesis in Microorganisms Being Used for Single Cell Oil Production. *Biochimie* **2004**, *86*, 807–815. [CrossRef] [PubMed]
12. John, U.; Beszteri, B.; Derelle, E.; Van de Peer, Y.; Read, B.; Moreau, H.; Cembella, A. Novel Insights into Evolution of Protistan Polyketide Synthases through Phylogenomic Analysis. *Protist* **2008**, *159*, 21–30. [CrossRef]
13. Freitag, M.; Beszteri, S.; Vogel, H.; John, U. Effects of Physiological Shock Treatments on Toxicity and Polyketide Synthase Gene Expression in Prymnesium parvum (Prymnesiophyceae). *Eur. J. Phycol.* **2011**, *46*, 193–201. [CrossRef]
14. Eichholz, K.; Beszteri, B.; John, U. Putative Monofunctional Type I Polyketide Synthase Units: A Dinoflagellate-Specific Feature? *PLoS ONE* **2012**, *7*, e48324. [CrossRef] [PubMed]
15. Armenta, R.E.; Valentine, M.C. Single-Cell Oils as a Source of Omega-3 Fatty Acids: An Overview of Recent Advances. *J. Am. Oil Chem. Soc.* **2013**, *90*, 167–182. [CrossRef]
16. Wallis, J.G.; Watts, J.L.; Browse, J. Polyunsaturated Fatty Acid Synthesis: What Will They Think of Next? *Trends Biochem. Sci.* **2002**, *27*, 467–473. [CrossRef]
17. Uttaro, A. Biosynthesis of Polyunsaturated Fatty Acids in Lower Eukaryotes. *IUBMB Life* **2006**, *58*, 563–571. [CrossRef] [PubMed]
18. Caramujo, M.-J.; Boschker, H.T.S.; Admiraal, W. Fatty Acid Profiles of Algae Mark the Development and Composition of Harpacticoid Copepods. *Freshw. Biol.* **2007**, *53*, 77–90. [CrossRef]
19. Pereira, H.; Barreira, L.; Figueiredo, F.; Custódio, L.; Vizetto-Duarte, C.; Polo, C.; Rešek, E.; Engelen, A.; Varela, J. Polyunsaturated Fatty Acids of Marine Macroalgae: Potential for Nutritional and Pharmaceutical Applications. *Mar. Drugs* **2012**, *10*, 1920–1935. [CrossRef]
20. de Carvalho, C.; Caramujo, M.-J. Fatty Acids as a Tool to Understand Microbial Diversity and Their Role in Food Webs of Mediterranean Temporary Ponds. *Molecules* **2014**, *19*, 5570–5598. [CrossRef] [PubMed]
21. Hixson, S.M.; Arts, M.T. Climate Warming Is Predicted to Reduce Omega-3, Long-Chain, Polyunsaturated Fatty Acid Production in Phytoplankton. *Glob. Chang. Biol.* **2016**, *22*, 2744–2755. [CrossRef] [PubMed]
22. Courchesne, N.M.D.; Parisien, A.; Wang, B.; Lan, C.Q. Enhancement of Lipid Production Using Biochemical, Genetic and Transcription Factor Engineering Approaches. *J. Biotechnol.* **2009**, *141*, 31–41. [CrossRef] [PubMed]
23. Ahmann, K.; Heilmann, M.; Feussner, I. Identification of a Δ4-Desaturase from the Microalga Ostreococcus lucimarinus. *Eur. J. Lipid Sci. Technol.* **2011**, *113*, 832–840. [CrossRef]
24. Vaezi, R.; Napier, J.; Sayanova, O. Identification and Functional Characterization of Genes Encoding Omega-3 Polyunsaturated Fatty Acid Biosynthetic Activities from Unicellular Microalgae. *Mar. Drugs* **2013**, *11*, 5116–5129. [CrossRef]

25. Kimura, K.; Okuda, S.; Nakayama, K.; Shikata, T.; Takahashi, F.; Yamaguchi, H.; Skamoto, S.; Yamaguchi, M.; Tomaru, Y. RNA Sequencing Revealed Numerous Polyketide Synthase Genes in the Harmful Dinoflagellate Karenia mikimotoi. *PLoS ONE* **2015**, *10*, e0142731. [CrossRef] [PubMed]
26. de Swaaf, M.E.; de Rijk, T.C.; van der Meer, P.; Eggink, G.; Sijtsma, L. Analysis of Docosahexaenoic Acid Biosynthesis in Cryphecodinium cohnii by 13C Labelling and Desaturase Inhibitor Experiments. *J. Biotechnol.* **2003**, *103*, 21–29. [CrossRef]
27. Van den Meersche, K.; Middelburg, J.J.; Soetaert, K.; van Rijswijk, P.; Boschker, H.T.S.; Heip, C.H.R. Carbon-Nitrogen Coupling and Algal-Bacterial Interactions during an Experimental Bloom: Modeling a ^{13}C Tracer Experiment. *Limnol. Oceanogr.* **2004**, *49*, 862–878. [CrossRef]
28. Ecker, J.; Scherer, M.; Schmitz, G.; Liebisch, G. A Rapid GC–MS Method for Quantification of Positional and Geometric Isomers of Fatty Acid Methyl Esters. *J. Chromatogr. B* **2012**, *897*, 98–104. [CrossRef] [PubMed]
29. Zhang, H.; Wu, C.; Wu, Q.; Dai, J.; Song, Y. Metabolic Flux Analysis of Lipid Biosynthesis in the Yeast Yarrowia lipolytica Using 13C-Labled Glucose and Gas Chromatography-Mass Spectrometry. *PLoS ONE* **2016**, *11*, e0159187. [CrossRef] [PubMed]
30. Zhao, J.; Shimizu, K. Metabolic Flux Analysis of Escherichia coli K12 Grown on 13C-Labeled Acetate and Glucose Using GC-MS and Powerful Flux Calculation Method. *J. Biotechnol.* **2003**, *101*, 101–117. [CrossRef]
31. Xiong, W.; Liu, L.; Wu, C.; Yang, C.; Wu, Q. 13C-Tracer and Gas Chromatography-Mass Spectrometry Analyses Reveal Metabolic Flux Distribution in the Oleaginous Microalga Chlorella protothecoides. *Plant Physiol.* **2010**, *154*, 1001–1011. [CrossRef] [PubMed]
32. Martzolff, A.; Cahoreau, E.; Cogne, G.; Peyriga, L.; Portais, J.-C.; Dechandol, E.; Le Grand, F.; Massou, S.; Gonçalves, O.; Pruvost, J.; et al. Photobioreactor Design for Isotopic Non-Stationary 13C-Metabolic Flux Analysis (INST 13C-MFA) under Photoautotrophic Conditions. *Biotechnol. Bioeng.* **2012**, *109*, 3030–3040. [CrossRef] [PubMed]
33. Cui, J.; Diao, J.; Sun, T.; Shi, M.; Liu, L.; Wang, F.; Chen, L.; Zhang, W. 13C Metabolic Flux Analysis of Enhanced Lipid Accumulation Modulated by Ethanolamine in Cryphecodinium cohnii. *Front. Microbiol.* **2018**, *9*, 956. [CrossRef] [PubMed]
34. Remize, M.; Planchon, F.; Loh, A.N.; Le Grand, F.; Bideau, A.; Le Goic, N.; Fleury, E.; Miner, P.; Corvaisier, R.; Volety, A.; et al. Study of Synthesis Pathways of the Essential Polyunsaturated Fatty Acid 20:5n-3 in the Diatom Chaetoceros muelleri Using 13C-Isotope Labeling. *Biomolecules* **2020**, *10*, 797. [CrossRef] [PubMed]
35. Remize, M.; Planchon, F.; Loh, A.N.; Le Grand, F.; Lambert, C.; Bideau, A.; Bidault, A.; Corvaisier, R.; Volety, A.; Soudant, P. Identification of Polyunsaturated Fatty Acids Synthesis Pathways in the Toxic Dinophyte Alexandrium minutum Using 13C-Labelling. *Biomolecules* **2020**, *10*, 1428. [CrossRef]
36. Grosse, J.; van Breugel, P.; Boschker, H.T.S. Tracing Carbon Fixation in Phytoplankton-Compound Specific and Total ^{13}C Incorporation Rates: ^{13}C Uptake into Macromolecules. *Limnol. Oceanogr. Methods* **2015**, *13*, 288–302. [CrossRef]
37. Menzel, R.; Ngosong, C.; Ruess, L. Isotopologue Profiling Enables Insights into Dietary Routing and Metabolism of Trophic Biomarker Fatty Acids. *Chemoecology* **2017**, *27*, 101–114. [CrossRef]
38. Wei, X.; Shi, B.; Koo, I.; Yin, X.; Lorkiewicz, P.; Suhail, H.; Rattan, R.; Giri, S.; McClain, C.J.; Zhang, X. Analysis of Stable Isotope Assisted Metabolomics Data Acquired by GC-MS. *Anal. Chim. Acta* **2017**, *980*, 25–32. [CrossRef]
39. Lima, V.F.; de Souza, L.P.; Williams, T.C.R.; Fernie, A.R.; Daloso, D.M. Gas Chromatography–Mass Spectrometry-Based 13C-Labeling Studies in Plant Metabolomics. In *Plant Metabolomics*; António, C.; Ed.; Methods in Molecular Biology; Springer New York: New York, NY, USA, 2018; Volume 1778, pp. 47–58. ISBN 978-1-4939-7818-2.
40. Eikrem, W.; Medlin, L.K.; Henderiks, J.; Rokitta, S.; Rost, B.; Probert, I.; Throndsen, J.; Edvardsen, B. *Haptophyta*. Handbook of the Protists; Archibald, J.M., Simpson, A.G.B., Slamovits, C.H., Margulis, L., Melkonian, M., Chapman, D.J., Corliss, J.O., Eds.; Springer International Publishing: Cham, Switzerland, 2017; pp. 1–61. ISBN 978-3-319-32669-6.
41. Volkman, J.K.; Jeffrey, S.W.; Nichols, P.D.; Rogers, G.I.; Garland, C.D. Fatty Acid and Lipid Composition of 10 Species of Microalgae Used in Mariculture. *J. Exp. Mar. Biol. Ecol.* **1989**, *128*, 219–240. [CrossRef]
42. Pernet, F.; Tremblay, R.; Demers, E.; Roussy, M. Variation of Lipid Class and Fatty Acid Composition of *Chaetoceros muelleri* and *Isochrysis* sp. Grown in a Semicontinuous System. *Aquaculture* **2003**, *221*, 393–406. [CrossRef]
43. Patil, V.; Källqvist, T.; Olsen, E.; Vogt, G.; Gislerød, H.R. Fatty Acid Composition of 12 Microalgae for Possible Use in Aquaculture Feed. *Aquacult Int.* **2007**, *15*, 1–9. [CrossRef]
44. Gladyshev, M.I.; Sushchik, N.N.; Makhutova, O.N. Production of EPA and DHA in Aquatic Ecosystems and Their Transfer to the Land. *Prostaglandins Other Lipid Mediat.* **2013**, *107*, 117–126. [CrossRef]
45. da Costa, F.; Le Grand, F.; Quéré, C.; Bougaran, G.; Cadoret, J.P.; Robert, R.; Soudant, P. Effects of Growth Phase and Nitrogen Limitation on Biochemical Composition of Two Strains of Tisochrysis lutea. *Algal. Res.* **2017**, *27*, 177–189. [CrossRef]
46. Huang, B.; Marchand, J.; Thiriet-Rupert, S.; Carrier, G.; Saint-Jean, B.; Lukomska, E.; Moreau, B.; Morant-Manceau, A.; Bougaran, G.; Mimouni, V. Betaine Lipid and Neutral Lipid Production under Nitrogen or Phosphorus Limitation in the Marine Microalga *Tisochrysis lutea* (Haptophyta). *Algal. Res.* **2019**, *40*, 101506. [CrossRef]
47. Kohli, G.S.; John, U.; Van Dolah, F.M.; Murray, S.A. Evolutionary Distinctiveness of Fatty Acid and Polyketide Synthesis in Eukaryotes. *ISME J.* **2016**, *10*, 1877–1890. [CrossRef] [PubMed]
48. Wang, S.; Zheng, L.; Cui, Z.; Chen, J.; Yang, B.; Han, X.; Liu, C. Cloning and Molecular Characterization of a Delta-6 Fatty Acid Desaturase Gene from *Isochrysis* sp. CCMM5001. *J. Appl. Phycol.* **2016**, *28*, 921–929. [CrossRef]
49. Joseph, J.D. Identification of 3, 6, 9, 12, 15-Octadecapentaenoic Acid in Laboratory-Cultured Photosynthetic Dinoflagellates. *Lipids* **1975**, *10*, 395–403. [CrossRef] [PubMed]

50. Kotajima, T.; Shiraiwa, Y.; Suzuki, I. Functional Screening of a Novel Δ15 Fatty Acid Desaturase from the Coccolithophorid Emiliania huxleyi. *Biochim. Biophys. Acta (BBA)-Mol. Cell Biol. Lipids* **2014**, *1841*, 1451–1458. [CrossRef] [PubMed]
51. Heydarizadeh, P.; Poirier, I.; Loizeau, D.; Ulmann, L.; Mimouni, V.; Schoefs, B.; Bertrand, M. Plastids of Marine Phytoplankton Produce Bioactive Pigments and Lipids. *Mar. Drugs* **2013**, *11*, 3425–3471. [CrossRef]
52. Nalder, T.D.; Miller, M.R.; Packer, M.A. Changes in Lipid Class Content and Composition of Isochrysis Sp. (T-Iso) Grown in Batch Culture. *Aquacult Int.* **2015**, *23*, 1293–1312. [CrossRef]
53. Zhong, Y.; Li, Y.; Xu, J.; Cao, J.; Zhou, C.; Yan, X. *Isolation of Chloroplasts from Marine Microalgae Isochrysis Galbana Parke Suitable for Organelle Lipid Composition Analysis*; In Review; Creative Commons: Mountain View, CA, USA, 2020.
54. Zhou, X.-R.; Robert, S.S.; Petrie, J.R.; Frampton, D.M.F.; Mansour, M.P.; Blackburn, S.I.; Nichols, P.D.; Green, A.G.; Singh, S.P. Isolation and Characterization of Genes from the Marine Microalga Pavlova salina Encoding Three Front-End Desaturases Involved in Docosahexaenoic Acid Biosynthesis. *Phytochemistry* **2007**, *68*, 785–796. [CrossRef]
55. Fraser, T.C.M.; Qi, B.; Elhussein, S.; Chatrattanakunchai, S.; Stobart, A.K.; Lazarus, C.M. Expression of the Isochrysis C18-Δ9 Polyunsaturated Fatty Acid Specific Elongase Component Alters Arabidopsis Glycerolipid Profiles. *Plant Physiol.* **2004**, *135*, 859–866. [CrossRef]
56. Tonon, T.; Harvey, D.; Larson, T.R.; Graham, I.A. Identification of a Very Long Chain Polyunsaturated Fatty Acid Δ4-Desaturase from the Microalga Pavlova lutheri. *FEBS Lett.* **2003**, *553*, 440–444. [CrossRef]
57. Robert, S.S.; Petrie, J.R.; Zhou, X.-R.; Mansour, M.P.; Blackburn, S.I.; Green, A.G.; Singh, S.P.; Nichols, P.D. Isolation and Characterisation of a Δ5-Fatty Acid Elongase from the Marine Microalga Pavlova salina. *Mar. Biotechnol.* **2009**, *11*, 410–418. [CrossRef]
58. Zhang, K.; Li, H.; Chen, W.; Zhao, M.; Cui, H.; Min, Q.; Wang, H.; Chen, S.; Li, D. Regulation of the Docosapentaenoic Acid/Docosahexaenoic Acid Ratio (DPA/DHA Ratio) in Schizochytrium limacinum B4D1. *Appl. Biochem. Biotechnol.* **2017**, *182*, 67–81. [CrossRef]
59. Zaslavsky, L.; Ciufo, S.; Fedorov, B.; Tatusova, T. Clustering Analysis of Proteins from Microbial Genomes at Multiple Levels of Resolution. *BMC Bioinform.* **2016**, *17*, 276. [CrossRef]
60. Kato, M.; Sakai, M.; Adachi, K.; Ikemoto, H.; Sano, H. Distribution of Betaine Lipids in Marine Algae. *Phytochemistry* **1996**, *42*, 1341–1345. [CrossRef]
61. Eichenberger, W.; Gribi, C. Lipids of Pavlova lutheri: Cellular Site and Metabolic Role of DGCC. *Phytochemistry* **1997**, *45*, 1561–1567. [CrossRef]
62. Meireles, L.A.; Guedes, A.C.; Malcata, F.X. Lipid Class Composition of the Microalga Pavlova lutheri: Eicosapentaenoic and Docosahexaenoic Acids. *J. Agric. Food Chem.* **2003**, *51*, 2237–2241. [CrossRef] [PubMed]
63. Armada, I.; Hachero-Cruzado, I.; Mazuelos, N.; Ríos, J.L.; Manchado, M.; Cañavate, J.P. Differences in Betaine Lipids and Fatty Acids between Pseudoisochrysis paradoxa VLP and Diacronema Vlkianum VLP Isolates (Haptophyta). *Phytochemistry* **2013**, *95*, 224–233. [CrossRef] [PubMed]
64. Walne, P.R. Experiments on the Large-Scale Culture of the Larvae Ostrea edulis. *J. Fish. Invest. Min. Agric. Fish. Lond.* **1966**, *2*, 25–53.
65. Hunter, W.R.; Jamieson, A.; Huvenne, V.A.I.; Witte, U. Sediment Community Responses to Marine vs. Terrigenous Organic Matter in a Submarine Canyon. *Biogeosciences* **2013**, *10*, 67–80. [CrossRef]
66. Berthelier, J.; Casse, N.; Daccord, N.; Jamilloux, V.; Saint-Jean, B.; Carrier, G. A Transposable Element Annotation Pipeline and Expression Analysis Reveal Potentially Active Elements in the Microalga Tisochrysis lutea. *BMC Genom.* **2018**, *19*, 378. [CrossRef]
67. John, U.; Beszteri, S.; Glöckner, G.; Singh, R.; Medlin, L.; Cembella, A.D. Genomic Characterisation of the Ichthyotoxic Prymnesiophyte Chrysochromulina polylepis, and the Expression of Polyketide Synthase Genes in Synchronized Cultures. *Eur. J. Phycol.* **2010**, *45*, 215–229. [CrossRef]
68. Marchler-Bauer, A.; Bo, Y.; Han, L.; He, J.; Lanczycki, C.J.; Lu, S.; Chitsaz, F.; Derbyshire, M.K.; Geer, R.C.; Gonzales, N.R.; et al. CDD/SPARCLE: Functional classification of proteins via subfamily domain architectures. *Nucleic Acids Res.* **2017**, *45*, D200–D203. [CrossRef]

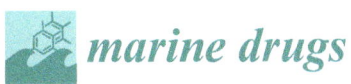

Article

Chitosan-Based Anti-Oxidation Delivery Nano-Platform: Applications in the Encapsulation of DHA-Enriched Fish Oil

Po-Kai Chang [1,†], Ming-Fong Tsai [1,†], Chun-Yung Huang [1], Chien-Liang Lee [2], Chitsan Lin [3], Chwen-Jen Shieh [4] and Chia-Hung Kuo [1,5,*]

1. Department of Seafood Science, National Kaohsiung University of Science and Technology, Kaohsiung 811, Taiwan; encorek30@gmail.com (P.-K.C.); l38982079@gmail.com (M.-F.T.); cyhuang@nkust.edu.tw (C.-Y.H.)
2. Department of Chemical and Materials Engineering, National Kaohsiung University of Science and Technology, Kaohsiung 807, Taiwan; cl_lee@nkust.edu.tw
3. Department of Marine Environmental Engineering, National Kaohsiung University of Science and Technology, Kaohsiung 811, Taiwan; ctlin@nkust.edu.tw
4. Biotechnology Center, National Chung Hsing University, Taichung 402, Taiwan; cjshieh@nchu.edu.tw
5. Center for Aquatic Products Inspection Service, National Kaohsiung University of Science and Technology, Kaohsiung 811, Taiwan
* Correspondence: kuoch@nkust.edu.tw; Tel.: +886-7-3617141 (ext. 23646); Fax: +886-7-3640456
† These authors contributed equally to this work.

Abstract: Refined cobia liver oil is a nutritional supplement (CBLO) that is rich in polyunsaturated fatty acids (PUFAs), such as DHA and EPA; however, PUFAs are prone to oxidation. In this study, the fabrication of chitosan-TPP-encapsulated CBLO nanoparticles (CS@CBLO NPs) was achieved by a two-step method, including emulsification and the ionic gelation of chitosan with sodium tripolyphosphate (TPP). The obtained nanoparticles were inspected by dynamic light scattering (DLS) and showed a positively charged surface with a z-average diameter of between 174 and 456 nm. Thermogravimetric analysis (TGA) results showed the three-stage weight loss trends contributing to the water evaporation, chitosan decomposition, and CBLO decomposition. The loading capacity (LC) and encapsulation efficiency (EE) of the CBLO loading in CS@CBLO NPs were 17.77–33.43% and 25.93–50.27%, respectively. The successful encapsulation of CBLO in CS@CBLO NPs was also confirmed by the Fourier transform infrared (FTIR) spectroscopy and X-ray diffraction (XRD) techniques. The oxidative stability of CBLO and CS@CBLO NPs was monitored by FTIR. As compared to CBLO, CS@CBLO NPs showed less oxidation with a lower generation of hydroperoxides and secondary oxidation products after four weeks of storage. CS@CBLO NPs are composed of two ingredients that are beneficial for health, chitosan and fish oil in a nano powdered fish oil form, with an excellent oxidative stability that will enhance its usage in the functional food and pharmaceutical industries.

Keywords: powdered fish oil; docosahexaenoic acid; chitosan nanoparticles; encapsulation efficiency; loading capacity; TGA; FTIR; oxidative stability

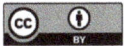

1. Introduction

Cobia (*Rachycentron canadum*) are a medium-sized migratory carnivorous fish that is widely distributed in tropical marine locations. Cobia has a high economic value and is a fish species that is popular for commercial aquaculture, with a global production of ~43,000 tons per year [1]. Cobia are mainly processed into fillets, with by-products of around 65% of the total weight generated [2,3]. Cobia liver is one of these waste products, accounting for 4% of the total weight and containing 46~48% fat; it is a potential raw material that could be used for producing fish oil. Cobia liver oil (CBLO) is rich in polyunsaturated fatty acids (PUFAs), such as DHA (Docosahexaenoicacid) and EPA (Eicosapentaenoic acid) [4]. DHA and EPA have been reported to possess anti-inflammatory and antidiabetic activities and can reduce the risk of cardiovascular disease, cancer, and Alzheimer's disease [5–7]. However, DHA and EPA are unstable due to the risk of oxidation, as the rate of oxidation increases with the number of double bonds in a fatty acid [8,9]. Oxidation exerts negative effects on flavor and nutritional value, thereby limiting the application of PUFA-enriched fish oil in nutritional supplements.

Reducing exposure to oxygen is one way to avoid the oxidation of fish oils. The encapsulation of lipophilic compounds in biocompatible materials with a nano-technique is a feasible means for achieving this purpose [10,11]. As a result, the encapsulation of CBLO can improve its stability, helping to avoid irradiation, oxidation, and thermal degradation while reducing the fishy smell. Chitosan, a cationic polysaccharide with an outstanding biocompatibility and biodegradability, is widely applied in the field of biomedicine [12,13]. The structure of chitosan comprises β(1,4)-linked D-glucosamine and N-acetyl-D-glucosamine; the pKa value of the primary amine is around 6.5, depending on the degree of N-deacetylation [14]. Chitosan is pH-sensitive due to the amino groups of D-glucosamine possessing a positive charge at pHs below 6, which cause chitosan to become a water-soluble cationic biopolymer. However, chitosan is insoluble in physiological conditions at neutral pH. Such characteristics make chitosan suitable for the encapsulation and delivery of lipophilic compounds [15,16]. In particular, chitosan exhibits many health benefits, helping one to resist ulcers, lowering cholesterol, reducing blood lipids, and helping in the prevention of coeliac disease [17,18]; based on the above benefits, chitosan is a suitable wall material that can be used for the encapsulation of drugs [19] and can help to achieving the purpose of controlled delivery [20].

Recently, several nanoencapsulation processes utilizing chitosan have been developed, such as ionic gelation [21], electrospinning [22], emulsion-homogenization [23], self-assembly [24], and antisolvent precipitation [25]. The ionic gelation method is the favorite among these, as it is non-toxic, non-solvent, and easily controllable. The ionic gelation technique is based on the electrostatic interaction between the positively charged amino groups of chitosan and the negatively charged groups of anions (such as sodium tripolyphosphate, TPP) to form a safety component, CS-TPP nanoparticles (CS NPs) [26,27]. CS NPs have been used for loading insulin and also applied in diabetes therapy [28]. Moreover, several food bioactive ingredients have been encapsulated in CS NPs, including curcumin [29], flavonoids [30], lutein [31], polyphenols [32], resveratrol [33], and vitamins (B9, B12, and C) [34]. Fish oils are rich in ω-3 PUFAs, which are highly prone to oxidation due to their higher content of unsaturated fatty acid undergoing lipid oxidation. The encapsulation of fish oil can protect unsaturated fatty acids against oxidation and help to avoid unwanted reactions [35]. However, as there is little literature available regarding CS NPs encapsulated fish oil, the effect of encapsulation on preventing the oxidation of ω-3 PUFAs is worthy of study.

In this study, the encapsulation of CBLO containing ω-3 PUFAs by chitosan at the nano-scale was explored. A two-step procedure (emulsification and ionic gelation) was performed to fabricate CS-TPP-encapsulated CBLO nanoparticles (CS@CBLO NPs). The characterizations of CS@CBLO NPs were investigated by scanning electron microscopy (SEM), dynamic light scattering (DLS), thermogravimetric analysis (TGA), X-ray diffraction (XRD), and Fourier transform infrared spectroscopy (FTIR). The effects of the initial CBLO content on the encapsulation efficiency (EE) and loading capacity (LC) were also investigated. Finally, the effect of CS@CBLO NPs on the oxidative stability of CBLO was evaluated.

2. Results and Discussion

2.1. Shape and Size of CS-TPP Encapsulated CBLO Nanoparticles

Refined cobia liver oil (CBLO) with an acid value of 0.15 mg KOH g^{-1} was used as the core material for encapsulation. The fatty acid profile of the CBLO is presented in Figure 1. The CBLO contained 24.52% total ω-3 PUFAs (18.85% DHA, 4.25% EPA, and 1.42% α-linolenic acid).

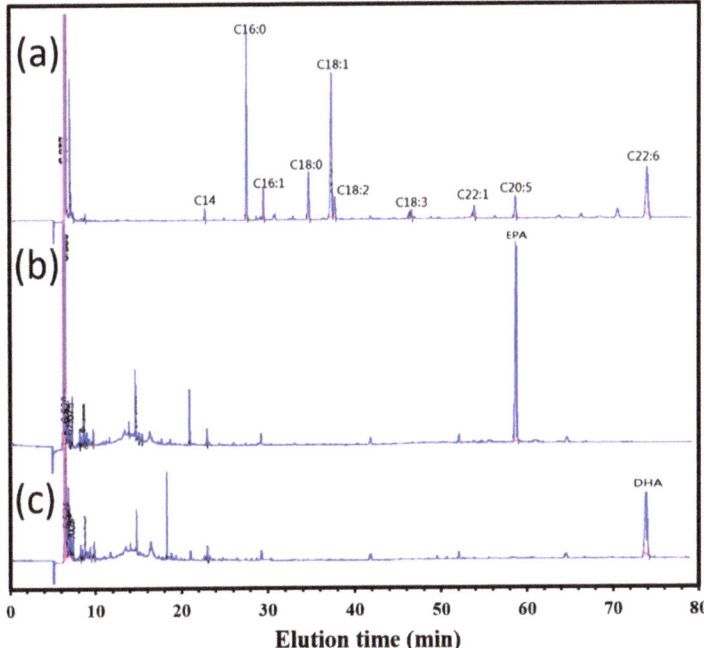

Figure 1. GC analysis of (**a**) the fatty acid profile of CBLO, (**b**) EPA standard, and (**c**) DHA standard.

The two-step method used for the fabrication of CS@CBLO NPs is illustrated in Scheme 1. The first step was emulsification; the chitosan was treated with the surfactant reagent Tween 80 for entrapment. CBLO gained an oil-in-water micelle structure. The second step was the solidification of the micelles by the ionic gelation of chitosan with TPP to form CS@CBLO NPs. The morphology of the obtained particles was observed by SEM. As shown in Figure 2a,b, both CS NPs and CS@CBLO NPs exhibit a spherical shape and nanosized structure. The particle sizes of CS NPs and CS@CBLO NPs measured by SEM were 726 ± 136 nm and 347 ± 118 nm, respectively. The smaller particle size of CS@CBLO NPs was due to the homogenization dispersing the hydrophobic CBLO in the solution and forming micelles with the surfactant. While the CS NPs were formed by the electrostatic interaction of chitosan and TPP, the CS@CBLO NPs were formed by the ionic gelation of chitosan absorbed on the micelle. The hydrophobic CBLO in the micelle reduced the aggregation of chitosan on the micelle surface and thus produced smaller particles.

The z-average diameter, PDI, and Zeta potential of CS NPs and CS@CBLO NPs were examined by DLS. Figure 3 shows that the z-average diameter of CS NPs is ~658 nm, while the z-average diameter of CS@CBLO NPs is between 174 and 456 nm. The DLS analysis was carried out in the aqueous environment; thus, the particle size would depend on the extent of the aggregation or swelling of the chitosan. Since the CBLO was entrapped inside the CS@CBLO NPs, the hydrophobicity of CBLO decreased the aggregation and/or the swelling of chitosan, resulting in the formation of smaller particles, meaning that the z-average diameter of CS@CBLO NPs decreased with the increasing ratio of CBLO to chitosan. This phenomenon was similar to that seen in other studies [36,37].

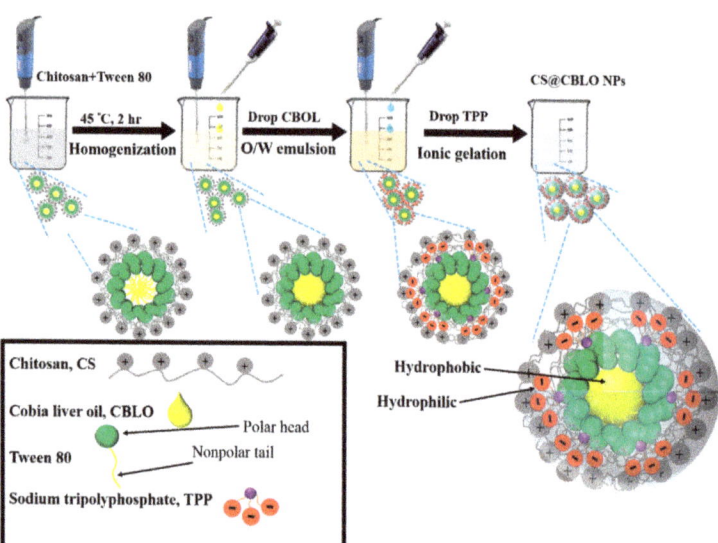

Scheme 1. The two-step method used for fabrication of CS@CBLO NPs via emulsification and ionic gelation.

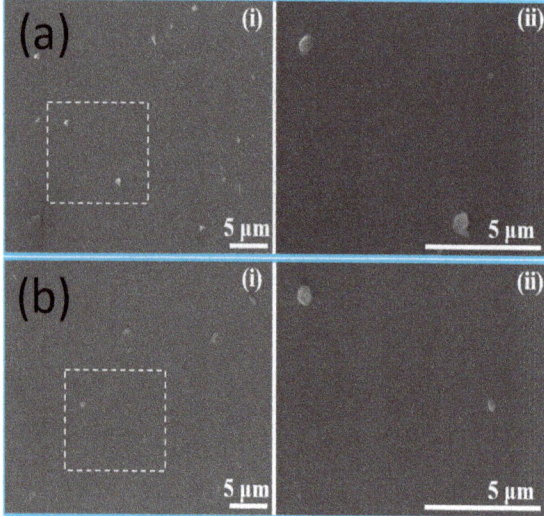

Figure 2. SEM images of (**a**) CS NPs and (**b**) CS@CBLO NPs (weight ratio of CBLO:chitosan at 1:1) at 2 kV. (**i**) and (**ii**) are the measured magnification at 5000× and 15,000×, respectively.

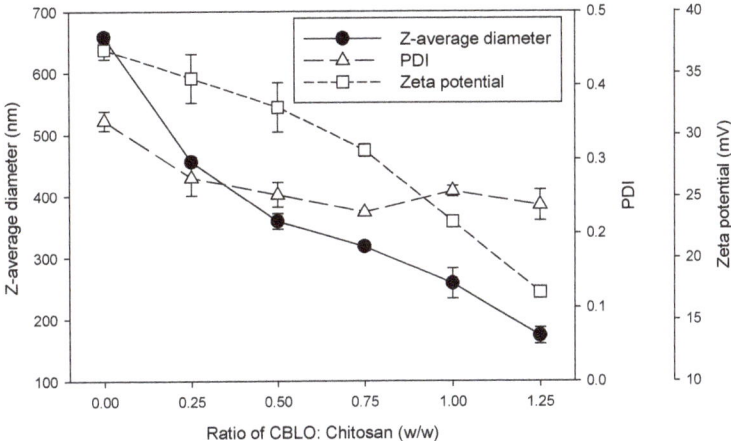

Figure 3. Z-average diameter, PDI and zeta potential of CS NPs and CS@CBLO NPs with different weight ratios of CBLO to chitosan. Data are the mean + standard deviation (n = 3).

PDI is a key parameter showing the quality of the size distribution of nanoparticles in suspensions. With a PDI lower than 0.3 and a single peak in the size distribution curve, it is considered to be monodisperse-sized dispersion [38]. In Figure 3, it can be seen that the highest PDI value was found to be 0.35 for CS NPs, while CS@CBLO NPs had a lower PDI value of 0.22–0.27. The results indicated that CS@CBLO NPs were a monodisperse dispersion with a low variability and no aggregation as compared to CS NPs. In addition, the zeta potential measurement is also shown in Figure 3. The zeta potential of CS NPs showed a positive charge of +36.9 mV contributed by the protonated amino group (NH_3^+) of chitosan. On the contrary, the zeta potential of CS@CBLO NPs decreased as the ratio of CBLO to chitosan increased. It has been reported that the zeta potential is related to the number of TPP and chitosan charge groups [39]. With the increasing CBLO, the relative proportion of TPP and chitosan decreased. Moreover, the reason for the decreasing zeta potential may be due to the shielding effect of CBLO reducing the surface charge of chitosan. Several studies have pointed out that when the chitosan encapsulated carvacrol [40], krill oil [36], and eugenol [41], the positively charged surface was reduced with the increasing initial content of the loaded drugs.

2.2. Thermogravimetric Analysis

TGA is a useful technique for studying the weight change of samples with increasing temperature. The degradation temperature (Td) is the temperature corresponding to the maximum rate of weight loss at each stage. The peak of Td can be clearly observed from the first derivative of the TGA curve with respect to temperature, called derivative thermogravimetry (DTG). As shown in Figure 4A, the weight of CS NPs and CS@CBLO NPs decreased as the temperature increased from 25 to 600 °C. The CS NPs showed two stages of weight loss (Figure 4A-i,B-i). The first and second stages of the weight loss of CS NPs were at temperature range of 31 to 114 °C and 171 to 293 °C, corresponding to water evaporation and chitosan decomposition, respectively. However, CS@CBLO NPs showed three stages of weight loss (Figure 4A-ii–vi,B-ii–vi). Compared to the TGA/DTG of CS NPs (Figure 4A-i,B-i), the third stage weight loss of CS@CBLO NPs in a temperature range of 293 to 415 °C was caused by CBLO decomposition. From the DTG thermograms, CS NPs exhibited two-stage degradation, at 65 °C and 250 °C, respectively (Figure 4B-i). However, the CS@CBLO NPs showed new Td at 368 °C (Figure 4B-ii–vi), corresponding to the Td of CBLO. The results confirmed that the encapsulation of CBLO into CS@CBLO NPs was successful.

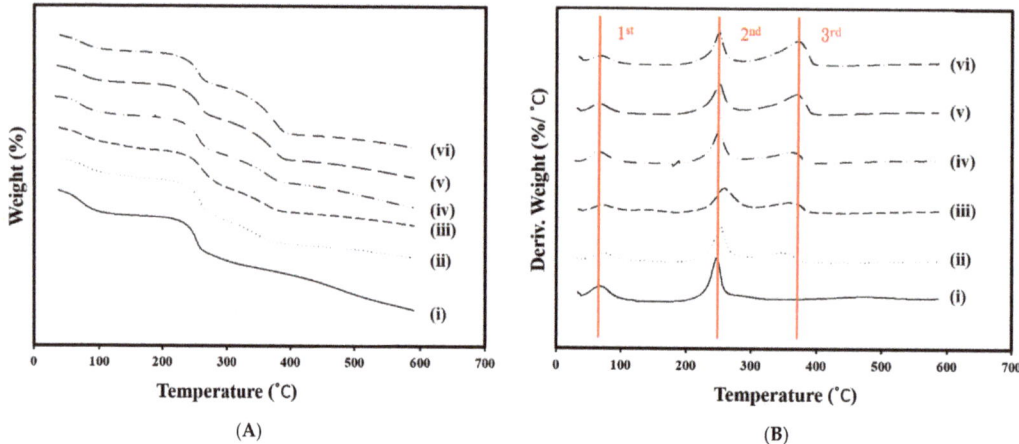

Figure 4. (**A**) TGA and (**B**) DTG thermograms of (**i**) CS NPs and (**ii**)–(**vi**) CS@CBLO NPs prepared using different weight ratios of CBLO to chitosan of (**ii**) 0.25:1, (**iii**) 0.50:1, (**iv**) 0.75:1, (**v**) 1.00:1, and (**vi**) 1.25:1.

2.3. Encapsulation Efficiency and Loading Capacity

The TGA/DGT technique can be used for quantitative analysis. The amount of CBLO loaded can be determined by the weight loss of CS@CBLO NPs at temperatures of 293–415 °C (Figure 4A-ii–vi), while the percentage of LC and EE of CBLO is calculated by Eqs. (1) and (2) in Section 3.5. According to the results of TGA, the LC and EE of CBLO are listed in Table 1. When the ratio of CBLO to chitosan increased from 0.25 to 1.25 (w/w), the percentage of LC increased from 17.77 to 33.43%. These results indicated that the percentage of LC depended on the initial CBLO concentration, which is consistent with the findings other studies—i.e., that the loading of krill oil, carvacrol, and eugenol in CS NPs is related to the initial concentration of the core material [36,41]. On the other hand, the EE ranged from 25.93% to 50.27%, and the maximum EE of 50.6% was obtained at the ratio of CBLO to chitosan of 0.25 (w/w). However, EE decreased with the increased ratio of CBLO to chitosan. The decrease in EE with the increasing of CBLO concentration indicated that CBLO loaded in CS@CBLO NPs is limited because the amount of chitosan is fixed. With an increasing CBLO concentration, the CBLO that can be encapsulated by chitosan gradually reaches saturation, resulting in a decrease in EE.

Table 1. The effect of different ratios of CBLO to chitosan on the loading capacity and encapsulation efficiency.

CBLO: Chitosan (w/w)	LC (%)	EE (%)
0.25:1.00	17.77 ± 0.09	50.27 ± 0.30
0.50:1.00	17.97 ± 0.02	29.53 ± 0.19
0.75:1.00	22.03 ± 0.22	25.93 ± 1.14
1.00:1.00	30.16 ± 0.48	29.40 ± 0.33
1.25:1.00	33.43 ± 0.37	28.47 ± 0.17

2.4. Characterization XRD and FTIR Spectroscopy

The crystal structure of chitosan powder, CS NPs, and CS@CBLO NPs was analyzed using the XRD technique. As Figure 5a shows, chitosan exhibits the main diffraction peak at 20.3°, indicating the high degree of crystallinity. After the electrostatic interaction with TPP, no peak was found in the diffractograms of CS NPs (Figure 5b). A quite flat diffraction pattern was obtained, indicating an amorphous structure. The width of the peaks in the XRD pattern is related to the grain size of the crystallites, and the broadened peaks are usually caused by imperfect crystals [42]. Therefore, the broad peak of CS NPs might be caused by ionic gelation with TPP, which did not allow a regular arrangement of the polymer network, leading to its amorphous structure [43]. Compared to chitosan and CS NPs, the characteristic peak of CS@CBLO NPs (Figure 5c) slightly shifted to 18.8° and was markedly sharp, confirming the presence of CBLO within CS NPs. This result also confirmed that the incorporation of CBLO caused a change in the packaging structure of chitosan-TPP.

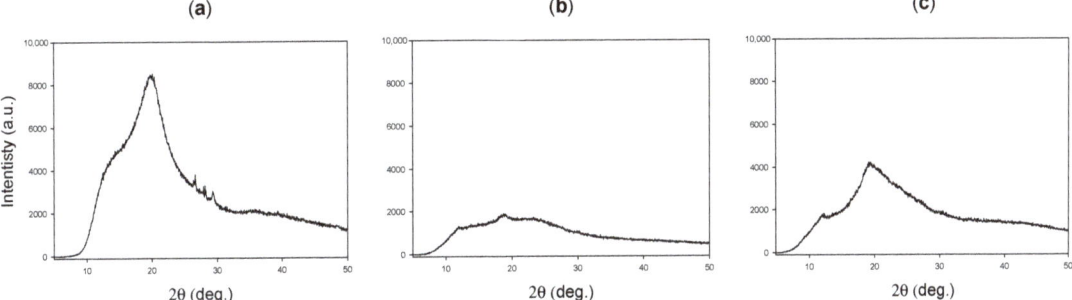

Figure 5. The XRD patterns of (a) chitosan powder, (b) CS NPs, and (c) CS@CBLO NPs.

The results of the FTIR showing the characteristic spectra of CBLO, CS NPs, and CS@CBLO NPs are presented in Figure 6. Figure 6a shows the characteristic peaks of CBLO appearing at 3473 cm^{-1} (C=O overtone), 3008 cm^{-1} (=CH stretching), 3000–2800 cm^{-1} (CH stretching), 1743 cm^{-1} (C=O stretching band), 1464 cm^{-1} (–CH$_2$–bending), 1377 cm^{-1} (–CH$_3$ bending), and 964 cm^{-1} (C=C stretching band). On the other hand, CS NPs shows the characteristic peaks of chitosan and TPP in Figure 6b. The characteristic peaks of CS NPs were found at 3467 cm^{-1} (OH stretching), 1655 cm^{-1} (amide I stretching), 1541 cm^{-1} (amide II stretching), 1155 cm^{-1} (P=O stretching), 1095 cm^{-1} (C–O–C stretching), and 899 cm^{-1} (P-O-P stretching). Compared to CBLO and CS NPs, all the characteristic peaks of both appeared in the FTIR spectra of CS@CBLO NPs (Figure 6c–g), indicating no modification or interaction between the CBLO and chitosan or TPP. In particular, the characteristic peaks of CS@CBLO NPs located at 2924–2854 cm^{-1} (CH stretching), and 1743 cm^{-1} (C=O stretching band), assigned to the methylene and carbonyl group of triglycerides, significantly increased in intensity with an increased ratio of CBLO to chitosan. This result not only reflected the presence of CBLO in CS@CBLO NPs but also showed the content of CBLO in CS@CBLO NPs. Compared to the results of LC in Table 1, the LC of CBLO increased with the increased ratio of CBLO to chitosan. Therefore, the peaks of CH stretching at 2924–2854 cm^{-1} and the C=O stretching band at 1743 cm^{-1} can be used as an indicator to represent the content of CBLO loaded into chitosan nanoparticles. With the analysis of XRD and FTIR, the two-step method through emulsification and ionic gelation is shown to be suitable for encapsulating CBLO in CS@CBLO NPs.

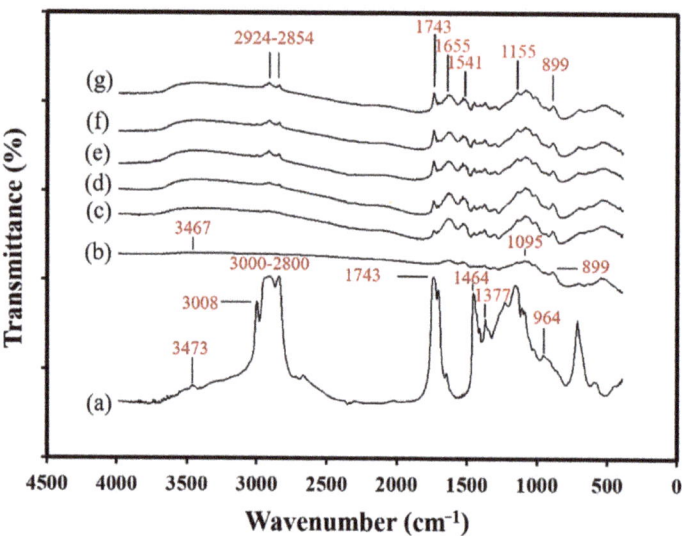

Figure 6. FTIR spectra of (**a**) CBLO, (**b**) CS NPs, and (**c**–**g**) CS@CBLO NPs prepared using different weight ratios of CBLO to chitosan of (**c**) 0.25:1, (**d**) 0.50:1, (**e**) 0.75:1, (**f**) 1.00:1, and (**g**) 1.25:1.

2.5. Oxidative Stability

The anti-oxidation capability to avoid CBLO oxidation is an important indicator for CS@CBLO NPs. CBLO is highly susceptible to oxidation due to its large number of PUFAs. In the early stage of oil oxidation, oxygen directly interacts with conjugated diene to form hydroperoxides [44]. FTIR spectroscopy has been used in the past to identify changes in functional groups in samples that have undergone lipid oxidation [45]. Non-oxidized oils show a narrow weak band in the region of 3400–3500 cm^{-1}, with maximum absorbance wavenumbers around 3470 cm^{-1}, which are assigned to the overtone of the glyceride ester carbonyl absorption [46]. However, the hydroperoxides generated in the oxidation process cause the maximum absorption to shift to lower wavenumbers [47]. The oxidative stability of CBLO and CS@CBLO NPs during the storage period was observed by FTIR. As Figure 7a shows, the FTIR spectra of CBLO obviously change with the storage time. The maximum absorbance wavenumbers shifted from 3473 to 3421 cm^{-1} as the storage time increased from 1 to 28 d. The peak shift of CBLO was due to the formation of hydroperoxides during storage. In contrast, the FTIR spectra of CS@CBLO NPs (Figure 7b,c) in the region of 3400–3500 cm^{-1} were more stable and without significant shifts or changes. This result indicated that CS@CBLO NPs had a lower hydroperoxide formation during storage compared to CBLO. The ratio of maximum absorbance wavenumber changes in the region of 3400–3500 cm^{-1} during storage can be seen in Figure 8. During the first two weeks of storage, CBLO showed little change, but by day 16 the formation of hydroperoxides caused a significant decrease in the ratio of the maximum absorbance wavenumber. At the same time, the ratio of maximum absorbance wavenumber for CS@CBLO NPs was only slightly decreased, supporting the notion that it had better antioxidative ability. On the other hand, the wavenumber at 967 cm^{-1} was associated with the bending vibrations of CH functional groups of isolated trans-olefins; the increase in trans double bonds during thermal oxidation can be observed by the increasing peak intensities at 967 cm^{-1} [48]. The wavenumbers at 973 and 976 cm^{-1} can be assigned to secondary oxidation products, such as aldehydes or ketones, supporting isolated trans-double bonds [49]. As Figure 9a shows, the peak intensities of CBLO at 967, 973, and 976 cm^{-1} increase with storage time, while the peak intensities of CS@CBLO NPs are almost flat with storage time. These results suggest that CBLO produced more trans double bonds and secondary oxidation products. Several studies have demonstrated that chitosan has good antioxidant properties, especially antioxidant activity, scavenging ability on hydroxyl radicals and chelating ability on ferrous ions [50–52]. In this paper, we clearly found that CS@CBLO NPs showed lower lipid hydroperoxides and secondary oxidation products, which might be attributed to chitosan providing good protection against CBLO oxidation.

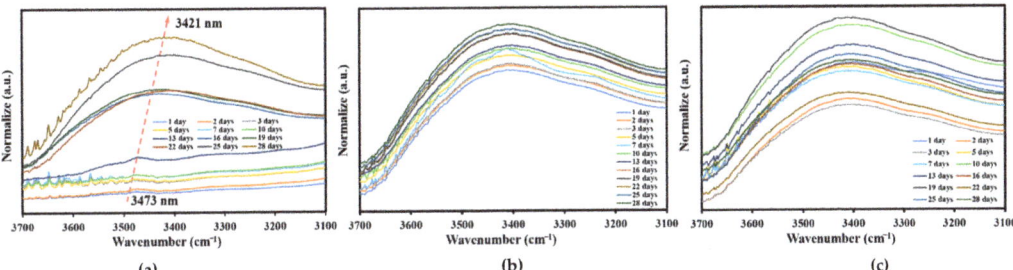

Figure 7. The changes of FTIR spectra at the region around 3400 to 3500 cm^{-1} during storage at room temperature for four weeks: (**a**) CBLO, (**b**,**c**) CS@CBLO NPs prepared using the weight ratios of CBLO to chitosan of (**b**) 1.00:1, and (**c**) 1.25:1.

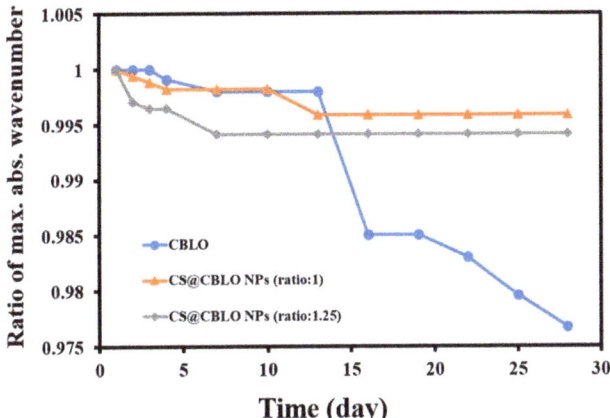

Figure 8. The ratio of maximum absorbance wavenumber in the region of 3400–3500 cm^{-1} during storage at room temperature for four weeks.

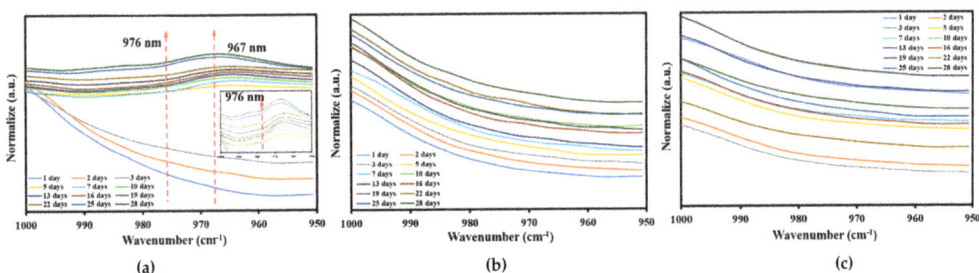

Figure 9. The changes in the FTIR spectra at the wavenumber of 967 and 976 cm^{-1} during storage at room temperature for four weeks: (**a**) CBLO, (**b**,**c**) CS@CBLO NPs prepared using the weight ratios of CBLO to chitosan of (**b**) 1.00:1, and (**c**) 1.25:1.

3. Materials and Methods

3.1. Materials

Crude cobia liver oil was extracted from cobia liver using homogenization in addition to the sonication method [53]. Briefly, 100 g of cobia liver was homogenized with 1 L hexane using a Polytron PT2100 homogenizer (Kinematica, Littau, Switzerland) equipped with a Polytron PT-DA 2120/2EC probe at 15,000 rpm for 2 min at room temperature, followed by treatment in an ultrasonic bath (40 kHz, Delta D400H, Taipei, Taiwan) for 1 h. The mixture was centrifuged at 3000 rpm for 5 min to remove the solid cobia liver. The supernatant was transferred to a rotary evaporator at 70 °C in order to remove the hexane and recover the oil. The refined cobia liver oil (CBLO) was obtained via degumming, neutralization, and bleaching, according to the procedures described previously [4]. The CBLO containing 24.52% total ω-3 PUFAs (18.85% DHA, 4.25% EPA, and 1.42% α-linolenic acid) was stored at −20 °C until further use. Fatty acid methyl esters of the standards of DHA and EPA and CBLO were prepared via saponification and methylation. The fatty acid composition was analyzed using the GC method by the Center for Aquatic Products Inspection Service, NKUST. cis-4,7,10,13,16,19-Docosahexaenoic acid was purchased from Acros (Fair Lawn, NJ, USA). cis-5,8,11,14,17-Eicosapentaenoic acid was purchased from TCI Co., LT. (Tokyo, Japan). Fatty acid methyl ester standards (Supelco 37 Component FAME Mix, Catalog No. 47885) and BF_3-methanol reagent (14% BF_3 in CH_3OH, w/v) were purchased from Sigma-Aldrich (St. Louis, MO, USA). Chitosan (degree of deacetylation of 94.42%) with an average molecular weight of 350 kDa was obtained from Charming & Beauty Co., Ltd. (Taipei, Taiwan). Tween 80 was purchased from Scharlau Chemical Reagent Co., Ltd. (Barcelona, Spain). Acetic acid was purchased from Riedel-de Haën (Seelze, Germany). The sodium tripolyphosphate (TPP) and sodium hydroxide were purchased from Wako Pure Chemical Industries (Osaka, Japan). Unless otherwise specified, all the reagents and chemicals used in this study were of analytical grade. All of the experiments were carried out using double-deionized water (18.2 Ω) using a machine from Merck Millipore.

3.2. Fabrication of CS-TPP Encapsulated CBLO Nanoparticles

The CS@CBLO NPs was prepared by a two-step method—i.e., via emulsification and ionic gelation [54]—with some modification. Briefly, chitosan powder was added to 1% (v/v) aqueous acetic acid solution at room temperature and stirred gently overnight to prepare the 1.5% (w/v) chitosan solution. The chitosan solution was centrifuged at 8000 rpm for 20 min, and the supernatant was collected for further use. Afterwards, 40 mL of chitosan solution was added to 0.5 g of Tween 80 and stirred at 45 °C for 2 h to obtain a transparent solution. The CBLO was gradually dropped into the transparent chitosan solution (40 mL) during homogenization (Polytron PT2100 with PT-DA 2112/2EC probe, Kinematica, Littau, Switzerland) at a speed of 13,000 rpm for 1 min and 16,500 rpm for 2 min to obtain an oil-in-water emulsion. Emulsions with different weight ratios of CBLO to chitosan (0:1, 0.25:1, 0.5:1, 0.75:1, 1:1, and 1.25:1, respectively) were prepared. After emulsification, 40 mL of TPP solution (0.5%, v/v) was gradually dropped into the emulsion under continuous stirring for 40 min. The formed particles were harvested using centrifugation at 10,000 rpm for 30 min, then subsequently washed several times with deionized water. Finally, the wet particles were dispersed in 25 mL of water by Q700 sonicator (Qsonica, CT, USA) to produce a homogeneous suspension. The ultrasonication was carried out in an ice bath operated at 30% amplitude for 2 min. The suspensions were immediately freeze-dried at −40 °C for 72 h to obtain the final product, CS@CBLO NPs, and were stored in dry conditions at room temperature.

3.3. Morphology of Nanoparticles

SEM was used to observe the morphology of the CS NPs and CS@CBLO NPs. One drop of the sample (50 μg/mL) was placed on a glass plate and dried at room temperature. The dried sample was sputter-coated with gold and then observed through an environmental scanning electron microscope (ESEM; FEI Quanta-200, Brno-Černovice, Czech Republic) under an accelerated voltage of 20 keV. The average particle size was measured from SEM images using an image analyzer (SigmaScan Pro 5, Chicago, IL, USA); in total, about 50 particles were measured.

3.4. Particle Size and Zeta Potential Measurement

The z-average diameter, polydispersity index (PDI), and zeta potential of CS NPs and CS@CBLO NPs were measured by dynamic light scattering (DLS) using a Brookhaven 90Plus nanoparticle size analyzer (Brookhaven Instruments, Holtsville, NY, USA). An approximately 2 mg sample was suspended in 5 mL of water using magnetic agitation for mono-dispersion, and then the sample was taken to fill the disposable zeta potential cuvettes for size distribution and surface charge analysis. All the tests were performed in triplicate.

3.5. Determination of Encapsulation Efficiency and Loading Capacity

To quantify the CBLO content in CS@CBLO NPs, the TGA/ DTG (derivative thermal gravimetric) techniques were employed for evaluating loading capacity (LC) and encapsulation efficiency (EE). Freeze dried CS NPs and CS@CBLO NPs were, respectively, analyzed by a TGA furnace at 25–600 °C with a heating rate of 10 °C/min under a nitrogen atmosphere. The percentage of weight loss of each composition during thermal decomposition obtained from TGA was used to determine the content of CBLO in CS@CBLO NPs. The equations for the calculation of the loading capacity (Equation (1)) and encapsulation efficiency (Equation (2)) are listed below:

$$LC = \frac{\text{Weight of loaded CBLO}}{\text{Weight of sample}} \times 100 \quad (1)$$

$$EE = \frac{\text{Weight of loaded CBLO}}{\text{Weight of initial CBLO}} \times 100 \quad (2)$$

3.6. Characterization using FTIR, TGA and XRD

The FTIR spectra of CBLO, CS NPs, and CS@CBLO NPs were measured by a Horiba FT-730 spectrometer (Kyoto, Japan). A sample of about 6 mg was mixed with 100 mg of KBr and then pressed in a standard device using a pressure of 6000 W to produce 13 mm-diameter pellets. For the CBLO spectral measurement, the liquid sample (~2 μL) was deposited onto a KBr disk. The spectra (4000–400 cm^{-1}) were recorded with a resolution of 4 cm^{-1} and 64 scans were performed per sample.

Thermogravimetric analysis (TGA) was performed with a TA2000/2960 thermogravimetric analyzer. Each freeze-dried sample (~5 mg) was placed into the TGA furnace and measurements were carried out under a nitrogen atmosphere with a heating rate of 10 °C/min from 25 to 600 °C.

X-ray diffraction (XRD) patterns of samples were recorded in the scanning mode on a Bruker D8ADVANCE diffractometer operated at a voltage of 40 kV and a current of 30 mA with Cu Kα radiation (λ = 1.5405 Å). The scanning angle (2θ) travelled from 5° to 50° with a scanning speed of 3° min^{-1}.

3.7. Oxidative Stability

The lipid hydroperoxides, which were the primary oxidation products, were examined by FTIR to evaluate the oxidation stability of CS@CBLO NPs according to the previous literature [46]. The CBLO and CS@CBLO NPs were stored at room temperature for 4 weeks and FTIR measurement was performed every 2 to 3 days. The FTIR spectrum was monitored at a specific wavenumber, around 3500 cm^{-1} to 3400 cm^{-1} for hydroperoxides (ROOH), 967 cm^{-1} for trans double bond and 973 or 976 cm^{-1} for secondary oxidation products, such as aldehydes or ketones supporting isolated trans-double bonds, in order to observe the oxidation stability of CBLO with or without encapsulation. The ratio of maximum absorbance wavenumber in the region of 3400–3500 cm^{-1} was defined as fn/fo. The fo was the initial maximum absorbance wavenumber and fn was the maximum absorbance wavenumber at each time point.

4. Conclusions

In this work, CS-TPP encapsulated CBLO nanoparticles (CS@CBLO NPs) were successfully fabricated using a two-step method via emulsification and ionic gelation. The particle size and its structure were revealed to be 347 nm and 174–456 nm, respectively, by scanning electron microscopy (SEM) and dynamic light scattering (DLS). The loading capacity (LC) and encapsulation efficiency (EE) of CBLO in CS@CBLO NPs were determined according to the TGA/DTG result at the degradation temperature of 368 °C. The LC and EE values were shown to be about 17.77~33.43% and 25.93~50.27%, respectively, when the ratio of CBLO to chitosan was in the range of 0.25–1.25. The oxidative stability of CS@CBLO NPs evaluated by FTIR showed that the CS@CBLO NPs could effectively prevent CBLO oxidation. The results demonstrated that the strategy of encapsulation using chitosan can effectively protect high-sensitivity materials from metamorphism. The CS@CBLO NPs combined two healthy ingredients, chitosan and fish oil, a kind of nano powdered fish oil; it can be conveniently used in various foods as a fortification of DHA and EPA to enhance their usage in the food and pharmaceutical industries.

Author Contributions: Conceptualization, C.-H.K.; methodology, P-K.C.; formal analysis, P.-K.C., C.-Y.H. and C.-L.L.; investigation, P-K.C. and M.-F.T.; resources, C.-Y.H., C.-L.L., C.L. and C.-J.S.; data curation, M.-F.T.; writing—original draft preparation, M.-F.T. and C.-H.K.; writing—review and editing, C.-H.K.; supervision, C.-H.K. All authors have read and agreed to the published version of the manuscript.

Funding: This research was funded by the Ministry of Science and Technology of Taiwan, grant number MOST 110-2221-E-992-009-.

Institutional Review Board Statement: Not applicable.

Informed Consent Statement: Not applicable.

Data Availability Statement: Data is contained within the article.

Acknowledgments: We are grateful to Center for Aquatic Products Inspection Service, NKUST, for providing analysis of fatty acid composition of CBLO.

Conflicts of Interest: The authors declare no conflict of interest in this research.

References

1. Sharma, S.R.; Dube, P.; Silpa, P.S.; Mini, K.G.; Pradeep, M.A.; Sanil, N.K. Coinfection with two strains of *Photobacterium damselae* subsp. damselae and *Vibrio harveyi* in cage farmed cobia, *Rachycentron canadum* (Linnaeus, 1766). *Aquac. Res.* **2021**, *52*, 1525–1537.
2. da Penha Franca, R.C.; Assis, C.R.D.; Santos, J.F.; Torquato, R.J.S.; Tanaka, A.S.; Hirata, I.Y.; Assis, D.M.; Juliano, M.A.; Cavalli, R.O.; de Carvalho, L.B., Jr. Bovine pancreatic trypsin inhibitor immobilized onto sepharose as a new strategy to purify a thermostable alkaline peptidase from cobia (*Rachycentron canadum*) processing waste. *J. Chromatogr. B* **2016**, *1033*, 210–217. [CrossRef]
3. Wang, Y.-H.; Kuo, C.-H.; Lee, C.-L.; Kuo, W.-C.; Tsai, M.-L.; Sun, P.-P. Enzyme-assisted aqueous extraction of cobia liver oil and protein hydrolysates with antioxidant activity. *Catalysts* **2020**, *10*, 1323. [CrossRef]
4. Kuo, C.H.; Liao, H.Z.; Wang, Y.H.; Wang, H.M.D.; Shieh, C.J.; Tseng, C.Y. Highly efficient extraction of EPA/DHA-enriched oil from cobia liver using homogenization plus sonication. *Eur. J. Lipid Sci. Technol.* **2017**, *119*, 1600466. [CrossRef]
5. Bird, J.K.; Calder, P.C.; Eggersdorfer, M. The role of n-3 long chain polyunsaturated fatty acids in cardiovascular disease prevention, and interactions with statins. *Nutrients* **2018**, *10*, 775. [CrossRef]
6. Oppedisano, F.; Macrì, R.; Gliozzi, M.; Musolino, V.; Carresi, C.; Maiuolo, J.; Bosco, F.; Nucera, S.; Caterina Zito, M.; Guarnieri, L. The anti-inflammatory and antioxidant properties of n-3 PUFAs: Their role in cardiovascular protection. *Biomedicines* **2020**, *8*, 306. [CrossRef] [PubMed]
7. Troesch, B.; Eggersdorfer, M.; Laviano, A.; Rolland, Y.; Smith, A.D.; Warnke, I.; Weimann, A.; Calder, P.C. Expert opinion on benefits of long-chain omega-3 fatty acids (DHA and EPA) in aging and clinical nutrition. *Nutrients* **2020**, *12*, 2555. [CrossRef] [PubMed]
8. Kazuo, M. Prevention of fish oil oxidation. *J. Oleo Sci.* **2019**, *68*, 1–11. [CrossRef]

9. Yang, K.-M.; Chiang, P.-Y. Variation quality and kinetic parameter of commercial n-3 PUFA-rich oil during oxidation via Rancimat. *Mar. Drugs* **2017**, *15*, 97. [CrossRef]
10. Hasan, M.; Elkhoury, K.; Kahn, C.J.; Arab-Tehrany, E.; Linder, M. Preparation, characterization, and release kinetics of chitosan-coated nanoliposomes encapsulating curcumin in simulated environments. *Molecules* **2019**, *24*, 2023. [CrossRef] [PubMed]
11. Gasa-Falcon, A.; Odriozola-Serrano, I.; Oms-Oliu, G.; Martín-Belloso, O. Nanostructured lipid-based delivery systems as a strategy to increase functionality of bioactive compounds. *Foods* **2020**, *9*, 325. [CrossRef]
12. Cicciù, M.; Fiorillo, L.; Cervino, G. Chitosan use in dentistry: A systematic review of recent clinical studies. *Mar. Drugs* **2019**, *17*, 417. [CrossRef] [PubMed]
13. Venkatesan, J.; Kim, S.-K. Chitosan composites for bone tissue engineering—An overview. *Mar. Drugs* **2010**, *8*, 2252–2266. [CrossRef] [PubMed]
14. Mohammed, M.A.; Syeda, J.; Wasan, K.M.; Wasan, E.K. An overview of chitosan nanoparticles and its application in non-parenteral drug delivery. *Pharmaceutics* **2017**, *9*, 53. [CrossRef]
15. Huang, K.-S.; Wang, C.-Y.; Yang, C.-H.; Grumezescu, A.M.; Lin, Y.-S.; Kung, C.-P.; Lin, I.-Y.; Chang, Y.-C.; Weng, W.-J.; Wang, W.-T. Synthesis and characterization of oil-chitosan composite spheres. *Molecules* **2013**, *18*, 5749–5760. [CrossRef] [PubMed]
16. Demisli, S.; Mitsou, E.; Pletsa, V.; Xenakis, A.; Papadimitriou, V. Development and study of nanoemulsions and nanoemulsion-based hydrogels for the encapsulation of lipophilic compounds. *Nanomaterials* **2020**, *10*, 2464. [CrossRef]
17. Cheung, R.C.F.; Ng, T.B.; Wong, J.H.; Chan, W.Y. Chitosan: An update on potential biomedical and pharmaceutical applications. *Mar. Drugs* **2015**, *13*, 5156–5186. [CrossRef]
18. Satitsri, S.; Muanprasat, C. Chitin and chitosan derivatives as biomaterial resources for biological and biomedical applications. *Molecules* **2020**, *25*, 5961. [CrossRef]
19. Raza, Z.A.; Khalil, S.; Ayub, A.; Banat, I.M. Recent developments in chitosan encapsulation of various active ingredients for multifunctional applications. *Carbohydr. Res.* **2020**, *492*, 108004. [CrossRef]
20. Aranaz, I.; Paños, I.; Peniche, C.; Heras, Á.; Acosta, N. Chitosan spray-dried microparticles for controlled delivery of venlafaxine hydrochloride. *Molecules* **2017**, *22*, 1980. [CrossRef]
21. Yan, J.; Guan, Z.-Y.; Zhu, W.-F.; Zhong, L.-Y.; Qiu, Z.-Q.; Yue, P.-F.; Wu, W.-T.; Liu, J.; Huang, X. Preparation of puerarin chitosan oral nanoparticles by ionic gelation method and its related kinetics. *Pharmaceutics* **2020**, *12*, 216. [CrossRef]
22. Muzzarelli, R.A. Biomedical exploitation of chitin and chitosan via mechano-chemical disassembly, electrospinning, dissolution in imidazolium ionic liquids, and supercritical drying. *Mar. Drugs* **2011**, *9*, 1510–1533. [CrossRef] [PubMed]
23. Agustinisari, I.; Mulia, K.; Nasikin, M. The effect of eugenol and chitosan concentration on the encapsulation of eugenol using whey protein–maltodextrin conjugates. *Appl. Sci.* **2020**, *10*, 3205. [CrossRef]
24. Bhalkaran, S.; Wilson, L.D. Investigation of self-assembly processes for chitosan-based coagulant-flocculant systems: A mini-review. *Int. J. Mol. Sci.* **2016**, *17*, 1662. [CrossRef] [PubMed]
25. Lammari, N.; Louaer, O.; Meniai, A.H.; Elaissari, A. Encapsulation of essential oils via nanoprecipitation process: Overview, progress, challenges and prospects. *Pharmaceutics* **2020**, *12*, 431. [CrossRef] [PubMed]
26. Kang, B.-S.; Lee, S.-E.; Ng, C.L.; Kim, J.-K.; Park, J.-S. Exploring the preparation of albendazole-loaded chitosan-tripolyphosphate nanoparticles. *Materials* **2015**, *8*, 486–498. [CrossRef]
27. Silva, M.M.; Calado, R.; Marto, J.; Bettencourt, A.; Almeida, A.J.; Gonçalves, L. Chitosan nanoparticles as a mucoadhesive drug delivery system for ocular administration. *Mar. Drugs* **2017**, *15*, 370. [CrossRef] [PubMed]
28. Avadi, M.R.; Sadeghi, A.M.M.; Mohammadpour, N.; Abedin, S.; Atyabi, F.; Dinarvand, R.; Rafiee-Tehrani, M. Preparation and characterization of insulin nanoparticles using chitosan and Arabic gum with ionic gelation method. *Nanomed. Nanotechnol. Biol. Med.* **2010**, *6*, 58–63. [CrossRef]
29. Omer, A.M.; Ziora, Z.M.; Tamer, T.M.; Khalifa, R.E.; Hassan, M.A.; Mohy-Eldin, M.S.; Blaskovich, M.A. Formulation of quaternized aminated chitosan nanoparticles for efficient encapsulation and slow release of curcumin. *Molecules* **2021**, *26*, 449. [CrossRef] [PubMed]
30. Wu, X.; Liu, C.; Chen, H.; Zhang, Y.; Li, L.; Tang, N. Layer-by-layer deposition of hyaluronan and quercetin-loaded chitosan nanoparticles onto titanium for improving blood compatibility. *Coatings* **2020**, *10*, 256. [CrossRef]
31. Arunkumar, R.; Prashanth, K.V.H.; Baskaran, V. Promising interaction between nanoencapsulated lutein with low molecular weight chitosan: Characterization and bioavailability of lutein in vitro and in vivo. *Food Chem.* **2013**, *141*, 327–337. [CrossRef] [PubMed]
32. Soltanzadeh, M.; Peighambardoust, S.H.; Ghanbarzadeh, B.; Mohammadi, M.; Lorenzo, J.M. Chitosan nanoparticles as a promising nanomaterial for encapsulation of pomegranate (*Punica granatum* L.) peel extract as a natural source of antioxidants. *Nanomaterials* **2021**, *11*, 1439. [CrossRef]
33. Miele, D.; Catenacci, L.; Sorrenti, M.; Rossi, S.; Sandri, G.; Malavasi, L.; Dacarro, G.; Ferrari, F.; Bonferoni, M.C. Chitosan oleate coated poly lactic-glycolic acid (PLGA) nanoparticles versus chitosan oleate self-assembled polymeric micelles, loaded with resveratrol. *Mar. Drugs* **2019**, *17*, 515. [CrossRef]
34. de Britto, D.; de Moura, M.R.; Aouada, F.A.; Mattoso, L.H.C.; Assis, O.B.G. N,N,N-trimethyl chitosan nanoparticles as a vitamin carrier system. *Food Hydrocolloid* **2012**, *27*, 487–493. [CrossRef]
35. Encina, C.; Vergara, C.; Giménez, B.; Oyarzún-Ampuero, F.; Robert, P. Conventional spray-drying and future trends for the microencapsulation of fish oil. *Trends Food Sci. Technol.* **2016**, *56*, 46–60. [CrossRef]

36. Haider, J.; Majeed, H.; Williams, P.A.; Safdar, W.; Zhong, F. Formation of chitosan nanoparticles to encapsulate krill oil (*Euphausia superba*) for application as a dietary supplement. *Food Hydrocolloid* **2017**, *63*, 27–34. [CrossRef]
37. Yoksan, R.; Jirawutthiwongchai, J.; Arpo, K. Encapsulation of ascorbyl palmitate in chitosan nanoparticles by oil-in-water emulsion and ionic gelation processes. *Colloid Surf. B* **2010**, *76*, 292–297. [CrossRef]
38. Sadeghi, R.; Etemad, S.G.; Keshavarzi, E.; Haghshenasfard, M. Investigation of alumina nanofluid stability by UV–vis spectrum. *Microfluid. Nanofluidics* **2015**, *18*, 1023–1030. [CrossRef]
39. Antoniou, J.; Liu, F.; Majeed, H.; Qi, J.; Yokoyama, W.; Zhong, F. Physicochemical and morphological properties of size-controlled chitosan-tripolyphosphate nanoparticles. *Colloid Surf. A* **2015**, *465*, 137–146. [CrossRef]
40. Keawchaoon, L.; Yoksan, R. Preparation, characterization and in vitro release study of carvacrol-loaded chitosan nanoparticles. *Colloid Surf. B* **2011**, *84*, 163–171. [CrossRef]
41. Woranuch, S.; Yoksan, R. Eugenol-loaded chitosan nanoparticles: I. Thermal stability improvement of eugenol through encapsulation. *Carbohydr. Polym.* **2013**, *96*, 578–585. [CrossRef]
42. Jingou, J.; Shilei, H.; Weiqi, L.; Danjun, W.; Tengfei, W.; Yi, X. Preparation, characterization of hydrophilic and hydrophobic drug in combine loaded chitosan/cyclodextrin nanoparticles and in vitro release study. *Colloids Surf. B Biointerfaces* **2011**, *83*, 103–107. [CrossRef] [PubMed]
43. Pati, F.; Adhikari, B.; Dhara, S. Development of chitosan–tripolyphosphate fibers through pH dependent ionotropic gelation. *Carbohydr. Res.* **2011**, *346*, 2582–2588. [CrossRef]
44. Repetto, M.; Semprine, J.; Boveris, A. Lipid peroxidation: Chemical mechanism, biological implications and analytical determination. *Lipid Peroxidation* **2012**, *1*, 3–30.
45. Guillén, M.D.; Ruiz, A.; Cabo, N. Study of the oxidative degradation of farmed salmon lipids by means of Fourier transform infrared spectroscopy. Influence of salting. *J. Sci. Food Agric.* **2004**, *84*, 1528–1534. [CrossRef]
46. Guillén, M.D.; Cabo, N. Usefulness of the frequency data of the Fourier transform infrared spectra to evaluate the degree of oxidation of edible oils. *J. Agric. Food Chem.* **1999**, *47*, 709–719. [CrossRef] [PubMed]
47. Guillén, M.D.; Cabo, N. Fourier transform infrared spectra data versus peroxide and anisidine values to determine oxidative stability of edible oils. *Food Chem.* **2002**, *77*, 503–510. [CrossRef]
48. Rohman, A.; Che Man, Y. Application of FTIR spectroscopy for monitoring the stabilities of selected vegetable oils during thermal oxidation. *Int. J. Food Prop.* **2013**, *16*, 1594–1603. [CrossRef]
49. Guillén, M.D.; Cabo, N. Some of the most significant changes in the Fourier transform infrared spectra of edible oils under oxidative conditions. *J. Sci. Food Agric.* **2000**, *80*, 2028–2036. [CrossRef]
50. Yasufuku, T.; Anraku, M.; Kondo, Y.; Hata, T.; Hirose, J.; Kobayashi, N.; Tomida, H. Useful extend-release chitosan tablets with high antioxidant activity. *Pharmaceutics* **2010**, *2*, 245–257. [CrossRef]
51. Avelelas, F.; Horta, A.; Pinto, L.F.; Cotrim Marques, S.; Marques Nunes, P.; Pedrosa, R.; Leandro, S.M. Antifungal and antioxidant properties of chitosan polymers obtained from nontraditional Polybius henslowii sources. *Mar. Drugs* **2019**, *17*, 239. [CrossRef] [PubMed]
52. Pati, S.; Chatterji, A.; Dash, B.P.; Raveen Nelson, B.; Sarkar, T.; Shahimi, S.; Atan Edinur, H.; Binti Abd Manan, T.S.; Jena, P.; Mohanta, Y.K. Structural characterization and antioxidant potential of chitosan by γ-irradiation from the carapace of horseshoe crab. *Polymers* **2020**, *12*, 2361. [CrossRef]
53. Kuo, C.-H.; Huang, C.-Y.; Chen, J.-W.; Wang, H.-M.D.; Shieh, C.-J. Concentration of docosahexaenoic and eicosapentaenoic acid from cobia liver oil by acetone fractionation of fatty acid salts. *Appl. Biochem. Biotechnol.* **2020**, *192*, 1–13. [CrossRef] [PubMed]
54. Hosseini, S.F.; Zandi, M.; Rezaei, M.; Farahmandghavi, F. Two-step method for encapsulation of oregano essential oil in chitosan nanoparticles: Preparation, characterization and in vitro release study. *Carbohydr. Polym.* **2013**, *95*, 50–56. [CrossRef] [PubMed]

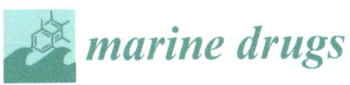

Article

Screening for Health-Promoting Fatty Acids in Ascidians and Seaweeds Grown under the Influence of Fish Farming Activities

Luísa Marques [1,*], Maria Rosário Domingues [2,3], Elisabete da Costa [2,3], Maria Helena Abreu [4], Ana Isabel Lillebø [1] and Ricardo Calado [1,*]

1. ECOMARE, CESAM—Centre for Environmental and Marine Studies, Department of Biology, University of Aveiro, Santiago University Campus, 3810-193 Aveiro, Portugal; lillebo@ua.pt
2. CESAM—Centre for Environmental and Marine Studies, Department of Chemistry, University of Aveiro, Santiago University Campus, 3810-193 Aveiro, Portugal; mrd@ua.pt (M.R.D.); elisabetecosta@ua.pt (E.d.C.)
3. Mass Spectrometry Centre, LAQV-REQUIMTE, Department of Chemistry, University of Aveiro, Santiago University Campus, 3810-193 Aveiro, Portugal
4. ALGAplus—Production and Trading of Seaweed and Derived Products Lda., 3830-196 Ílhavo, Portugal; helena.abreu@algaplus.pt
* Correspondence: luisa.marques@ua.pt (L.M.); rjcalado@ua.pt (R.C.); Tel.: +351-967-676-182 (L.M.); +351-917-989-010 (R.C.)

Abstract: The present study aimed to contrast the fatty acid (FA) profile of ascidians (Ascidiacea) and seaweeds (sea lettuce, *Ulva* spp. and bladderwrack, *Fucus* sp.) occurring in a coastal lagoon with versus without the influence of organic-rich effluents from fish farming activities. Our results revealed that ascidians and seaweeds from these contrasting environments displayed significant differences in their FA profiles. The n-3/n-6 ratio of Ascidiacea was lower under the influence of fish farming conditions, likely a consequence of the growing level of terrestrial-based ingredients rich on n-6 FA used in the formulation of aquafeeds. Unsurprisingly, these specimens also displayed significantly higher levels of 18:1(n-7+n-9) and 18:2n-6, as these combined accounted for more than 50% of the total pool of FAs present in formulated aquafeeds. The dissimilarities recorded in the FAs of seaweeds from these different environments were less marked ($\approx$5%), with these being more pronounced in the FA classes of the brown seaweed *Fucus* sp. (namely PUFA). Overall, even under the influence of organic-rich effluents from fish farming activities, ascidians and seaweeds are a valuable source of health-promoting FAs, which confirms their potential for sustainable farming practices, such as integrated multi-trophic aquaculture.

Keywords: aquafeeds; EPA; DHA; n-3/n-6 ratio; n-3 PUFA; IMTA

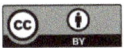

1. Introduction

Marine organisms are commonly perceived as a rich source of n-3 fatty acids (FA) [1–4] whose consumption ensures health-promoting benefits against cardiovascular and neurological diseases. Additionally, consumers also acknowledge the anti-inflammatory, anti-coagulation, anti-oxidative properties (among others) of n-3 FA originating from seafood, making them paramount for human nutrition [5–8]. As a result of the fast-growing trend of the world population [8,9] and the high request for nutritious and healthy marine food [1,10,11], aquaculture activities are facing a major challenge in recent years to keep up with an ever-growing demand. Proportionally, there is also a growing focus on the improvement of aquaculture efficiency, as well as the promotion of environmentally and financially sustainable practices [12–15]. As an example of this ongoing effort, one can refer to the reduction of the levels of marine-based ingredients, such as fishmeal and fish oil, in the formulation of aquafeeds for marine species aquaculture (namely finfish and shrimp) [11,16]. Indeed, a growing proportion of marine-based ingredients have been partially replaced by land-based ingredients (e.g., wheat, soy, corn) [17–19] and oils (e.g., palm oil, soybean oil, sunflower oil) [20,21]. Nonetheless, aquafeeds for marine species production still include marine-based ingredients to achieve desirable FA profiles [22]. These marine-based ingredients, particularly fish oil, are a source of essential FAs, such as n-3 long-chain polyunsaturated FAs (PUFA) 20:5n-3 eicosapentaenoic acid (EPA), and 22:6n-3 docosahexaenoic acid (DHA), which are paramount to ensure the healthy development of species being farmed, and as such, safeguard that these remain a valid source of these important nutrients in human diets [23,24]. Consequently, the aquaculture industry has evolved to develop productive frameworks that target the co-production of extractive species that impair the loss of valuable nutrients (such as n-3 long-chain PUFA); this approach has been termed integrated multi-trophic aquaculture (IMTA) and has gained a growing interest in the scientific community [25–28]. These productive systems benefit from the simultaneous farming of species occupying different trophic levels to sequester, recycle and remove excess nutrients originating from uneaten and undigested feed, as well as excretion products [29] present in aquaculture effluents that shape the biochemical content of co-farmed species [10]. Extractive species produced under organic-rich effluents (Org) are responsive to their surrounding environment and experience more or less pronounced shifts in their biochemical composition [2,30,31]. Consequently, FA analysis has become an excellent tool to trace the biochemical fingerprint of aquaculture effluents in aquatic environments and their species [32,33].

Ascidians are marine filter-feeders commonly investigated for marine natural products development, such as anti-cancer and anti-malarial drugs [34]. Knowledge on ascidians' FA profiling is still poorly explored. However, some studies have already confirmed that ascidians present a high n-3/n-6 ratio [3,35] and high values of EPA and DHA [36], establishing ascidians as a potential new bioresource for n-3 fatty acids-rich marine lipids [3,37,38]. Hassanzadeh [38] concluded that the FA profile of ascidians presented similar values to that of fish oil and, therefore, considered ascidians as a good alternative for fish oil in the formulation of aquafeeds. Additionally, ascidian's biomass may even successfully replace fishmeal in the formulation of aquafeeds [39,40].

The use of seaweeds has been thoroughly explored in IMTA systems [26,41,42]. Seaweed production under this productive framework is receiving growing attention for mass production given their nutritional value and profile in natural bioactive metabolites (particularly with antioxidant properties) [41,43]. Similar to ascidians, seaweeds are considered an important source of n-3 long-chain PUFA, especially α-linolenic acid (ALA; 18:3n-3) and EPA [4,44], with their potential as ingredients for aquafeed formulations also being increasingly acknowledged [45]. Although the lipid content in seaweed is relatively low (1.27% to 9.13%) [46], these organisms feature high n-3/n-6 ratios, making them an appealing source of a valuable source of essential FA in health-promoting diets [47].

The present study aimed to compare the FA profile of ascidians (Ascidiacea) and seaweeds (sea lettuce, *Ulva* spp. and bladderwrack, *Fucus* sp.) sampled in a coastal lagoon with versus without the influence of organic-rich effluents from fish farming activities. Additionally, the FA profile of ascidians is also contrasted with that of the most commercially used fish aquafeed employed in the studied location to investigate whether these filter-feeding marine organisms somehow mimicked the FA profile of those aquafeeds when grown under the influence of organic-rich effluents originating from fish farms.

2. Results

2.1. Ascidiacea

The FA profile of Ascidiacea revealed a total of 42 different FA (Supplementary Information Table S1). Nonetheless, 4 FAs alone represented more than 50% of the total pool of FAs (Table 1).

Table 1. Fatty acid profile of ascidians (Ascidiacea) and seaweeds (sea lettuce, *Ulva* spp. and bladderwrack, *Fucus* sp.) sampled in locations with versus without the influence of organic-rich effluents from fish farming activities (+Org or −Org, respectively), as well as the formulated fish feed (FF) most commonly supplied in fish farming activities in the study location. Values are expressed as a percentage of the total pool of fatty acids and are averages of five replicates ($n = 5$) ± SD. Only fatty acids accounting for at least 5% of the total pool of fatty acids in one of the biological matrices surveyed are presented. SFA: saturated fatty acids, MUFA: monounsaturated fatty acids, PUFA: polyunsaturated fatty acids.

	Ascidiacea		*Ulva* spp.		*Fucus* sp.		Fish Feed
	+Org	−Org	+Org	−Org	+Org	−Org	
14:0	0.94 ± 0.17	1.45 ± 0.12	0.68 ± 0.22	0.64 ± 0.17	8.04 ± 0.64	8.47 ± 0.27	1.53 ± 0.35
16:0	11.50 ± 1.31	12.56 ± 0.67	37.74 ± 1.14	38.05 ± 1.86	16.17 ± 1.29	15.03 ± 0.62	17.25 ± 0.68
16:1n-9	5.78 ± 0.62	5.37 ± 0.29	3.33 ± 0.27	2.67 ± 0.27	0.25 ± 0.04	0.29 ± 0.03	3.62 ± 0.18
16:4n-3	n.d	n.d	5.18 ± 0.33	4.27 ± 0.67	0.59 ± 0.06	0.59 ± 0.05	n.d
18:0	4.87 ± 1.23	5.89 ± 0.53	6.58 ± 3.99	8.70 ± 2.29	4.34 ± 1.61	1.77 ± 0.16	6.51 ± 1.09
18:1n-7+n-9	20.27 ± 1.80	11.98 ± 0.95 **	15.23 ± 1.21	15.19 ± 1.22	26.50 ± 2.28	21.34 ± 1.51 *	35.97 ± 0.43
18:2n-6	5.85 ± 1.62	2.26 ± 0.08 *	4.41 ± 0.19	2.74 ± 0.41	6.82 ± 0.38	7.45 ± 0.21 *	16.86 ± 0.19
18:3n-3	2.16 ± 0.22	2.38 ± 0.48	8.95 ± 0.70	7.85 ± 0.57 *	6.96 ± 0.41	8.87 ± 0.51 **	2.85 ± 0.07
18:4n-3	1.54 ± 0.61	3.61 ± 0.69	9.72 ± 0.65	10.10 ± 0.72	3.70 ± 0.36	5.55 ± 0.62	0.62 ± 0.05
20:4n-6	2.43 ± 0.37	3.11 ± 0.27	n.d	n.d	14.08 ± 1.17	15.03 ± 0.22	0.47 ± 0.03
20:5n-3	17.77 ± 2.90	20.44 ± 1.00	0.61 ± 0.13	1.25 ± 1.14	7.66 ± 0.74	9.95 ± 0.39 **	2.13 ± 0.11
22:6n-3	8.75 ± 1.00	11.85 ± 1.01 **	n.d	n.d	n.d	n.d	4.59 ± 0.32
$\sum n$-3	32.03 ± 3.62	40.07 ± 1.54 *	27.35 ± 1.87	27.61 ± 2.30	19.16 ± 1.54	25.24 ± 1.42 **	11.43 ± 0.51
$\sum n$-6	9.02 ± 1.25	6.94 ± 0.46 *	5.00 ± 0.24	3.45 ± 0.44 **	22.42 ± 1.59	24.18 ± 0.07 *	18.09 ± 0.23
$\sum n$-3/$\sum n$-6	3.66 ± 0.98	5.79 ± 0.37 *	5.46 ± 0.25	8.04 ± 0.36 **	0.85 ± 0.03	1.04 ± 0.06 **	0.63 ± 0.03
$\sum$SFA	19.52 ± 2.36	22.39 ±1.00 *	46.30 ± 3.35	48.78 ± 3.37	29.35 ± 3.48	26.02 ± 0.50	25.72 ± 1.42
$\sum$MUFA	32.99 ± 0.92	19.95 ± 1.39 **	20.88 ± 1.62	20.07 ± 1.66	29.07 ± 2.32	24.42 ± 1.48 *	44.77 ± 0.81
$\sum$PUFA	42.81 ± 2.65	48.48 ± 1.80 *	32.82 ± 1.94	31.19 ± 2.73	41.58 ± 3.08	49.43 ± 1.42 **	29.52 ± 0.64

nd: not detected; * $p < 0.05$; ** $p < 0.001$. $\sum$SFA: 14:0, 15:0, 16:0, 17:0, 18:0, 20:0, 21:0, 22:0, 24:0; $\sum$MUFA: 15:1, 16:1, 16:1n-7, 16:1n-9, 17:1, 17:1n-9, 18:1n-7+n-9, 20:1, 20:1n-7, 22:1n-11, 22:1n-9, 24:1n-9; $\sum$PUFA: 16:2, 16:2n-6, 16:3n-6, 16:4n-3, 18:2, 18:2n-6, 18:3n-6, 18:3n-3, 18:4n-3, 20:2, 20:2n-6, 20:3n-6, 20:3n-3, 20:4n-6, 20:4n-3, 20:5n-3, 22:4, 22:4, 22:5n-6, 22:5n-3, 22:6n-3.

PERMANOVA test revealed the existence of significant differences in the FA profiles ($p = 0.006$) and FA classes ($p = 0.011$) of Ascidiacea from the two locations surveyed (Table 2). Furthermore, statistical differences were also recorded between all FA classes (Table 1). Concerning the n-3/n-6 ratio, significant differences were detected between both sampling locations ($p = 0.002$) (Table 1), with higher values being recorded for Ascidiacea sampled at −Org (5.77) (Figure 1). In general, all FAs presented a higher relative abundance at −Org, with the exception of FA octadecenoic acid 18:1(n-7+n-9), 18:2, 18:2n-6, and 20:1n-9, which displayed higher abundances at +Org. The FAs EPA and DHA were the two most well-represented FAs (17.8% for +Org and 20.4% for −Org; 8.8% for +Org and 11.9% for −Org, respectively) (Table 1). Furthermore, the relative abundance of FAs 18:1(n-7+n-9), 18:2n-6, and DHA differed significantly between the two locations (Table 1).

Table 2. The results of the permutational multivariate analysis of variance (PERMANOVA) of fatty acids and fatty acid classes of ascidians (Ascidiacea) and seaweeds (sea lettuce, *Ulva* spp. and bladderwrack, *Fucus* sp.) sampled in locations with versus without the influence of organic-rich effluents from fish farming activities (+Org or −Org, respectively). Significant differences were considered at $p < 0.05$ (represented in bold); P(perm): p-values based on more than 999 permutations.

	Permanova +Org vs. −Org	
	Fatty Acids	Fatty Acids Classes
Ascidiacea	0.006	0.011
Ulva spp.	0.021	0.341
Fucus sp.	0.013	0.013

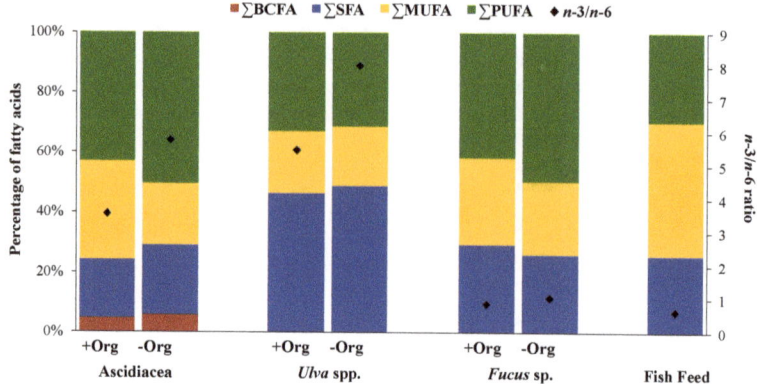

Figure 1. Fatty acid classes expressed as a percentage of the total pool of fatty acids (only values above 1% were considered) of ascidians (Ascidiacea) and seaweeds (sea lettuce, *Ulva* spp. and bladderwrack, *Fucus* sp.) sampled in locations with versus without the influence of organic-rich effluents from fish farming activities (+Org or −Org, respectively), as well as the formulated fish feed (FF) most commonly supplied in fish farming. BCFA: branched fatty acids, SFA: saturated fatty acids, MUFA: monounsaturated fatty acids, PUFA: polyunsaturated fatty acids.

Branched FAs (BCFA) represented the least abundant FA class identified in specimens sampled from both locations (4.6% for +Org; 5.5% for −Org) (Figure 1). Saturated FAs (SFA) and PUFA demonstrated higher values in specimens from −Org (22.3% and 48.5%, respectively). In addition, monounsaturated FAs (MUFA) values were higher at +Org (33% for +Org and 20.7% for −Org) (Figure 1). Similarity Percentage Species Contributions (SIMPER) analysis (Table 3A) showed that the FA profiles of Ascidiacea originating from the two locations displayed an average dissimilarity of 10.6%, with more than 50% cumulative dissimilarities being explained by the following FAs: eicosenoic acid 20:1n-9, 18:1(n-7+n-9), linoleic acid—LA 18:2n-6, and stearidonic acid—SDA 18:4n-3.

2.2. Seaweeds

A total of 17 and 24 different FAs were identified for *Ulva* spp. and *Fucus* sp., respectively (Supplementary Information Table S1) (Table 1). The FAs palmitic acid 16:0 and 18:1(n-7+n-9) were dominant in both seaweeds (37.7% for +Org and 38.1% for −Org; 15.2% for +Org and 15.2% for −Org, respectively). However, some contrasts worth highlighting were also recorded, such as the relative abundance of arachidonic acid (AA) 20:4n-6 and EPA in *Fucus* sp. (14.1% for +Org and 15.0% for −Org; 7.7% for +Org and 10.0% for −Org; respectively) that were either not detected or present at trace levels (respectively) in *Ulva* spp. Statistically significant differences were detected in 18:3n-3 for *Ulva* spp. ($p = 0.025$), while for *Fucus* sp. FAs 18:1(n-7+n-9), 18:2n-6, 18:3n-3, and EPA all differed significantly ($p = 0.003$, $p = 0.013$, $p < 0.001$, $p < 0.001$, respectively). PERMANOVA test showed statistical differences in the mean FA profiles of seaweeds originating from the two sampling locations ($p = 0.021$ for *Ulva* spp.; $p = 0.013$ for *Fucus* sp.), yet only significant differences were seen in the FA classes of *Fucus* sp. ($p = 0.013$) (Table 2), with significant differences being recorded between MUFA and PUFA ($p = 0.005$, $p < 0.001$, respectively) of specimens of this brown seaweed originating from the two sampling locations (Table 1). The n-3/n-6 ratio also exhibited significant differences between both sampling locations ($p < 0.001$ for *Ulva* spp., $p < 0.001$ for *Fucus* sp.) (Table 1), with higher values being recorded for seaweeds at −Org. The prevailing FA class in *Ulva* spp. was SFA (46.3% for +Org and 48.8% for −Org) (Figure 1), while PUFA registered higher values for *Fucus* sp. (41.6% for +Org; 49.4% for −Org). The non-metric multidimensional scaling (MDS) plot (Figure 2) revealed a distinct separation between the two seaweeds and the two sampling sites, with similarity values of 59% grouping both FA profiles.

Table 3. Summary of SIMPER analysis listing the fatty acids that most contributed to discriminate: (**A**) ascidians (Ascidiacea) and seaweeds (sea lettuce, *Ulva* spp. and bladderwrack, *Fucus* sp.) sampled in locations with versus without the influence of organic-rich effluents from fish farming activities (+Org or −Org, respectively); and (**B**) ascidians from +Org or −Org with the formulated fish feed (FF) most commonly supplied in fish farming activities in the study location. Cut-off percentage: 50%.

						Dissimilarity						
(**A**)		Ascidiacea				*Ulva* spp.				*Fucus* sp.		
		+Org vs. −Org 10.62%				+Org vs. −Org 5.29%				+Org vs. −Org 5.48%		
−Org vs. +Org		+ORW	−ORW	Contrib%		+Org	−Org	Contrib%		+Org	−Org	Contrib%
	20:1n-9	2.21	1.03	15.81	18:0	2.48	2.93	23.19	18:0	2.05	1.33	22.78
	18:1n-7+n-9	4.50	3.46	13.92	18:2n-6	2.10	1.65	14.23	18:1n-7+n-9	5.14	4.62	16.65
	18:2n-6	2.40	1.50	11.94	22:5n-3	1.54	1.91	11.59	18:4n-3	1.92	2.35	13.56
	18:4n-3	1.22	1.89	8.98	20:5n-3	0.78	1.04	9.76				
(**B**)					Ascidiacea							
		+Org vs. FF 31.06%				−Org vs. FF 36.35%						
Org vs. FF		+Org	FF	Contrib%		−Org	FF	Contrib%				
	20:5n-3	4.21	1.46	13.91	20:5n-3	4.52	1.46	13.33				
	18:2n-6	2.40	4.11	8.65	18:2n-6	1.50	4.11	11.34				
	20:4n-6	1.55	0	7.87	18:1n-7+n-9	3.46	6.00	11.06				
	18:1n-7+n-9	4.5	6.00	7.58	18:4n-3	1.89	0	8.24				
	22:1n-11	0	1.36	7.05	20:4n-6	1.76	0	7.68				
	18:4n-3	1.22	0	6.18								

SIMPER analysis (Table 3A) revealed that the FA profiles of *Ulva* spp. and *Fucus* sp. display comparable values of dissimilarities between +Org and −Org (5.29% and 5.48%, respectively), with FA 18:0 contributing the most for such differences.

2.3. Fish Feed

A total of 26 FAs were identified in fish feed (Supplementary Information Table S1) (Table 1). MUFA was the most abundant FA class for fish feed (44.8%) (Figure 1) with a major contribution of FA 18:1(n-7+n-9) (36.0%) (Table 1). SFA and PUFA presented similar values (25.7% and 29.5%, respectively). The n-3/n-6 ratio obtained was 0.63, indicating higher amounts of n-6 FAs. The MDS plot (Figure 2) revealed that the FA profile of fish feed is more similar to the FA profile of Ascidiacea from +Org than from −Org. SIMPER analysis of the FA profiles of fish feed and Ascidiacea (Table 3B) revealed higher dissimilarities with specimens originating from −Org. For Ascidiacea, EPA was the main responsible for such differences.

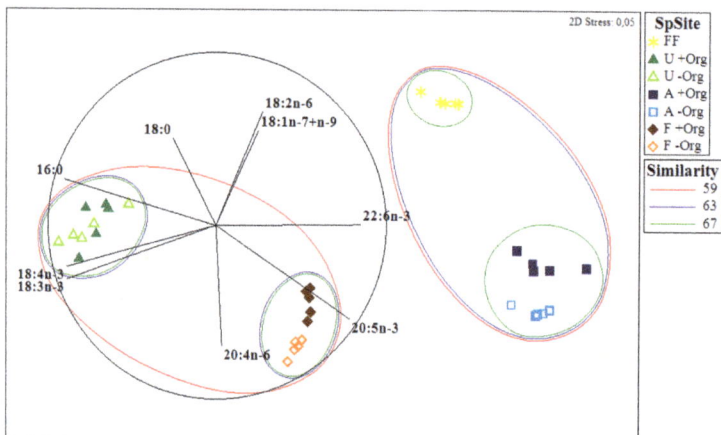

Figure 2. Multidimensional scaling (MDS) ordination plot comparing the fatty acid profiles between specimens of ascidians (Ascidiacea) (A) and seaweeds (sea lettuce, *Ulva* spp. (U) and bladderwrack, *Fucus* sp. (F)) sampled in locations with versus without the influence of organic-rich effluents from fish farming activities (+Org or −Org, respectively) and the formulated fish feed (FF) most commonly supplied in fish farming activities in the study location.

3. Discussion

To the authors' best knowledge, the present study is the first approach reported in the scientific literature to screen for health-promoting FAs in ascidians grown under the influence of fish farming organic-rich effluents. From the total pool of FA identified in Ascidiacea (42 FAs), only 4 of these biomolecules (16:0, 18:1(n-7+n-9), EPA, and DHA) represented average values above 10% of the total pool of FA. These findings share similarities with those reported from previous works screening the FA profile of ascidians [37,48–50]. The FAs 18:1(n-7+n-9) and 18:2n-6 also displayed higher values in +Org, near twice the ones recorded for −Org. Considering that these FAs accounted for 53% of the fish aquafeed FA pool, it is likely that ascidians may selectively retain these FAs in their tissues. The higher levels of n-3 FAs present in the −Org resulted in a higher n-3/n-6 ratio, with FAs 18:4n-3, EPA, and DHA being the main contributors to this trend. This finding is consistent with Monmai et al. [35], as these authors verified that in the edible ascidian *Halocynthia aurantium* n-3 FAs were present in much higher levels than n-6 FAs. Likewise, Zhao and Li [37] documented that tunics and inner body tissues of ascidians *Halocynthia roretzi*, *Styela plicata*, *Ascidia* sp. and *Ciona intestinalis* presented higher levels of n-3 FAs.

Ulva spp. and *Fucus* sp. presented some similarities in their FA profiles, with 16:0 and 18:1(n-7+n-9) displaying the highest relative abundances in the total pool of FAs recorded in both locations. This finding is in line with previous studies [51–53]. Our results on the profiling of unsaturated FAs (MUFA+PUFA) are fully aligned with those reported by Herbreteau et al. [54], who reported the FA composition of five species of seaweeds and verified that unsaturated FAs accounted for more than 50% of the total pool of FAs, with this proportion reaching up to 75% for *Fucus* sp. Silva et al. [55] focused on ten brown seaweeds also verifying important amounts of unsaturated FAs. In addition, our study recorded 46% to 49% of SFA in *Ulva* spp., unlike Lopes et al. [4] who have reported about half of these values for the same seaweed species (≈24%). Yet, the values of FA classes reported for *Fucus* sp. by Lopes et al. [4] are very much in line with the ones reported in the present work. Several studies [4,55,56] have mentioned that despite lipid content representing a minor fraction of seaweeds, it features levels of n-3 PUFAs worth being investigated. Our results validated the presence of EPA in *Fucus* sp., but not DHA, and no traces of either of these FAs were detected in *Ulva* spp. These latter values correlate fairly well with Pereira et al., [57] with *Ulva* spp. also presenting higher proportions of FA 18:3n-3, and thus, further supporting the idea that seaweeds do display an n-3/n-6 "healthy" ratio.

Several studies [1,5,6,30,58] have reported an increase in the use of n-6 PUFA-rich land-based ingredients and oils in aquafeed formulations sometimes leading to an inverted n-3/n-6 ratio in fish aquafeeds. Under organic-rich effluents, the biochemical profile of extractive species will most likely be shaped by the prevalence of these ingredients [16]. However, the availability of natural nutrients [59], sampling location, and season [55], amongst other factors, must be taken into consideration when profiling the FAs of marine species, as they too can modulate their biochemical profile and findings being reported results must be interpreted with care. Kim et al. [52] demonstrated how temperature, salinity, light, and nitrogen levels influence the level and profile of lipids present in the brown seaweed *Fucus serratus*. Similar findings were reported by Glencross [23] who emphasized how the hydrological source is a primary factor weighing in on the differences in FA requirements. This trend can extend to a multitude of marine organisms of interest for production under an IMTA framework, such as polychaetes [60,61], isopods [62], bivalves [63,64], and several fish species [65].

In conclusion, the present study demonstrated that Ascidiacea presented high values of EPA (17.8% in +Org; 20.4% in −Org) and DHA (8.8% in +Org; 11.9% in −Org) and can be considered as a potential new bioresource for n-3 long-chain FAs. The organic-rich effluent originating from fish farming systems can indeed shape the lipid profile of extractive species being employed in IMTA frameworks, whether as a consequence of direct consumption of available organic nutrients in dissolved and particulate form, as in the case of ascidians, or indirectly from de novo FA synthesis as in the case of seaweeds uptaking dissolved inorganic nutrients. The use of extractive species to maximize the use of ingredients present in formulated aquafeeds employed to farm marine finfish and shrimp can be considered as a pathway towards more sustainable and efficient aquaculture practices and have the potential to generate biomass with the potential to deliver important biomolecules for multiple biotechnological applications [66]. Our findings clearly point towards the need to further investigate the biochemical profile, particularly the FA profile of extractive species used in IMTA systems, as an approach to sequester valuable health-promoting FAs that will otherwise be lost to the aquatic environment through the effluents of fish farms.

4. Materials and Methods

4.1. Study Areas

Ria de Aveiro is a shallow coastal lagoon in the west margin of mainland Portugal that inholds the Vouga river estuary and presents a complex and irregular geometry. This coastal lagoon has four main channels emerging from the sea entrance: S. Jacinto-Ovar, Espinheiro, Ílhavo, and Mira channel (Figure 3). The first sampling location surveyed was located at Mira channel (40°36′51″ N, 8°44′25″ W) without the influence of organic-rich effluents from fish farming activities and is herein referred as −Org. The second sampling location surveyed was located at a land-based semi-intensive fish farm (40°36′43″ N, 8°40′43″ W) supplied by Ílhavo channel's waters. An IMTA framework is employed in this location, on which European seabass and Gilthead seabream are produced in earthen ponds and seaweeds are produced in tanks supplied with organic-rich waters from these earthen ponds. This location will be referred to as +Org. Both channels of this coastal lagoon present strong salinity gradients with very low values at their upper reaches. Salinity, temperature, dissolved oxygen, and pH were registered in situ at the time of sampling. Environmental parameters are summarized as Supplementary Information (Table S2).

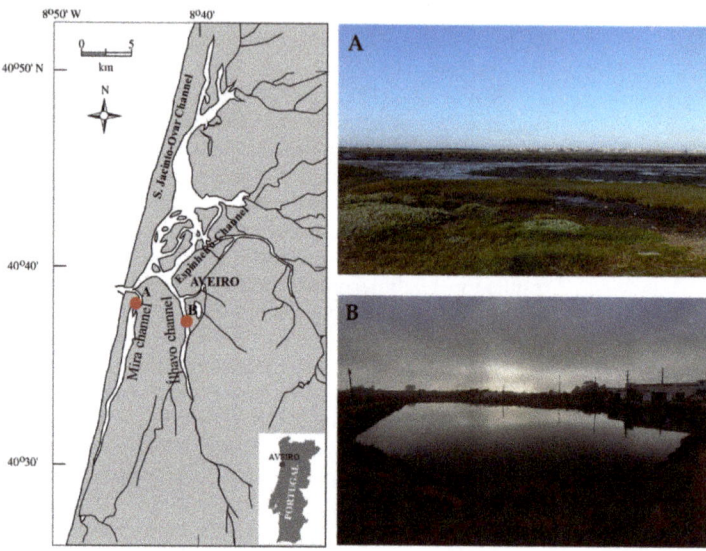

Figure 3. Sampling locations at Ria de Aveiro coastal lagoon (Portugal): (**A**) located in Mira channel (40°36′51″ N, 8°44′25″ W) and without the influence of organic-rich effluents from fish farming activities (−Org); and (**B**) located at a land-based semi-intensive fish farm (40°36′43″ N, 8°40′43″ W) supplied by Ílhavo channel's waters employing an IMTA framework where seaweeds are produced in tanks supplied with organic-rich waters from earthen ponds stocked with fish (+Org).

4.2. Sample Collection

4.2.1. Ascidiacea

Ascidians were collected manually from both locations described above. The taxonomic identification of ascidians is complex, and producers are unable to readily sort them by species, namely if they target the production of small sized specimens (when key diagnosing morphological features are incipient). While *Styela plicata* and *Ciona intestinalis* were certainly present among the ascidians collected, it is not impossible to rule out the presence of other species without using molecular tools (e.g., DNA barcodes) or taxonomic identification by experts. As such, ascidians were pooled into composite samples and will be simply termed as Ascidiacea. All specimens were left to depurate for 48 h after being sampled, in order to safeguard that their guts were emptied and, as such, avoid any bias on their FA profile from dietary prey. All specimens were depurated using filtered seawater (GFFC, glass microfiber filter 1.2 μm, Ø47 mm) from their sampling locations. After depuration all specimens were washed thoroughly using tap water to eliminate any impurities and all five composite samples of 3 individuals each (of similar sizes) were selected per sampling location. All samples were freeze-dried and stored at -20 °C. Prior to FA analysis, samples were grounded into a fine powder using a mortar and pestle.

4.2.2. Seaweeds

Specimens from the genus *Ulva* (Chlorophyceae) and *Fucus* (Phaeophyceae) were collected from the same locations as ascidians (−Org and +Org). As already detailed above for ascidians, more than one species of *Ulva* can be present in one or both of the sampling locations surveyed in the present work. As such, all collected sea lettuce samples were termed as *Ulva* spp. Concerning the samples of bladderwrack collected in the present work, all specimens of this brown seaweed could be easily identified to the species level (*Fucus vesiculosus*), but to keep consistency with the identification level of the green seaweed, it will be addressed as one species of the genus *Fucus*. All seaweeds were washed using tap water to eliminate impurities and excess water was dried from samples. Five composite samples of five seaweeds each were separated by species and location, freeze-dried and stored at -20 °C. As for ascidians, seaweeds biomass was also grounded into a fine powder using a mortar and pestle.

4.2.3. Fish Feed

The FA profile of the formulated fish feed (Standard Orange 4; SORGAL, Sociedade de óleos e rações, SA) supplied at the fish farm operating under an IMTA framework was determined using 250 mg of feed per each of the five replicates analyzed (Table S3 for detailed composition). All storage and processing of these samples prior to FA analysis were identical to those described above for ascidians and seaweeds.

4.3. Total Lipid Extraction

Lipid extraction was performed by adding 3.75 mL of a mixture of methanol/chloroform (2:1, v/v) to 150 mg of ascidians and 250 mg of seaweeds (five biological replicates per biological matrix tested) in a glass test tube with a Teflon-lined screw cap. Samples were then homogenized and incubated in ice on a rocking platform shaker (Stuart Scientific STR6, Bibby, UK) for 2 h and 30 min. The mixture was centrifuged at 2000 rpm for 10 min., and after the organic phase was collected. The biomass residue was re-extracted two times with 2 mL of methanol and 1 mL of chloroform. Afterward, water was added (2.3 mL) to the total collected organic phase, centrifuged at 2000 rpm for 10 min and the organic (lower) phase was recovered. Solvents were dried under a stream of nitrogen gas. Total lipid extract was estimated by gravimetry. Lipid extracts were stored in dark vials and stored at -20 °C before analysis by gas chromatography-mass spectrometry (GC–MS). Reagents were purchased from Fisher Scientific Ltd. (Loughborough, UK). All other reagents were purchased from major commercial suppliers. Milli-Q water (Synergy, Millipore Corporation, Billerica, MA, USA) was used.

4.4. Fatty Acid Profiling

Fatty acid methyl esters (FAMEs) were prepared using a methanolic solution of potassium hydroxide (2.0 M) as described by Melo et al. [67]. Subsequently, 2.0 µL of a hexane solution containing FAMEs were analyzed by GC–MS on an Agilent Technologies 6890 N Network (Santa Clara, CA, USA) equipped with a DB–FFAP column. The column was 30 m long, had 0.32 mm of internal diameter, and a film thickness of 0.25 µm (123-3232, J&W Scientific, Folsom, CA, USA). The GC equipment was connected to a Mass Selective Detector (Agilent 5973 Network) operating with an electron impact mode at 70 eV and scanning the range m/z 50–550 in a 1 s cycle in a full scan mode acquisition. The carrier gas Helium was used at a flow rate of 1.4 mL min^{-1}. The elution relied on an increasing temperature gradient: 80 °C for 3 min, a linear increase to 160 °C at 25 °C min^{-1}, followed by a linear increase at 2 °C min^{-1} to 210 °C, then at 30 °C min^{-1} to 250 °C, standing at 250 °C for 10 min Identification of FAs was performed considering retention times and mass spectrometry spectra of FA standards (Supelco 37 Component Fame Mix, Sigma-Aldrich, St. Louis, MO, USA), as well as through mass spectrum comparison with those in Wiley 275 library and AOCS Lipid Library. The relative amounts of FAs were calculated by the percent area method with proper normalization, considering the sum of all areas of the identified FAs. The results were expressed as means $\pm$ SD.

4.5. Statistical Analysis

Data from FA profiles were square-rooted transformed, and a Bray-Curtis matrix was assembled. A one-way PERMANOVA was used to test for differences between the FA profiles (for both all individual FAs, as well as FA classes) of Ascidiacea and seaweeds originating from +Org and −Org, with "sampling location" being used as a fixed factor. The statistical significance of variance components was tested using 999 permutations of unrestricted permutations of data, with an a priori chose significance level of $\alpha = 0.05$. Individual differences in the relative abundance of FA (whose values recorded > 5% of the total pool of FA in at least one of the biological matrices surveyed), FA classes, $\sum n$-3, $\sum n$-6, and the $\sum n$-3/$\sum n$-6 ratio from +Org and −Org were compared by either a t-test or the non-parametric Mann-Whitney U rank comparisons if samples were not normally distributed. A MDS was used to graphically visualize overall patterns and relationships between the different biological matrices survey. A SIMPER analysis was used to determine which FAs contributed the most to similarities and dissimilarities within Ascidiacea and seaweeds, at a cut-off of 50%. All analyses were performed using the PRIMER 6 + PERMANOVA© software (software package from Plymouth Marine Laboratory, Plymouth, UK).

Supplementary Materials: The following are available online at https://www.mdpi.com/article/10.3390/md19080469/s1, Table S1: Fatty acid profile of ascidians (Ascidiacea) and seaweeds (sea lettuce, *Ulva* spp. and bladderwrack, *Fucus* sp.) sampled in locations with versus without the influence of organic-rich effluents from fish farming activities (+Org or −Org, respectively), as well as the formulated fish feed (FF) most commonly supplied in fish farming activities in the study location. Values are expressed as a percentage of the total pool of fatty acids and are averages of five replicates (n=5) ± SD. BCFA: Branched fatty acids, SFA: saturated fatty acids, MUFA: monounsaturated fatty acids, PUFA: polyunsaturated fatty acids. n.d: not detected; Table S2: Summary of the environmental parameters measured at the time of sampling in locations with versus without the influence of organic-rich waters from fish farming activities (+Org or −Org, respectively). Values are expressed as a percentage and are averages of three replicates (n=6) ± SD; Table S3: Nutritional composition of the formulated fish feed provided to the fish at the fish farming location (+Org).

Author Contributions: Funding acquisition, A.I.L. and R.C.; investigation, L.M.; methodology, L.M. and E.d.C.; resources, M.R.D. and M.H.A.; supervision, A.I.L. and R.C.; validation, M.R.D., E.d.C., M.H.A., A.I.L. and R.C.; writing—original draft, L.M.; writing—review and editing, L.M., A.I.L. and R.C.. All authors have read and agreed to the published version of the manuscript.

Funding: This research was funded by project "AquaMMIn—Development and validation of a modular integrated multitrophic aquaculture system for marine and brackish water species" (MAR-02.01.01-FEAMP-0038) co-funded by Portugal 2020 and the European Union through Mar2020, the Operational Programme (OP) for the European Maritime and Fisheries Fund (EMFF) in Portugal. We also acknowledge FCT (Portuguese Foundation for Science and Technology) for the financial support to L. Marques through a PhD grant (PD/BD/127918/2016). Thanks, are also due to CESAM (UIDP/50017/2020+UIDB/50017/2020), to FCT/MEC through national funds, and the co-funding by the FEDER, within the PT2020 Partnership Agreement and Compete 2020.

Institutional Review Board Statement: Not applicable.

Data Availability Statement: The data presented in this study are included in the corresponding sections throughout the manuscript.

Acknowledgments: The authors are grateful to ALGAplus-Produção e Comércio de algas e seus derivados, Lda. for supplying the ascidians and seaweeds samples for this work.

Conflicts of Interest: The authors declare no conflict of interest.

References

1. Strobel, C.; Jahreis, G.; Kuhnt, K. Survey of n-3 and n-6 polyunsaturated fatty acids in fish and fish products. *Lipids Health Dis.* **2012**, *11*, 144. [CrossRef]
2. Marques, B.; Lillebø, A.I.; Ricardo, F.; Nunes, C.; Coimbra, M.A.; Calado, R. Adding value to ragworms (*Hediste diversicolor*) through the bioremediation of a super-intensive marine fish farm. *Aquac. Environ. Interact.* **2018**, *10*, 79–88. [CrossRef]
3. Zhao, Y.; Wang, M.; Lindström, M.E.; Li, J. Fatty acid and lipid profiles with emphasis on n-3 fatty acids and phospholipids from *Ciona intestinalis*. *Lipids* **2015**, *50*, 1009–1027. [CrossRef]
4. Lopes, D.; Melo, T.; Rey, F.; Meneses, J.; Monteiro, F.L.; Helguero, L.A.; Abreu, M.H.; Lillebø, A.I.; Calado, R.; Domingues, M.R. Valuing bioactive lipids from green, red and brown macroalgae from aquaculture, to foster functionality and biotechnological applications. *Molecules* **2020**, *25*, 3883. [CrossRef]
5. Simopoulos, A.P. The importance of the ratio of omega-6/omega-3 essential fatty acids. *Biomed. Pharmacother.* **2002**, *56*, 365–379. [CrossRef]
6. Candela, C.G.; López, L.M.B.; Kohen, V.L. Importance of a balanced omega 6/omega 3 ratio for the maintenance of health. *Nutr. Recomm. Nutr. Hosp.* **2011**, *26*, 323–329. [CrossRef]

7. Swanson, D.; Block, R.; Mousa, S.A. Omega-3 fatty acids EPA and DHA: Health benefits throughout life. *Adv. Nutr.* **2012**, *3*, 1–7. [CrossRef]
8. Béné, C.; Barange, M.; Subasinghe, R.; Pinstrup-Andersen, P.; Merino, G.; Hemre, G.I.; Williams, M. Feeding 9 billion by 2050—Putting fish back on the menu. *Food Secur.* **2015**, *7*, 261–274. [CrossRef]
9. FAO. *The State of World Fisheries and Aquaculture*; FAO: Rome, Italy, 2020; ISBN 9789251326923.
10. Abreu, M.H.; Pereira, R.; Sassi, J.F. Marine algae and the global food industry. In *Marine Algae Biodiversity, Taxonomy, Environmental Assessment, and Biotechnology*; CRC Press: Boca Raton, FL, USA, 2014; pp. 300–319. [CrossRef]
11. Olsen, Y. Resources for fish feed in future mariculture. *Aquac. Environ. Interact.* **2011**, *1*, 187–200. [CrossRef]
12. Engle, C.; Abramo, L.R.D.; Slater, M.J. Global Aquaculture 2050. *J. World Aquac. Soc.* **2017**, *48*, 3–6. [CrossRef]
13. Alexander, K.A.; Angel, D.; Freeman, S.; Israel, D.; Johansen, J.; Kletou, D.; Meland, M.; Pecorino, D.; Rebours, C.; Rousou, M.; et al. Improving sustainability of aquaculture in Europe: Stakeholder dialogues on Integrated Multi-trophic Aquaculture (IMTA). *Environ. Sci. Policy* **2016**, *55*, 96–106. [CrossRef]
14. Hasan, M.; Halwart, M. *Fish as Feed Inputs for Aquaculture: Practices, Sustainability and Implications*; FAO: Rome, Italy, 2009; ISBN 9789251064191.
15. Custódio, M.; Villasante, S.; Calado, R.; Lillebø, A.I. Valuation of ecosystem services to promote sustainable aquaculture practices. *Rev. Aquac.* **2020**, *12*, 392–405. [CrossRef]
16. Hodar, A.R.; Vasava, R.; Joshi, N.H. Fish meal and fish oil replacement for aquafeed formulation by using alternative sources: A review. *J. Exp. Zool. India* **2020**, *23*, 13–21.
17. Apper-bossard, E.; Feneuil, A.; Wagner, A.; Respondek, F. Use of vital wheat gluten in aquaculture feeds. *Aquat. Biosyst.* **2013**, *9*, 21. [CrossRef]
18. Metwalli, A.A.A. Effects of partial and total substitution of fish meal with corn gluten meal on growth performance, nutrients utilization and some blood constituents of the Nile tilapia *Oreochromis niloticus*. *Egypt J. Aquat. Biol. Fish.* **2013**, *17*, 91–100.
19. Iqbal, M.; Yaqub, A.; Ayub, M. Partial and full substitution of fish meal and soybean meal by canola meal in diets for genetically improved farmed tilapia (*O. niloticus*): Growth performance, carcass composition, serum biochemistry, immune response, and intestine histology. *J. Appl. Aquac.* **2021**, 1–26. [CrossRef]
20. Soller, F.; Roy, L.A.; Davis, D.A. Replacement of fish oil in plant-based diets for Pacific white shrimp, *Litopenaeus vannamei*, by stearine fish oil and palm oil. *Fundam. Stud.* **2018**, *50*, 186–203. [CrossRef]
21. Ayisi, C.L.; Zhao, J.; Wu, J. Replacement of fish oil with palm oil: Effects on growth performance, innate immune response, antioxidant capacity and disease resistance in Nile tilapia (*Oreochromis niloticus*). *PLoS ONE* **2018**, *13*, e0196100. [CrossRef]
22. Makkar, H.P.; Tran, G.; Heuzé, V.; Giger-Reverdin, S.; Lessire, M.; Lebas, F.; Ankers, P. Seaweeds for livestock diets: A review. *Anim. Feed Sci. Technol.* **2016**, *212*, 1–17. [CrossRef]
23. Glencross, B.D. Exploring the nutritional demand for essential fatty acids by aquaculture species. *Rev. Aquac.* **2009**, *1*, 71–124. [CrossRef]
24. Broadhurst, C.L.; Wang, Y.; Crawford, M.A.; Cunnane, S.C.; Parkington, J.E.; Schmidt, W.F. Brain-specific lipids from marine, lacustrine, or terrestrial food resources: Potential impact on early African *Homo sapiens*. *Comp. Biochem. Physiol. Part B Biochem. Mol. Biol.* **2002**, *131*, 653–673. [CrossRef]
25. Ju, B.; Jiang, A.; Xing, R.; Chen, L.; Teng, L. Optimization of conditions for an integrated multi-trophic aquaculture system consisting of sea cucumber *Apostichopus japonicus* and ascidian *Styela clava*. *Aquac. Int.* **2016**, *25*, 265–286. [CrossRef]
26. Chatzoglou, E.; Kechagia, P.; Tsopelakos, A.; Miliou, H.; Slembrouck, J. Co-culture of *Ulva* sp. and *Dicentrarchus labrax* in Recirculating Aquaculture System: Effects on growth, retention of nutrients and fatty acid profile. *Aquat. Living Resour.* **2020**, *33*, 19. [CrossRef]
27. Marques, B.; Calado, R.; Lillebø, A.I. New species for the biomitigation of a super-intensive marine fish farm effluent: Combined use of polychaete-assisted sand filters and halophyte aquaponics. *Sci. Total Environ.* **2017**, *599–600*, 1922–1928. [CrossRef]
28. Jerónimo, D.; Lillebø, A.I.; Cremades, J.; Cartaxana, P.; Calado, R. Recovering wasted nutrients from shrimp farming through the combined culture of polychaetes and halophytes. *Sci. Rep.* **2021**, *11*, 1–16. [CrossRef] [PubMed]
29. Cripps, S.J.; Bergheim, A. Solids management and removal for intensive land-based aquaculture production systems. *Aquac. Eng.* **2000**, *22*, 33–56. [CrossRef]
30. Sprague, M.; Dick, J.R.; Tocher, D.R. Impact of sustainable feeds on omega-3 long-chain fatty acid levels in farmed Atlantic salmon. *Sci. Rep.* **2016**, *6*, 21892. [CrossRef]
31. Aguado-Giménez, F.; Hernández, M.D.; Cerezo-Valverde, J.; Piedecausa, M.A.; García-García, B. Does flat oyster (*Ostrea edulis*) rearing improve under open-sea integrated multi-trophic conditions? *Aquac. Int.* **2014**, *22*, 447–467. [CrossRef]
32. White, C.A.; Woodcock, S.H.; Bannister, R.J.; Nichols, P.D. Terrestrial fatty acids as tracers of finfish aquaculture waste in the marine environment. *Rev. Aquac.* **2017**, *11*, 133–148. [CrossRef]
33. Fernandez-Jover, D.; Arechavala-Lopez, P.; Martinez-Rubio, L.; Tocher, D.R.; Bayle-Sempere, J.T.; Lopez-Jimenez, J.A.; Martinez-Lopez, F.; Sanchez-Jerez, P. Monitoring the influence of marine aquaculture on wild fish communities: Benefits and limitations of fatty acid profiles. *Aquac. Environ. Interact.* **2011**, *2*, 39–47. [CrossRef]
34. Palanisamy, S.K.; Rajendran, N.M.; Marino, A. Natural products diversity of marine ascidians (Tunicates; Ascidiacea) and successful drugs in clinical development. *Nat. Prod. Bioprospect.* **2017**, *7*, 1–111. [CrossRef] [PubMed]

35. Monmai, C.; Go, S.H.; Shin, I.-S.; You, S.G.; Lee, H.; Kang, S.B.; Park, W.J. Immune-enhancement and anti-inflammatory activities of fatty acids extracted from *Halocynthia aurantium* tunic in RAW264.7 cells. *Mar. Drugs* **2018**, *16*, 309. [CrossRef]
36. Dagorn, F.; Dumay, J.; Wielgosz-Collin, G.; Rabesaotra, V.; Viau, M.; Monniot, C.; Biard, J.-F.; Barnathan, G. Phospholipid distribution and phospholipid fatty acids of the tropical tunicates *Eudistoma* sp. and *Leptoclinides uniorbis*. *Lipids* **2010**, *45*, 253–261. [CrossRef]
37. Zhao, Y.; Li, J. Ascidian bioresources: Common and variant chemical compositions and exploitation strategy—examples of *Halocynthia roretzi*, *Styela plicata*, *Ascidia* sp. and *Ciona intestinalis*. *Zeitschrift fur Naturforsch* **2016**, *71*, 165–180. [CrossRef] [PubMed]
38. Hassanzadeh, M. Unique marine organism: Identification of some methods for biomaterial production. *Chem. Eng. Trans.* **2014**, *37*, 385–390. [CrossRef]
39. Choi, D.G.; Kim, J.; Yun, A.; Cho, S.H.; Jeong, H.S.; Lee, K.W.; Kim, H.S.; Kim, P.Y.; Ha, M.S. Dietary substitution effect of fishmeal with tunic meal of sea squirt, *Halocynthia roretzi*, Drasche, on growth and soft body composition of juvenile abalone, *Haliotis discus*, Reeve 1846. *J. World Aquac. Soc.* **2018**, *49*, 1095–1104. [CrossRef]
40. Jang, B.; Kim, P.Y.; Kim, H.S.; Lee, K.W.; Kim, H.J.; Choi, D.G.; Cho, S.H.; Min, B.; Kim, K.; Han, H. Substitution effect of sea tangle (ST) (*Laminaria japonica*) with tunic of sea squirt (SS) (*Halocynthia roretzi*) in diet on growth and carcass composition of juvenile abalone (*Haliotis discus*, Reeve 1846). *Aquac. Nutr.* **2017**, *24*, 586–593. [CrossRef]
41. Giangrande, A.; Pierri, C.; Arduini, D.; Borghese, J.; Licciano, M.; Trani, R.; Corriero, G.; Basile, G.; Cecere, E.; Petrocelli, A.; et al. An innovative IMTA system: Polychaetes, sponges and macroalgae co-cultured in a Southern Italian in-shore mariculture plant (Ionian Sea). *J. Mar. Sci. Eng.* **2020**, *8*, 733. [CrossRef]
42. Vega, J.; Álvarez-Gómez, F.; Güenaga, L.; Figueroa, F.L.; Gómez-Pinchetti, J.L. Antioxidant activity of extracts from marine macroalgae, wild-collected and cultivated, in an integrated multi-trophic aquaculture system. *Aquaculture* **2020**, *522*, 735088. [CrossRef]
43. Ashkenazi, D.Y.; Israel, A.; Abelson, A. A novel two-stage seaweed integrated multi-trophic aquaculture. *Rev. Aquac.* **2019**, *11*, 246–262. [CrossRef]
44. Da Costa, E.; Domingues, P.; Melo, T.; Coelho, E.; Pereira, R.; Calado, R.; Abreu, M.H.; Domingues, M.R. Lipidomic signatures reveal seasonal shifts on the relative abundance of high-valued lipids from the brown algae *Fucus vesiculosus*. *Mar. Drugs* **2019**, *17*, 335. [CrossRef]
45. Wan, A.H.L.; Davies, S.J.; Soler-Vila, A.; Fitzgerald, R.; Johnson, M.P. Macroalgae as a sustainable aquafeed ingredient. *Rev. Aquac.* **2019**, *11*, 458–492. [CrossRef]
46. Pirian, K.; Jeliani, Z.Z.; Arman, M.; Sohrabipour, J.; Yousefzadi, M. Proximate analysis of selected macroalgal species from The Persian Gulf as a nutritional resource. *Trop. Life Sci. Res.* **2020**, *31*, 1–17. [CrossRef]
47. Moreira, A.S.P.; da Costa, E.; Melo, T.; Sulpice, R.; Cardoso, S.M.; Pitarma, B.; Pereira, R.; Abreu, M.H.; Domingues, P.; Calado, R.; et al. Seasonal plasticity of the polar lipidome of *Ulva rigida* cultivated in a sustainable integrated multi-trophic aquaculture. *Algal Res.* **2020**, *49*, 101958. [CrossRef]
48. Jeong, B.Y.; Ohshima, T.; Koizumi, C. Hydrocarbon chain distribution of ether phospholipids of the ascidian *Halocynthia roretzi* and the sea urchin *Strongylocentrotus intermedius*. *Lipids* **1996**, *31*, 9–18. [CrossRef] [PubMed]
49. Sri Kumaran, N.; Bragadeeswaran, S. Nutritional composition of the colonial ascidian *Eudistoma viride* and *Didemnum psammathodes*. *Biosci. Biotechnol. Res. Asia* **2014**, *11*, 331–338. [CrossRef]
50. Maoufoud, S.; Abdelmjid, A.; Abboud, Y.; Tarik, A. Chemical composition of fatty acids and sterols from tunicates *Cynthia savignyi*, *Cynthia squamulata* and from the brown alga *Cystoseira tamariscifolia*. *Phys. Chem. News* **2009**, *47*, 115–119.
51. Schmid, M.; Guihéneuf, F.; Stengel, D.B. Fatty acid contents and profiles of 16 macroalgae collected from the Irish Coast at two seasons. *J. Appl. Phycol.* **2014**, *26*, 451–463. [CrossRef]
52. Kim, M.-K.; Dubacq, J.-P.; Thomas, J.-C.; Giraud, G. Seasonal variations of triacylglycerols and fatty acids in *Fucus serratus*. *Phytochemistry* **1996**, *43*, 49–55. [CrossRef]
53. Morais, T.; Cotas, J.; Pacheco, D.; Pereira, L. Seaweeds compounds: An ecosustainable source of comestic ingredients? *Cosmetics* **2021**, *8*, 8. [CrossRef]
54. Herbreteau, F.; Coiffard, L.J.M.; Derrien, A.; De Roeck-Holtzhauer, Y. The fatty acid composition of five species of macroalgae. *Bot. Mar.* **1997**, *40*, 25–28. [CrossRef]
55. Silva, G.; Pereira, R.B.; Valentão, P.; Paula, B. Distinct fatty acid profile of ten brown macroalgae. *Brazilian J. Pharmacogn.* **2013**, *23*, 608–613. [CrossRef]
56. Kendel, M.; Wielgosz-Collin, G.; Bertrand, S.; Roussakis, C.; Bourgougnon, N.B.; Bedoux, G. Lipid composition, fatty acids and sterols in the seaweeds *Ulva armoricana*, and *Solieria chordalis* from brittany (France): An analysis from nutritional, chemotaxonomic, and antiproliferative activity perspectives. *Mar. Drugs* **2015**, *13*, 5606–5628. [CrossRef] [PubMed]
57. Pereira, H.; Barreira, L.; Figueiredo, F.; Custódio, L.; Vizetto-Duarte, C.; Polo, C.; Rešek, E.; Aschwin, E.; Varela, J. Polyunsaturated fatty acids of marine macroalgae: Potential for nutritional and pharmaceutical applications. *Mar. Drugs* **2012**, *10*, 1920–1935. [CrossRef]
58. van Vliet, T.; Katan, B. Lower ratio of n-3 to n-6 fatty acids in cultured than in wild fish. *Am. J. Clin. Nutr.* **1990**, *51*, 1–2. [CrossRef]
59. Pedersen, M.F.; Borum, J. Nutrient control of estuarine macroalgae: Growth strategy and the balance between nitrogen requirements and uptake. *Mar. Ecol. Prog. Ser.* **1997**, *161*, 155–163. [CrossRef]

60. García-Alonso, J.; Müller, C.T.; Hardege, J.D. Influence of food regimes and seasonality on fatty acid composition in the ragworm. *Aquat. Biol.* **2008**, *4*, 7–13. [CrossRef]
61. Luis, O.J.; Passos, A.M. Seasonal changes in lipid content and composition of the polychaete *Nereis* (*Hediste*) *diversicolor*. *Comp. Biochem. Physiol. Part B Biochem.* **1995**, *111*, 579–586. [CrossRef]
62. Prato, E.; Danieli, A.; Maffia, M.; Biandolino, F. Lipid contents and fatty acid compositions of *Idotea baltica* and *Sphaeroma serratum* (Crustacea: Isopoda) as indicators of food sources. *Zool. Stud.* **2012**, *51*, 38–50.
63. Chetoui, I.; Rabeh, I.; Bejaoui, S.; Telahigue, K.; Ghribi, F.; El Cafsi, M. First seasonal investigation of the fatty acid composition in three organs of the Tunisian bivalve *Mactra stultorum*. *Grasas y Aceites* **2019**, *70*, 291. [CrossRef]
64. Ezgeta-Balić, D.; Najdek, M.; Peharda, M.; Blažina, M. Seasonal fatty acid profile analysis to trace origin of food sources of four commercially important bivalves. *Aquaculture* **2012**, *334–337*, 89–100. [CrossRef]
65. Zlatanos, S.; Laskaridis, K. Seasonal variation in the fatty acid composition of three Mediterranean fish—sardine (*Sardina pilchardus*), anchovy (*Engraulis encrasicholus*) and picarel (*Spicara smaris*). *Food Chem.* **2007**, *103*, 725–728. [CrossRef]
66. Vieira, H.; Leal, M.C.; Calado, R. Fifty shades of blue: How blue biotechnology is shaping the bioeconomy. *Trends Biotechnol.* **2020**, *38*, 940–943. [CrossRef] [PubMed]
67. Melo, T.; Alves, E.; Azevedo, V.; Martins, A.S.; Neves, B.M.; Domingues, P.; Calado, R.; Abreu, M.H.; Domingues, M.R. Lipidomics as a new approach for the bioprospecting of marine macroalgae—Unraveling the polar lipid and fatty acid composition of *Chondrus crispus*. *Algal Res.* **2015**, *8*, 181–191. [CrossRef]

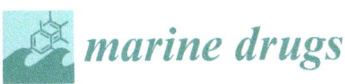

Article

The Negative Relationship between Fouling Organisms and the Content of Eicosapentaenoic Acid and Docosahexaenoic Acid in Cultivated Pacific Oysters, *Crassostrea gigas*

Megumu Fujibayashi [1,*], Osamu Nishimura [2] and Takashi Sakamaki [2]

1. Faculty of Engineering, Kyushu University, Fukuoka 819-0395, Japan
2. Department of Civil and Environmental Engineering, Graduate School of Engineering, Tohoku University, Miyagi 980-8579, Japan; osamu.nishimura.d2@tohoku.ac.jp (O.N.); takashi.sakamaki.a5@tohoku.ac.jp (T.S.)
* Correspondence: m.fujibayashi@civil.kyushu-u.ac.jp; Tel.: +81-92-802-3423

Abstract: Bivalves serve as an important aquaculture product, as they are the source of essential fatty acids, such as eicosapentaenoic acid (EPA) and docosahexaenoic acid (DHA), in our diet. However, their cultivation in the wild can be affected by fouling organisms that, in turn, affect their EPA and DHA content. The effects of fouling organisms on the EPA and DHA contents of cultivated bivalves have not been well documented. We examined the effects of fouling organisms on the EPA and DHA contents and condition index of cultured oysters, *Crassostrea gigas*, in an aquaculture system. We sampled two-year-old oysters from five sites in Shizugawa Bay, Japan, in August 2014. Most of the fouling organisms were sponges, macroalgae, and *Mytilus galloprovincialis*. A significant negative relationship existed between the DHA content in *C. gigas* and the presence of sponges and macroalgae. A lower *C. gigas* EPA content corresponded to a higher *M. galloprovincialis* fouling mass and a lower *C. gigas* condition index. This can be explained by dietary competition between *C. gigas* and *M. galloprovincialis* for diatoms, which were the main producer of EPA in our study sites. Our findings indicate that fouling organisms likely reduce the EPA and DHA content in cultivated oysters. Therefore, our results suggest that the current efforts to remove fouling organisms from oyster clusters is an effective strategy to enhance the content of EPA and DHA in oysters.

Keywords: dietary resource; *Mytilus galloprovincialis*; *Crassostrea gigas*; diatom; competition; biofouling; EPA; DHA

1. Introduction

Bivalve aquaculture is common in coastal areas worldwide and is highly important for food production and ecosystem services [1]. In particular, oysters are a major bivalve aquaculture species; they comprised ~30% of global marine mollusc aquaculture in 2016 [2]. In general, shellfish aquaculture does not require artificial food supplements for the cultured organisms and is considered more environmentally friendly and sustainable than other feeding aquaculture species, such as finfish [3].

Bivalves are a rich source of highly unsaturated fatty acids, such as eicosapentaenoic acid (EPA) and docosahexaenoic acid (DHA) [4]. Consuming an adequate amount of these omega-3 fatty acids is important for human health because they have important roles in regulating biological functions [5,6]. These fatty acids are mainly synthesised by aquatic algae and are transferred to humans via the food chain [7,8]. However, due to the increasing demand for these essential fatty acids due to population growth, an estimation of the global supply of EPA and DHA for humans has indicated that adequate amounts of these fatty acids cannot be provided sustainably [9]. Therefore, the provision of EPA and DHA by aquaculture will become more important [4].

Biofouling is one of the most critical issues in suspended bivalve farming and substantially raises the costs of maintaining culture equipment and farming operations [10,11]. The biomass of fouling organisms devalues the products and increases the weight of culture equipment, creating difficulties in maintenance and farming operations [12]. Fouling organisms growing on bivalve shells are generally considered to negatively affect bivalve growth and survival [13,14] by weakening the water movement around the cultured bivalves and reducing the advective influx of food resources to them [12,15,16]. Moreover, numerical modelling studies on carrying capacity in bivalve aquaculture have demonstrated that food limitations owing to the overharvesting of the cultivated species can suppress growth of the cultivated species [17,18]. This implies that dietary competition with fouling suspension-feeding organisms may decrease the growth rate of these organisms. In fact, dietary competition has been highlighted as one of the main mechanisms of negative effects on the growth of cultivated species in laboratory experiments [19]. Since EPA and DHA are obtained from dietary sources, dietary competition may lead to a reduction of EPA and DHA in cultivated species. However, to our knowledge, no study has yet evaluated the effect of fouling organisms on the content of EPA and DHA in cultivated species.

Crassostrea gigas is one of the most economically important cultured oyster species in Northeast Asia [20]. Fouling marine organisms on oyster shells comprise various taxonomic groups, such as molluscs, bryozoans, barnacles, sponges, algae, ascidians, hydrozoans, and polychaetes [21–23]. Although the positive effects of fouling organisms on the growth of *C. gigas* have been reported in one case, fouling organisms can negatively affect the growth of *C. gigas* by food and space competition and require additional cost for maintenance to operators [23]. The objective of this study was to examine how fouling organisms affect the content of EPA and DHA in *C. gigas*. Furthermore, body condition, which is expressed as the relative weight of whole soft tissue to shell volume, is considered an important index of the product value of the cultivated oyster [24]. We collected oysters and fouling organisms from oyster farming sites in a temperate bay, located in Northeast Japan, and analysed the fatty acid composition and body condition of the *C. gigas* oysters.

2. Results

The wet weight of fouling organisms ranged from 567 to 4177 g cluster^{-1} (Figure 1), and the mean value was 1795 g cluster^{-1}. The relative weight of fouling organisms by taxonomic group differed between the 15 sampled clusters (Figure 2). The major components were generally sponges and macroalgae, which contributed 3–53% of the total wet weight of the clusters, and the mean value was 29.7%. *M. galloprovincialis* was the second most dominant fouling organism, ranging from 2 to 32% of the total wet weight of the clusters, and the mean value was 14.7%. Other organisms, consisting of mainly polychaetes, cirripedians, and decapod crustaceans, made a minor contribution to the clusters in our study sites (below 0.5%).

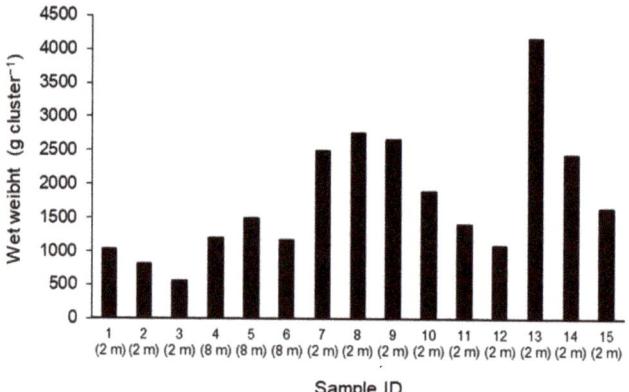

Figure 1. Total wet weight of fouling organisms of each sample. The values given in parentheses represent collecting water depth.

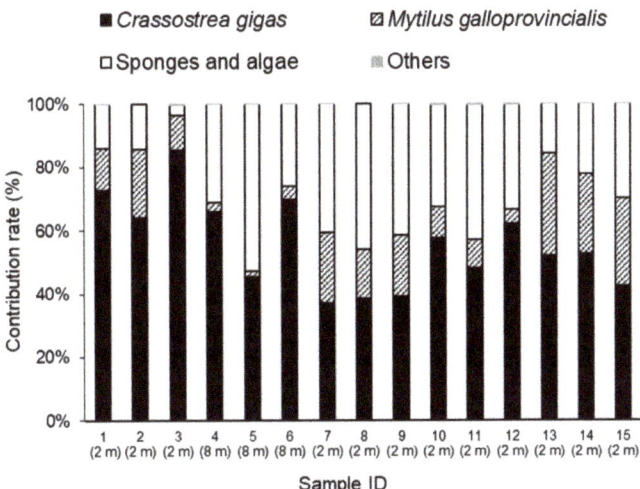

Figure 2. The contribution of each component within the sampled clusters from each sampling site. The "Other" component comprised mainly polychaetes, cirripedians, and decapod crustaceans. The mean values of *Crassostrea gigas*, *Mytilus galloprovincialis*, sponge and algae, and others are 55.5, 14.7, 29.7, and 0.1%, respectively. The values given in parentheses represent collecting water depth.

The condition index and content of EPA in *C. gigas* individuals were negatively correlated with the wet weight of *M. galloprovincialis* (Table 1). Negative correlations were also detected between the DHA content in *C. gigas* individuals and the wet weight of sponges and macroalgae (Table 1). For the relative weight of fouling organisms, *M. galloprovincialis* correlated negatively with EPA content in *C. gigas* individuals and CI (Table 1). Sponges and algae correlated negatively with the total wet weight, EPA with clusters, DHA with individuals, and DHA with clusters of *C. gigas*. The CI of *C. gigas* and *M. galloprovincialis* had a significant positive relationship with the EPA content (Figure 3). In addition, a significant positive relationship between CI and DHA was detected for *C. gigas* (Figure 3). The EPA content in *C. gigas* showed a significant positive relationship with the ratios of palmitoleic acid (16:1ω7) to palmitic acid (16:0) in *C. gigas* (Figure 4).

Table 1. The r values of the correlation analysis between cultivated oysters and the main fouling organisms. Spearman rank correlation analysis was applied for *Mytilus galloprovincialis* and Pearson's correlation analysis was applied for sponges and algae.

Fouling Organisms	unit	*Crassostrea gigas*					
		Total Wet Weight g cluster^{-1}	CI -	EPA	DHA	EPA	DHA
				mg g^{-1}		g cluster^{-1}	
		Wet weight					
Mytilus galloprovincialis	g cluster^{-1}	0.204	**−0.743 ****	**−0.689 ****	−0.154	−0.250	−0.061
Sponges and algae	g cluster^{-1}	−0.189	−0.409	−0.475	**−0.642 ****	−0.409	−0.357
		Wet weight ratios to oyster					
Mytilus galloprovincialis	g g^{-1}	−0.071	**−0.661 ****	**−0.646 ****	−0.310	−0.421	−0.236
Sponges and algae	g g^{-1}	**−0.649 ****	−0.259	−0.312	**−0.585 ***	**−0.697 ****	**−0.732 ****

Bold represents a significant relationship, *: $p < 0.05$, **: $p < 0.01$.

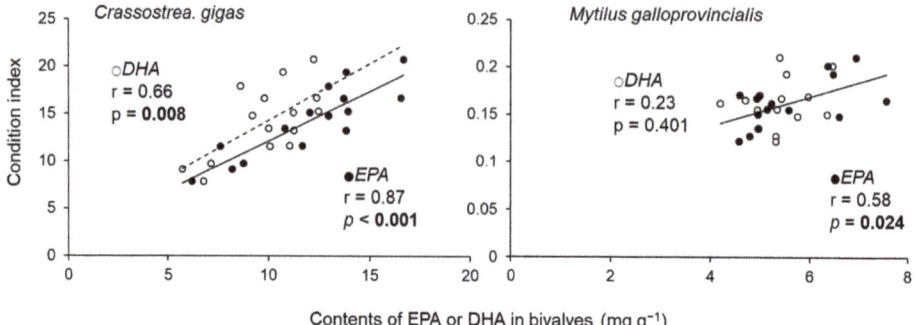

Figure 3. The relationship between the condition index and EPA or DHA content in *Crassostrea gigas* and *Mytilus galloprovincialis*. Each plot is the average of five individuals from each cluster.

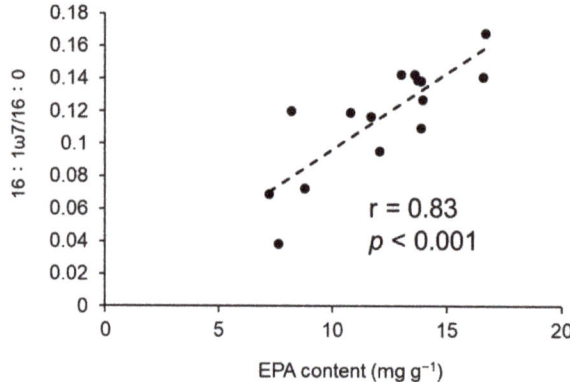

Figure 4. The correlation of the EPA content and the ratios of palmitoleic acid (16:1ω7) to palmitic acid (16:0) in *Crassostrea gigas*. Each plot is the average of five individuals from each cluster.

3. Discussion

The main fouling species of *C. gigas* aquaculture in the studied bay were sponges, algae, and *M. galloprovincialis* regardless of sampling site and depth, a finding that was partially inconsistent with some previous aquaculture studies conducted in Japan, which reported that mussels were dominant [25–27]. Mazouni et al. [28] reported that the predominant fouling organisms on *C. giga* clusters were ascidians. Royer et al. [29] reported that *C. gigas* clusters were mostly fouled by barnacles. Rodriguez et al. [22] found that ascidians, bryozoans, sponges, hydrozoans, and algae were the predominant colonisers on oyster farming beds, indicating that biofouling communities differ compositionally, even for the same host species [30]. This can be explained by the difference of environmental factors and climate among previous reports and the current study. Spatiotemporally variable factors, such as water temperature [22], the season [28], and larval supply from the benthic community [31], influence the settlement, abundance, and community structure in oyster farms.

While the negative effects of fouling organisms on oysters have been widely reported [23,32], some studies have indicated no significant effect of fouling organisms on cultivated oysters [29,33]. These inconsistent findings may indicate that the effects of fouling organisms on host oysters are species-specific and depend on focal factors (e.g., growth rate, survival rate, etc.) [30]. Similarly, in this study, the effects of sponges, macroalgae, and *M. galloprovincialis* on the fatty acid content and condition of *C. gigas* were different.

Sponges and macroalgal mixtures seem to have decreased the DHA content of *C. gigas* individuals. It is known that *C. gigas* have a poor ability to carry out biosynthesis of DHA [34,35]. Thus, the reduction of DHA in *C. gigas* implies that the dietary intake of DHA sources was reduced. DHA is abundant in some algal classes, such as dinoflagellates [36] and haptophyta [37]. For Shizugawa bay near farm A in July 2017, dinoflagellates were detected; however, haptophyta were not observed (Sakamaki, unpublished data, Table S1). Since sponges are suspension feeders [38], dietary competition for dinoflagellates between oysters and sponges is one of the possible mechanisms for the reduction of DHA in oysters. However, sponges generally ingest smaller particles, and their main dietary sources are known to be bacteria [39]. In addition, sponges can meet their dietary requirements through ingesting particles of <1 μm in diameter [40]. Therefore, competition is unlikely to explain the reduction of DHA in oysters, because most dinoflagellates are larger than 1 μm in diameter.

For macroalgae, allelopathy could be a possible mechanism for the reduction of DHA in oysters. Brown algae and *Ulva* spp., which were dominant macroalgae in our oyster aquaculture, have been demonstrated to significantly reduce the growth of dinoflagellates through allelopathy [41,42]. This hypothesis could explain the reduction of DHA in oysters if we assume that the allelopathy was more effective for dinoflagellates. In fact, species-specific allelopathy effects have been demonstrated, including *Ulva* and dinoflagellates [43]. However, further research is needed to clarify the mechanisms behind the DHA reduction in *C. gigas* when sponges and macroalgae act as fouling organisms.

A mixture of sponges and macroalgae also seem to have reduced the amount of EPA and DHA in *C. gigas* clusters. Since a negative relationship between the total weight of *C. gigas* in a cluster and the relative weight of the sponge and macroalgal mixture was detected, the observed reduction of EPA and DHA in the oyster clusters can be explained by the reduction of the total biomass of the oysters, as the relative weight of the sponges and macroalgae increased.

M. galloprovincialis seem to have decreased the EPA content and CI of *C. gigas*. Although *C. gigas* can biosynthesise EPA from its precursors, its conversion efficiency is not enough to meet its requirement, and the EPA content in *C. gigas* mainly represents dietary EPA [35]. Thus, the amount of EPA in *C. gigas* seemed to depend mainly on their dietary intake, rather than on their own biosynthesis. Although EPA is abundant in diatoms, Cryptophyceae, and Rhodophyceae [36], the main EPA source for the assessed *C. gigas* was diatoms, because diatoms were dominant near our study sites (Sakamaki, unpublished data, Table S1). Furthermore, the observed significant positive relationship between EPA and 16:1n7/16:0 in oysters (Figure 5), which have been used as diatom markers, indicated that the main origin of EPA in the oysters were diatoms [44]. Pernet et al. [45] reported high bivalve growth rates during diatom bloom periods, and a feeding experiment by Piveteau et al. [46] also demonstrated an increase in the condition index of *C. gigas* when feeding on diatoms. In addition, a positive relationship was found between the EPA content and growth of a mussel species, *M. edulis* [47]. This was further demonstrated by the significant positive relationships between CI and EPA content in both bivalve species in our study. These findings support the idea that diatoms are a high-quality dietary source for both *C. gigas* and *M. galloprovincialis* and also indicate that there is probably a high competition potential for diatoms between *C. gigas* and *M. galloprovincialis*. Therefore, the condition index of *C. gigas* can be reduced as a result of competition with *M. galloprovincialis* for diatoms, with a consequent reduction of EPA acquisition.

Although these species have the potential to compete for diatoms, the CI of *M. galloprovincialis* was not negatively affected by the presence of *C. gigas*. This indicates that the dietary competition between *C. gigas* and *M. galloprovincialis* is not balanced. Although both *C. gigas* and *M. galloprovincialis* preferentially selected larger particles (>5 μm) in their diet, they did not necessarily need to compete, because *M. galloprovincialis* can also utilise smaller particles (<2 μm), which are not retained by *C. gigas* [48]. In fact, the invasion of *C. gigas* did not negatively affect local populations of the mussels *M. edulis* in Limfjord,

Denmark, even though *C. gigas* were considered to have a competitive advantage owing to their higher filtration rate [49]. Contrary to this, our results clearly demonstrated that *M. galloprovincialis* has an advantage in dietary competition over *C. gigas*. There are two possible reasons for this. First, more than 97% of the EPA was distributed in particles of >2 μm near farm A in Shizugawa Bay [50], and dietary segregation by utilising small particles (<2 μm) by *M. galloprovincialis* was not valid in our study fields. The second reason was the vertical distribution of *C. gigas* and *M. galloprovincialis* in the cluster. *M. galloprovincialis* develops on the shells of *C. gigas* in Shizugawa Bay since oyster spats are artificially settled on the surface of scallop shells and grow before the scallop shells are put in the bay. As *M. galloprovincialis* settles on the surfaces of *C. gigas* shells, *M. galloprovincialis* has a spatial advantage in terms of feeding on diatoms before *C. gigas*. A portion of the diatoms ingested by the bivalves can survive [51], indicating that the faecal material of *M. galloprovincialis*, including diatoms, may supply the *C. gigas*, which are located inside the cluster. However, faecal material generally contains less EPA than suspended matter [50]. Therefore, *M. galloprovincialis* fouling on *C. gigas* could have substantial negative effects on the *C. gigas* in oyster aquaculture farms, in terms of EPA acquisition.

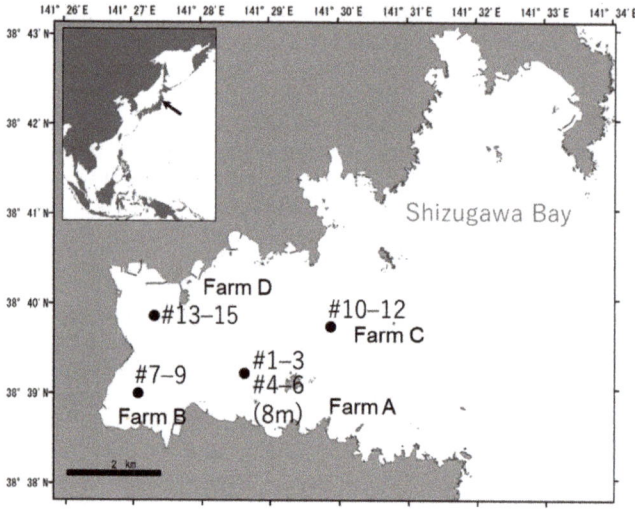

Figure 5. The location of sampling points in Shizugawa Bay, Japan.

Although our data indicated that fouling organisms possibly reduce the EPA and DHA content of *C. gigas*, it should be noted that other environmental factors can also affect the EPA and DHA content of *C. gigas*. For instance, water temperature [52] and the reproductive cycle [53] are known to affect fatty acid profiles of oysters. In addition, the total amount and quality of supplied food sources, especially diatoms and dinoflagellate, may influence the EPA and DHA content in *C. gigas*. In this study, *C. gigas* were all collected with two-year-old oysters with similar sizes on the same day, which indicates that the effects of water temperature and the reproductive cycle can be assumed to not produce the difference of EPA and DHA content. Unfortunately, as we did not investigate the supplied food at each sampling point, further study is required to understand the effect of food availability. Furthermore, the fatty acid content of oysters changes spatially and seasonally [54,55], and this could be associated with composition and the amounts of fouling organisms. Therefore, long-term monitoring in different sites is an effective way for the comprehensive understanding of the effects of fouling organisms on the EPA and DHA content in cultivated species.

Although EPA and DHA are essential fatty acids for humans [5,6], the effect of fouling organisms on the EPA and DHA content in cultivated host species has not been comprehensively evaluated before. Our findings demonstrated a reduction of EPA and DHA in the cultivated oyster *C. gigas* likely due to fouling organisms. This can devalue the quality of the oysters as an aquaculture product. Removing fouling mussels is empirically known to reduce their negative impact on oyster growth [25,27]. Our results support the idea that the current efforts to remove fouling mussels from oyster clusters in the study region [56], which include hot water treatment and physical removal, are expected to enhance the content of EPA and DHA in the oysters.

4. Materials and Methods

4.1. Study Site

This study was conducted in the inner part of Shizugawa bay, located on the northeast side of Honshu Island, Japan (38.65° N, 141.50° E; Figure 5). The area of the bay is 46.8 km^2, and the average and the maximum depth at the bay mouth is 30 and 54 m, respectively. In our observations in 2015, the annual range of seawater temperatures at a depth of 2 m was approximately 5–21 °C. The Pacific oyster *C. gigas* is one of the major aquaculture products in this bay, and longline oyster suspension facilities are distributed in the inner parts of the bay, in which the depth ranges from approximately 10–30 m. Oyster spats are artificially settled on scallop shells. Then, oyster clusters growing on scallop shells are tied at ~0.4 m intervals to ropes of approximately 8 to 10 m in length, and the ropes are vertically suspended from ~100 m longlines that are horizontally sustained by floating buoys. There are ~400 oyster farming longline facilities in the bay, which is based on the information provided by a local fishery cooperative.

4.2. Field Sampling

To assess the composition of the fouling organism communities, oyster clusters growing on scallop shells were collected from four oyster farms in the inner part of the bay in August 2014 (Figure 5). The seawater temperature at a depth of 2 m in farm A was 20–21 °C. At all sampling farms, two-year-old oysters were cultured (the oysters were hatched in summer 2012). One oyster cluster (Figure 6) was collected from ~2 m depth from each of the three ropes that were randomly selected at each farm. Since vertical distribution of fouling organisms are expected to be different [23], three clusters were collected from ~8 m depth at farm A. Thus, 15 oyster clusters were sampled in total. Immediately after sample collection, the oyster clusters, including oysters, mussels, sponges and algae, and others, were disassembled by hand and sorted into four groups. Because sponges and macroalgae were attached together tightly and intricately, these two groups could not be separated. Thus, sponges and macroalgae were treated as one group. The macroalgae were mainly composed of *Ulva* and brown algae. Each group of sessile fouling organisms was measured for abundance and wet biomass. For the wet weight measurement, the samples were carefully dried with paper towels to minimise errors and then weighed using an electronic scale. For the sampled oysters, all individuals were measured for length, width, shell height, and whole-body wet weight. The soft tissues were then obtained by dissection and measured for wet weight. The shells were weighed after air drying. For each sampled cluster, to remove the effect of individual size on the fatty acid analysis, tissue samples were selected from five individuals with similar shell lengths (103.3 ± 12.3 mm, mean ± SD) and preserved in a freezer at −30 °C for later fatty acid analysis. Similarly, for the *M. galloprovincialis* mussels, which were predominant among the sessile fouling organisms, five individuals were randomly selected from each cluster sample with similar shell lengths (46.8 ± 6.8 mm, mean ± SD), and the shell size, wet weight of the soft tissue, and dry weight of the shell were measured. The soft tissue samples of the mussels were preserved in a freezer for later fatty acid analysis.

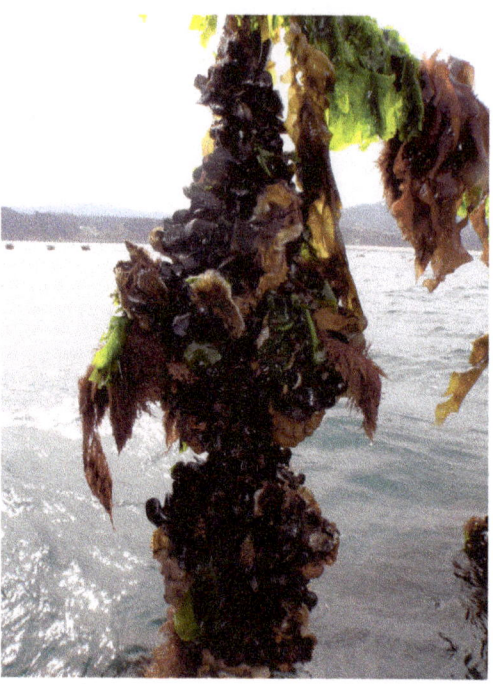

Figure 6. Two oyster clusters fouled by sponges, macroalgae, *M. galloprovincialis,* and other organisms. This photo was taken at farm B in February 2017.

4.3. Fatty Acid Analysis

Since the whole body of the oyster is eaten by humans, we evaluated the fatty acid contents of oysters from the whole body. First, the soft tissue samples of the oysters and mussels were freeze-dried. Then, the whole body was powdered and homogenised in a blender. The 'one-step method' described by Abdulkadir and Tsuchiya [57] was applied for lipid extraction and derivatisation from the freeze-dried samples. Approximately 100 mg of freeze-dried sample was moved to a 50 mL glass tube. One millilitre of internal standard (1 mg tricosanoic acid per ml hexane), 4 mL hexane, and 2 mL 14% boron trifluoride methanol were added to the test tube, and nitrogen gas was added to fill the head space. The glass tubes were heated at 100 °C in a water bath for 2 h, then cooled to room temperature, and 1 mL hexane and 2 mL ultrapure water were added. The samples were shaken vigorously and centrifuged for 3 min at 2500 rpm (M-4000, KUBOTA Corp., Tokyo, Japan). The upper layer of hexane, which contained fatty acid methyl esters (FAME), was then placed in a 1.5 mL GC vial.

For quantification of the fatty acids, 1 µL FAME solution was injected into a gas chromatograph with an FID detector (GC-2014, Shimadzu, Kyoto, Japan) equipped with a capillary column (Select FAME, 100 m × 0.25 mm i.d., Agilent Technologies, Tokyo, Japan). The analytical conditions followed those outlined by Fujibayashi et al. [58]. The peak of each fatty acid was identified by comparison with the retention time of commercial standard mixtures (Supelco37, PUFA No.3, Bacterial FAME, Supelco®, Darmstadt, Germany). The amount of each fatty acid (milligram fatty acid per dry weight of animal) was calculated by following the method of Abdulkadir and Tsuchiya [57], with the internal standard (i.e., tricosanoic acid).

4.4. Data Analysis

We applied two condition indices (CI1 and CI2) in this study. CI1 and CI2 have been generally applied for oysters and other bivalve species, including mussels [24,59,60].

The oyster body condition index (CI1), which was developed by Lawrence and Scott [50], was calculated by

$$CI1 = (Dfw\ (g))/(Ww\ (g) - Shw\ (g)) \times 100$$

where Dfw is the dry weight of soft tissue, which was measured after freeze drying, Ww is the total wet weight of the shell and soft tissue without any fouling organisms, and Shw is the dried shell weight. CI1 expresses the ratio of the dry weight of soft tissue to the internal shell volume, with the assumption that the density of soft tissue is almost the same as that of seawater. This assumption has been validated in oysters [24]. However, there has been no attempt to verify this for *M. galloprovincialis*, and Lucas and Beninger [59] pointed out that it is unlikely that the underlying assumptions are applicable to all bivalves. Therefore, we considered CI2 more appropriate for *M. galloprovincialis* in this study.

For mussels, the following condition index was applied [60]:

$$CI2 = (Dfw\ (g))/(Shw\ (g))$$

To examine the effects of fouling organisms on the CI and content of EPA and DHA in the cultivated oysters, correlation analysis was conducted by SPSS software (IBM, ver.20). All data were explored for normality using a Kolmogorov–Smirnov test and normality was not supported for the wet weight and relative weight of *M. galloprovincialis*. Then, Spearman rank correlation analysis was applied for *M. galloprovincialis*, and Pearson's correlation analysis was applied for other fouling organisms. Fouling organisms were expressed as the total wet weight (g cluster^{-1}). Furthermore, relative weight to oysters (g g^{-1}) was also calculated since relative weight of fouling organisms can be expected to affect *C. gigas*. For the content of EPA and DHA, the concentration in each individual (mg g^{-1}) and total amount in a cluster (g cluster^{-1}) were evaluated and applied in the correlation analysis.

Supplementary Materials: The following are available online at https://www.mdpi.com/article/10.3390/md19070369/s1, Table S1: Composition of phytoplankton taxa collected near farm A in July 2017 (cell L^{-1}).

Author Contributions: Conceptualisation, M.F., O.N. and T.S.; methodology, M.F. and T.S.; investigation, M.F. and T.S.; chemical analysis, M.F. and T.S.; writing—original draft preparation, M.F. and T.S.; writing—review and editing, M.F., O.N. and T.S.; visualisation, M.F.; supervision, O.N.; project administration, O.N.; funding acquisition, O.N. All authors have read and agreed to the published version of the manuscript.

Funding: This work was financially supported by the Environment Research and Technology Development Fund of the Ministry of the Environment, Japan (grant number S-13), the Japanese Institute of Fisheries Infrastructure and Communities, and KAKENHI (grant number JP17H01885, 19KT0006).

Institutional Review Board Statement: Not applicable.

Informed Consent Statement: Not applicable.

Data Availability Statement: The data are included in the manuscript.

Acknowledgments: We thank K. Goto, T. Kudo, N. Chiba, A. Kato, C. Maruo, H. Kanzaki, and Y. Zheng for assistance with the field and laboratory work. We thank R. Filgueira for their valuable comments on the manuscript.

Conflicts of Interest: The authors declare no conflict of interest.

References

1. Shumway, S.E. *Shellfish Aquaculture and the Environment*; Wiley-Blackwell: Oxford, UK, 2011.
2. FAO. *The State of World Fisheries and Aquaculture 2018 Meeting the Sustainable Development Goals*; FAO: Rome, Italy, 2018.
3. Gibbs, M.T. Sustainability performance indicators for suspended bivalve aquaculture activities. *Ecol. Indic.* **2007**, *7*, 94–107. [CrossRef]

4. Tan, K.; Ma, H.; Li, S. Bivalves as future source of sustainable natural omega-3 polyunsaturated fatty acids. *Food Chem.* **2020**, *311*, 125907. [CrossRef] [PubMed]
5. Simopoulos, A.P. Omega-3 fatty acids in health and disease and in growth and development. *Am. J. Clin. Nutr.* **1991**, *54*, 438–463. [CrossRef] [PubMed]
6. Swanson, D.; Block, R.; Mousa, S.A. Omega-3 fatty acids EPA and DHA: Health benefits throughout life. *Adv. Nutr.* **2012**, *3*, 1–7. [CrossRef]
7. Arts, M.T.; Ackman, R.G.; Holub, B.J. "Essential fatty acids" in aquatic ecosystems: A crucial link between diet and human health and evolution. *Can. J. Fish. Aquat. Sci.* **2001**, *58*, 122–137. [CrossRef]
8. Harwood, J.L. Algae: Critical sources of very long-chain polyunsaturated fatty acids. *Biomolecules* **2019**, *9*, 708. [CrossRef]
9. Salem, N., Jr.; Eggersdorfer, M. Is the world supply of omega-3 fatty acids adequate for optimal human nutrition? *Curr. Opin. Clin. Nutr. Metab. Care* **2015**, *18*, 147–154. [CrossRef]
10. Adams, C.M.; Shumway, S.E.; Whitlatch, R.B.; Getchis, T. Biofouling in marine molluscan shellfish aquaculture: A survey assessing the business and economic implications of mitigation. *J. World Aquac. Soc.* **2011**, *42*, 242–252. [CrossRef]
11. Fitridge, I.; Dempster, T.; Guenther, J.; de Nys, R. The impact and control of biofouling in marine aquaculture: A review. *Biofouling* **2012**, *28*, 649–669. [CrossRef]
12. Lodeiros, C.J.; Himmelman, J.H. Influence of fouling on the growth and survival of the tropical scallop, *Euvola* (Pecten) *ziczac* (L. 1758) in suspended culture. *Aquac. Res.* **1996**, *27*, 749–756. [CrossRef]
13. Taylor, J.J.; Southgate, P.C.; Rose, R.A. Fouling animals and their effect on the growth of silver-lip pearl oysters, *Pinctada maxima* (Jameson) in suspended culture. *Aquaculture* **1997**, *153*, 31–40. [CrossRef]
14. Kripa, V.; Mohamed, K.S.; Velayudhan, T.S. Seasonal fouling stress on the farmed pearl oyster, *Pinctada fucata*, from southeastern Arabian Sea. *J. World Aquac. Soc.* **2012**, *43*, 514–525. [CrossRef]
15. Claereboudt, M.; Bureau, D.; Côté, J.; Himmelman, J.H. Fouling development and its effect on the growth of juvenile giant scallops (*Placopecten magellanicus*) in suspended culture. *Aquaculture* **1994**, *121*, 327–342. [CrossRef]
16. Lodeiros, C.J.M.; Himmelman, J.H. Identification of environmental factors affecting growth and survival of the tropical scallop *Euvola* (Pecten) *ziczac* in suspended culture in the Golfo de Cariaco, Venezuela. *Aquaculture* **2000**, *182*, 91–114. [CrossRef]
17. Filgueira, R.; Grant, J. A Box Model for ecosystem-level management of mussel culture carrying capacity in a coastal bay. *Ecosystems* **2009**, *12*, 1222–1233. [CrossRef]
18. Filgueira, R.; Guyondet, T.; Comeau, L.A.; Grant, J. A fully-spatial ecosystem-DEB model of oyster (*Crassostrea virginica*) carrying capacity in the Richibucto Estuary, Eastern Canada. *J. Mar. Syst.* **2014**, *136*, 42–54. [CrossRef]
19. Daigle, R.M.; Herbinger, C.M. Ecological interactions between the vase tunicate (*Ciona intestinalis*) and the farmed blue mussel (*Mytilus edulis*) in Nova Scotia, Canada. *Aquat. Invasions* **2009**, *4*, 177–187. [CrossRef]
20. Qi, H.; Song, K.; Li, C.; Wang, W.; Li, B.; Li, L.; Zhang, G. Construction and evaluation of a high-density SNP array for the Pacific oyster (*Crassostrea gigas*). *PLoS ONE* **2017**, *12*, e0174007. [CrossRef]
21. Alagarswami, K.; Chellam, A. On fouling and boring organisms and mortality of pearl oysters in the farm at Veppalodai, Gulf of Mannar. *Indian J. Fish.* **1976**, *23*, 10–22.
22. Rodriguez, L.F.; Ibarra-Obando, S.E. Cover and colonization of commercial oyster (*Crassostrea gigas*) shells by fouling organisms in San Quintin Bay, Mexico. *J. Shellfish Res.* **2008**, *27*, 337–343. [CrossRef]
23. Arakawa, K.Y. Competitors and fouling organisms in the hanging culture of the Pacific oyster, *Crassostrea gigas* (Thunberg). *Mar. Behav. Physiol.* **1990**, *17*, 67–94. [CrossRef]
24. Lawrence, D.R.; Scott, G.I. The determination and use of condition index of oysters. *Estuaries* **1982**, *5*, 23–27. [CrossRef]
25. Sato, S.; Takeda, T. Studies on the organisms attaching to raft cultured oysters. I. On the extermination of the mussels (*Mytilus edulis* L.). *Bull. Tohoku Reg. Fish. Res. Lab.* **1952**, *1*, 63–67.
26. Fuzita, S.; Fujita, T.; Ito, M. On mussels, *Mytilus edulis*, attached to the oyster rafts in Miyako Bay-II. *Aquac. Sci.* **1996**, *14*, 47–50. (In Japanese)
27. Sato, H. Elimination of purple sea mussel in oyster cultivation. *Bull. Fukuoka Fish. Mar. Technol. Res. Cent.* **1999**, *9*, 57–60. (In Japanese)
28. Mazouni, N.; Gaertner, J.C.; Deslous-Paoli, J.M. Composition of biofouling communities on suspended oyster cultures: An in situ study of their interactions with the water column. *Mar. Ecol. Prog. Ser.* **2001**, *214*, 93–102. [CrossRef]
29. Royer, J.; Ropert, M.; Mathieu, M.; Costil, K. Presence of spionid worms and other epibionts in Pacific oysters (*Crassostrea gigas*) cultured in Normandy, France. *Aquaculture* **2006**, *253*, 461–474. [CrossRef]
30. Lacoste, E.; Gaertner-Mazouni, N. Biofouling impact on production and ecosystem functioning: A review for bivalve aquaculture. *Rev. Aquac.* **2015**, *7*, 187–196. [CrossRef]
31. De Nys, R.; Ison, O. Biofouling. In *The Pearl Oyster*; Southgate, P., Lucas, J., Eds.; Elsevier: Oxford, UK, 2008.
32. Watts, J.C.; Carroll, J.M.; Munroe, D.M.; Finelli, C.M. Examination of the potential relationship between boring sponges and pea crabs and their effects on eastern oyster condition. *Dis. Aquat. Org.* **2018**, *130*, 25–36. [CrossRef] [PubMed]
33. Sala, A.; Lucchetti, A. Low-cost tool to reduce biofouling in oyster longline culture. *Aquac. Eng.* **2008**, *39*, 53–58. [CrossRef]
34. Pennarun, A.L.; Prost, C.; Haure, J.; Demaimay, M. Comparison of two microalgal diets. 1. Influence on the biochemical and fatty acid compositions of raw oysters (*Crassostrea gigas*). *J. Agric. Food Chem.* **2003**, *51*, 2006–2010. [CrossRef] [PubMed]

35. Da Costa, F.; Robert, R.; Quéré, C.; Wikfors, G.H.; Soudant, P. Essential fatty acid assimilation and synthesis in larvae of the bivalve *Crassostrea gigas*. *Lipids* **2005**, *50*, 503–511. [CrossRef] [PubMed]
36. Cobelas, M.A.; Lechado, J.Z. Lipids in microalgae. A review 1. Biochemistry. *Grasas Aceites* **1989**, *40*, 118–145.
37. Mitani, E.; Nakayama, F.; Matsuwaki, I.; Ichi, I.; Kawabata, A.; Kawachi, M.; Kato, M. Fatty acid composition profiles of 235 strains of three microalgal divisions within the NIES Microbial Culture Collection. *Microb. Resour. Syst.* **2017**, *33*, 19–29.
38. Gili, J.M.; Coma, R. Benthic suspension feeders: Their paramount role in littoral marine food webs. *Trends Ecol. Evol.* **1998**, *13*, 316–321. [CrossRef]
39. Coma, R.; Ribes, M.; Gili, J.M.; Hughes, R.N. The ultimate opportunists: Consumers of seston. *Mar. Ecol. Prog. Ser.* **2001**, *219*, 305–308. [CrossRef]
40. Stuart, V.; Klumpp, D.W. Evidence for food-resources partitioning by kelpbed filter feeders. *Mar. Ecol. Prog. Ser.* **1984**, *16*, 27–37. [CrossRef]
41. Accoroni, S.; Percopo, I.; Cerino, F.; Romagnoli, T.; Pichierri, S.; Perrone, C.; Totti, C. Allelopathic interactions between the HAB dinoflagellate *Ostreopsis* cf. *ovata* and macroalgae. *Harmful Algae* **2015**, *49*, 149–155.
42. Gharbia, H.B.; Yahia, O.K.D.; Cecchi, P.; Masseret, E.; Amzil, Z.; Herve, F.; Rovillon, G.; Nouri, H.; M'Rabet, C.; Couet, D.; et al. New insights on the species-specific allelopathic interactions between macrophytes and marine HAB dinoflagellates. *PLoS ONE* **2017**, *12*, e0187963. [CrossRef]
43. Sun, Y.Y.; Zhou, W.J.; Wang, H.; Guo, G.L.; Su, Z.X.; Pu, Y.F. Antialgal compounds with antialgal activity against the common red tide microalgae from a green algae *Ulva pertusa*. *Ecotoxicol. Environ. Saf.* **2018**, *157*, 61–66. [CrossRef]
44. Fujibayashi, M.; Nishimura, O.; Tanaka, H. Evaluation of Food Sources Assimilated by Unionid Mussels Using Fatty Acid Trophic Markers in Japanese Freshwater Ecosystems. *J. Shellfish Res.* **2016**, *35*, 231–235. [CrossRef]
45. Pernet, F.; Malet, N.; Pastoureaud, A.; Vaquer, A.; Quéré, C.; Dubroca, L. Marine diatoms sustain growth of bivalves in a Mediterranean lagoon. *J. Sea Res.* **2012**, *68*, 20–32. [CrossRef]
46. Piveteau, F.; Gandemer, G.; Baud, J.P.; Demaimay, M. Changes in lipid and fatty acid compositions of European oysters fattened with *Skeletonema costatum* diatom for six weeks in ponds. *Aquac. Int.* **1999**, *7*, 341–355. [CrossRef]
47. Alkanani, T.; Parrish, C.C.; Thompson, R.J.; McKenzie, C.H. Role of fatty acids in cultured mussels, *Mytilus edulis*, grown in Notre Dame Bay, Newfoundland. *J. Exp. Mar. Biol. Ecol.* **2007**, *348*, 33–45. [CrossRef]
48. Rahman, M.A.; Henderson, S.; Miller-Ezzy, P.A.; Li, X.X.; Qin, J.G. Analysis of the seasonal impact of three marine bivalves on seston particles in water column. *J. Exp. Mar. Biol. Ecol.* **2020**, *522*, 151251. [CrossRef]
49. Holm, M.W.; Davids, J.K.; Dolmer, P.; Holmes, E.; Nielsen, T.T.; Vismann, B.; Hansen, B.W. Coexistence of Pacific oyster *Crassostrea gigas* (Thunberg, 1793) and blue mussels *Mytilus edulis* Linnaeus, 1758 on a sheltered intertidal bivalve bed? *Aquat. Invasions* **2016**, *11*, 155–165. [CrossRef]
50. Sakamaki, T.; Hayashi, K.; Zheng, Y.; Fujibayashi, M.; Nishimura, O. Effects of oyster age on the selective filter-feeding and chemical composition of biodeposits: Insights from fatty acid analysis. *Mar. Ecol. Prog. Ser.* **2020**, *644*, 75–89. [CrossRef]
51. Barillé, L.; Cognie, B. Revival capacity of diatoms in bivalve pseudofaeces and faeces. *Diatom Res.* **2000**, *15*, 11–17. [CrossRef]
52. Flores-Vergara, C.; Cordero-Esquivel, B.; Cerón-Ortiz, A.N.; Arredondo-Vega, B.O. Combined effects of temperature and diet on growth and biochemical composition of the Pacific oyster *Crassostrea gigas* (Thunberg) spat. *Aquac. Res.* **2004**, *35*, 172–183. [CrossRef]
53. Hurtado, M.A.; Racotta, I.S.; Arcos, F.; Morales-Bojórquez, E.; Moal, J.; Soudant, P.; Palacios, E. Seasonal variations of biochemical, pigment, fatty acid, and sterol compositions in female *Crassostrea corteziensis* oysters in relation to the reproductive cycle. *Comp. Biochem. Physiol. B* **2012**, *163*, 172–183. [CrossRef]
54. Isono, C.; Maruta, H.; Ma, Y.; Ganeko, N.; Miyake, T.; Yamashita, H. Seasonal variations in major components of *Crassostrea gigas* from Seto Inland Sea. *Fish. Sci.* **2020**, *86*, 1087–1099. [CrossRef]
55. Dagorn, F.; Couzinet-Mossion, A.; Kendel, M.; Beninger, P.G.; Rabesaotra, V.; Barnathan, G.; Wielgosz-Collin, G. Exploitable lipids and fatty acids in the invasive oyster *Crassostrea gigas* on the French Atlantic coast. *Mar. Drugs* **2016**, *14*, 104. [CrossRef]
56. Hatakeyama, Y.; Kawahata, T.; Fujibayashi, M.; Nishimura, O.; Sakamaki, T. Sources and oxygen consumption of particulate organic matter settling in oyster aquaculture farms: Insights from analysis of fatty acid composition. *Estuar. Coast. Shelf Sci.* **2021**, *254*, 107328. [CrossRef]
57. Abdulkadir, S.; Tsuchiya, T. One-step method for quantitative and qualitative analysis of fatty acids in marine animal samples. *J. Exp. Mar. Biol. Ecol.* **2008**, *354*, 1–8. [CrossRef]
58. Fujibayashi, M.; Ogino, M.; Nishimura, O. Fractionation of the stable carbon isotope ratio of essential fatty acids in zebrafish *Danio rerio* and mud snails *Bellamya chinensis*. *Oecologia* **2016**, *180*, 589–600. [CrossRef]
59. Lucas, A.; Beninger, P.G. The use of physiological condition indices in marine bivalve aquaculture. *Aquaculture* **1985**, *44*, 187–200. [CrossRef]
60. Orban, E.; Di Lena, G.; Nevigato, T.; Casini, I.; Marzetti, A.; Caproni, R. Seasonal changes in meat content, condition index and chemical composition of mussels (*Mytilus galloprovincialis*) cultured in two different Italian sites. *Food Chem.* **2002**, *77*, 57–65. [CrossRef]

Article

Fish Oil Increases Diet-Induced Thermogenesis in Mice

Tomomi Yamazaki [1,*], Dongyang Li [1,2] and Reina Ikaga [1]

1. Department of Nutrition and Metabolism, National Institute of Health and Nutrition, National Institutes of Biomedical Innovation, Health and Nutrition, 1-23-1 Toyama, Shinjuku-ku, Tokyo 162-8636, Japan; g1670612@edu.cc.ocha.ac.jp (D.L.); reina017@nibiohn.go.jp (R.I.)
2. The Graduate School of Humanities and Sciences, Ochanomizu University, 2-1-1 Otsuka, Bunkyo-ku, Tokyo 112-8610, Japan
* Correspondence: tomo0322@nibiohn.go.jp; Tel.: +81-3-3203-5725

Abstract: Increasing energy expenditure (EE) is beneficial for preventing obesity. Diet-induced thermogenesis (DIT) is one of the components of total EE. Therefore, increasing DIT is effective against obesity. We examined how much fish oil (FO) increased DIT by measuring absolute values of DIT in mice. C57BL/6J male mice were given diets of 30 energy% fat consisting of FO or safflower oil plus butter as control oil (Con). After administration for 9 days, respiration in mice was monitored, and then the data were used to calculate DIT and EE. DIT increased significantly by 1.2-fold in the FO-fed mice compared with the Con-fed mice. Body weight gain was significantly lower in the FO-fed mice. FO increased the levels of uncoupling protein 1 (*Ucp1*) mRNA and UCP1 protein in brown adipose tissue (BAT) by 1.5- and 1.2-fold, respectively. In subcutaneous white adipose tissue (subWAT), the levels of *Ucp1* mRNA and UCP1 protein were increased by 6.3- and 2.7-fold, respectively, by FO administration. FO also significantly increased the expression of markers of browning in subWAT such as fibroblast growth factor 21 and cell death-inducing DNA fragmentation factor α-like effector a. Thus, dietary FO seems to increase DIT in mice via the increased expressions of *Ucp1* in BAT and induced browning of subWAT. FO might be a promising dietary fat in the prevention of obesity by upregulation of energy metabolism.

Keywords: brown adipose tissue; browning; energy expenditure; n-3 fatty acid; uncoupling protein; white adipose tissue

1. Introduction

Obesity results when energy intake continuously exceeds energy expenditure (EE). Total daily energy expenditure (TEE) is comprised of multiple components such as basal metabolic rate, diet-induced thermogenesis (DIT) and physical activity-related EE [1]. DIT is defined as an increase in EE above that of the fasting state and is related to digestion, intestinal absorption of nutrients and storage of these nutrients [2]. One of the methods to prevent overweight and obesity is to increase energy consumption by upregulation of DIT [3].

Brown adipose tissue (BAT) is the main site for the induction of DIT and cold-induced thermogenesis, which significantly contributes to controlling body temperature and EE [4]. Although BAT is considered to be abundant in small rodents and human infants and decreases with aging in human [5], recent studies showed that functional BAT was identified in adult human [6,7]. The thermogenic ability of BAT is principally dependent on uncoupling protein 1 (UCP1) [8,9]. UCP1 facilitates uncoupling of mitochondrial substrate oxidation from ATP production, which leads to energy release as heat from free fatty acid oxidation [4].

UCP1-ablated mice consumed less oxygen than wild-type mice during the eating period, that is, DIT was UCP1-dependent [10]. UCP1-deficient mice maintained in a room at 23 °C developed obesity with age; therefore, UCP1 may play an important role against obesity [11]. UCP1 gene polymorphism (−3826 A/G) showed lowered capacity of thermic effect in response to dietary intake in healthy boys aged 8–11 years [12]. Thus, the function of UCP1 and activity promoting the activation of BAT greatly contribute to the increase of DIT.

BAT is strongly activated by exposure to cold and by pharmacological effects, such as that of β3-adrenergic receptor agonist [6,13,14]. Moreover, it has been reported that BAT is activated by food ingredients such as capsinoids, thereby contributing to a reduction in body fat [15,16]. Fish oil (FO) also has anti-obesity effects in humans [17–19]. FO contains a high content of n-3 polyunsaturated fatty acids, eicosapentaenoic acid (EPA) and docosahexaenoic acid (DHA), which must be obtained from the diet or synthesized from alpha-linolenic acid in the body [20–22]. DHA and EPA bind to peroxisome proliferator-activated receptor (PPAR) α and thereby activate PPARα [23,24], which is highly expressed in BAT [25]. PPARα binds to the PPAR response element of the *Ucp1* gene to increase mRNA expression of *Ucp1* [26].

Recently, beige adipose tissue, which is produced by the browning of white adipose tissue (WAT), has been reported as a third type of adipose tissue in addition to WAT and BAT [27–29]. Beige adipocytes are strongly induced by some environmental conditions and external cues such as exposure to cold and some pharmacological treatments, and they have potent thermogenic ability similar to that of classical brown adipocytes [30]. FO treatment leads to the browning of WAT, increases thermogenic genes such as *Ucp1* [31–33], stimulates thermogenesis, as measured by rectal temperature [34,35], and increases EE without changes in food intake [36]. These studies only suggest the possibility that FO influences DIT, however, and how much FO actually increases DIT is still unknown.

We recently developed a new technique to measure absolute DIT values in mice by applying a methodology used in the measurement of DIT in human to mice using a respiratory chamber [37]. In the present study, we showed how much FO increased DIT through activation of BAT and browning of WAT. An increase in DIT may have potential impact on anti-obesity and therapy for diabetes [6,7,38], and the evidence shown in this study indicates that FO might be a promising dietary fat.

2. Results
2.1. Effects of Fish Oil Supplementation on DIT, EE, Activity and RER

Energy metabolism of mice was measured after 9 days of feeding of each experimental diet. The measurements of O_2 consumption, CO_2 production and activity (defined as the count per minute of any movement made by mouse) of the mice were carried out over a 22-h period. The DIT of the control fat (Con)-fed mice began to increase as soon as they started eating, was maintained at a high level during the dark period, and then decreased toward the end of the dark period (Figure 1a). However, DIT increased again after the start of the light period. Similar changes were observed in the FO-fed mice (Figure 1a). When comparing the DIT in the Con- and FO-fed mice every hour, DIT in the FO-fed mice was significantly higher at 0000 and 0300. EE in the dark period and light period was not different in the Con- and FO-fed mice (Dark: Con, 7615 ± 76 cal/h/kg$^{0.75}$; FO, 7582 ± 87 cal/h/kg$^{0.75}$; Light: Con, 6712 ± 83 cal/h/kg$^{0.75}$; FO, 6641 ± 92 cal/h/kg$^{0.75}$). However, DIT in the dark period was higher in the FO-fed mice than that in the Con-fed mice (Dark: Con, 1275 ± 22 cal/h/kg$^{0.75}$; FO, 1541 ± 32 cal/h/kg$^{0.75}$, $p < 0.01$; Light: Con, 1509 ± 47 cal/h/kg$^{0.75}$; FO, 1674 ± 46 cal/h/kg$^{0.75}$). There was no difference in activity every hour between the two groups (Figure 1b). Activity in the dark period and light period was not different in the Con- and FO-fed mice (Dark: Con, 238.2 ± 13.2 count/min; FO, 221.2 ± 23.4 count/min; Light: Con, 95.4 ± 5.8 count/min; FO, 96.5 ± 11.7 count/min). The respiratory exchange ratio (RER) in the FO-fed mice was higher at 0600 and 1300 than that in the Con-fed mice, but there was no significant difference at other times (Figure 1c). RER in the dark period and light period was not different in the Con- and FO-fed mice (Dark: Con, 0.881 ± 0.010; FO, 0.901 ± 0.006; Light: Con, 0.860 ± 0.005; FO, 0.893 ± 0.009). The total energy intake during DIT measurement was almost the same in the Con- and the FO-fed mice (Figure 2a). Total DIT over 22 h was calculated from the area under each curve. Total DIT in the FO-fed mice was 1.2-fold higher than that in the Con-fed mice (Figure 2b). TEE over 22 h was also calculated from the area under each curve. The values of activity and TEE between the two groups were not different (Figure 2c,d). DIT (%) versus calorie intake was calculated by dividing total DIT by total calorie intake and is indicated as $DIT_{/intake}$ in Figure 2e. $DIT_{/intake}$ was 11.2% for the FO-fed mice, which was 1.2-fold higher than that for the Con-fed mice. DIT (%) versus TEE was calculated by dividing total DIT by TEE and is indicated as $DIT_{/TEE}$ in Figure 2f. $DIT_{/TEE}$ for the FO-fed mice was 22.3%, which was also 1.2-fold higher than that for the Con-fed mice.

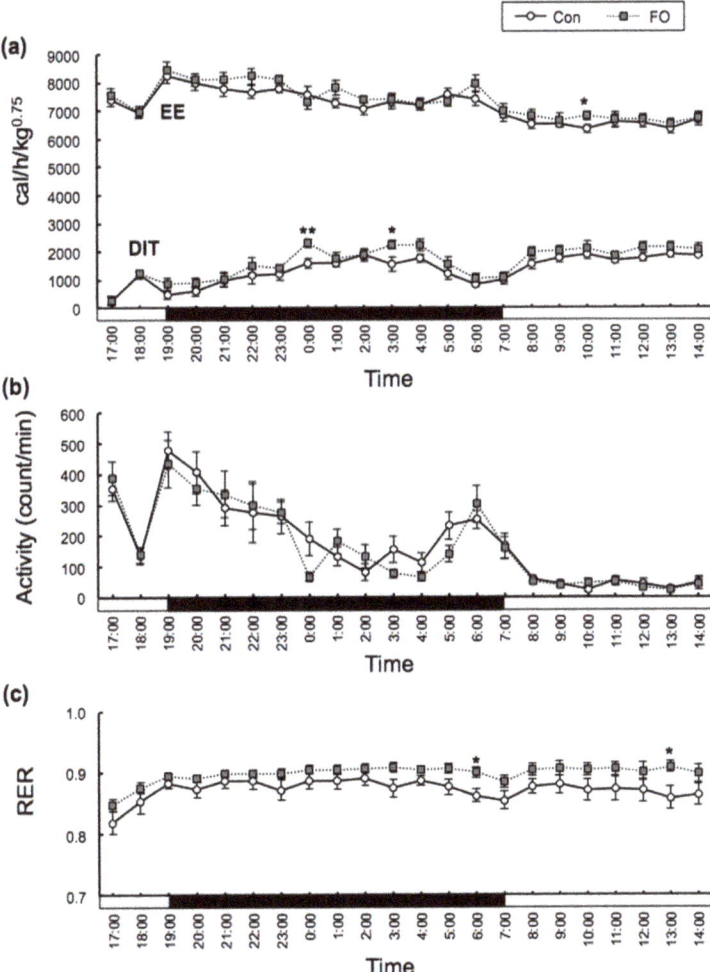

Figure 1. Time course of diet-induced thermogenesis (DIT), energy expenditure (EE), activity and respiratory exchange ratio (RER) in the control fat (Con)- and fish oil (FO)-fed male mice. The measurements were carried out over a 22-h period. The data of EE (upper lines), DIT (lower lines) (**a**), activity (**b**) and RER (**c**) are shown for every hour. White circles and gray squares represent data from the Con- and the FO-fed mice, respectively. The black and white bars on the x axis represent dark and light cycles, respectively. Values are mean ± SEM (n = 7). * $p < 0.05$, ** $p < 0.01$ vs. Con-fed mice. Significant differences between two groups were tested by Student *t*-test.

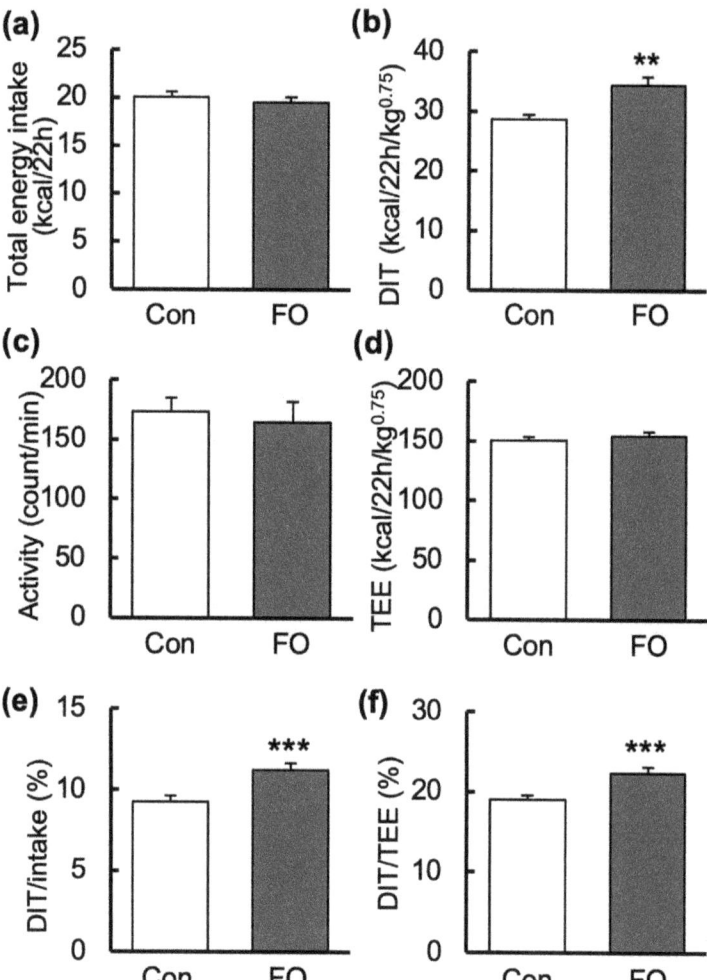

Figure 2. Values of total energy intake, diet-induced thermogenesis (DIT), activity and total energy expenditure (TEE) during DIT measurement in the control fat (Con)- and fish oil (FO)-fed male mice. Total energy intake (**a**) at measurement of energy metabolism was estimated by subtracting the food weight at the completion of measurement from the initial food weight measurement. The values of total DIT (**b**), activity (**c**) and TEE (**d**) were calculated from measurements taken over 22 h under the fed condition. DIT/intake (**e**) and DIT/TEE (**f**) were calculated by dividing total DIT by total calorie intake and by TEE, respectively. White and gray columns represent data from the Con- and FO-fed mice, respectively. Values are mean ± SEM (n = 7). ** $p < 0.01$, *** $p < 0.001$ vs. Con-fed mice. Significant differences between two groups were tested by Student *t*-test.

2.2. Body Weight and Tissue Weights of Con- and FO-Fed Mice

The mean energy intake was similar between the Con- and the FO-fed mice during the 10-day administration period (Con, 17.6 ± 0.8 kcal/day; FO, 17.7 ± 0.6 kcal/day, $p = 0.97$). Although final body weight (BW) was not different between the Con- and FO-fed mice, the BW gain in the FO-fed mice was significantly lower than that in the Con-fed mice during the 10-day period (Con, 10.3 ± 1.4%; FO, 6.6 ± 1.0%, $p < 0.05$). The weights of subcutaneous WAT (subWAT) in the FO-fed mice were not different from those in the

FO-fed mice (p = 0.07, Table 1). However, the weights of epididymal WAT and mesenteric WAT in the FO-fed mice were lower than those in the Con-fed mice. The weight of BAT was not affected by FO supplementation.

Table 1. BW and weights of tissues in Con- and FO-fed mice.

BW/Tissues	Con-Fed	FO-Fed
BW at start (g)	23.1 ± 0.4	23.1 ± 0.2
Final BW (g)	25.9 ± 0.5	25.2 ± 0.4
BAT (g)	0.087 ± 0.006	0.083 ± 0.007
Subcutaneous WAT(g)	0.329 ± 0.029	0.251 ± 0.026
Epididymal WAT (g)	0.462 ± 0.041	0.326 ± 0.018 *
Mesenteric WAT (g)	0.149 ± 0.024	0.081 ± 0.008 *
Liver (g)	1.19 ± 0.03	1.22 ± 0.04

Values are mean ± SEM (n = 7). * $p < 0.05$ vs. Con-fed mice. Significant differences between two groups were tested by Student t-test. BW: body weight; Con: control; FO: fish oil; BAT: brown adipose tissue; WAT: white adipose tissue.

2.3. Serum Chemicals of Con- and FO-Fed Mice

Because the weights of the epididymal WAT and mesenteric WAT in the FO-fed mice were lower than those in the Con-fed mice, we analyzed serum concentrations of glucose, non-esterified fatty acid (NEFA), triglyceride (TG) and total cholesterol (TC). The concentrations of serum glucose in the Con- and the FO-fed mice were the same (Table 2). However, the serum concentrations of NEFA, TG and TC in the FO-fed mice were significantly lower than those in the Con-fed mice (Table 2).

Table 2. Serum chemicals of Con- and FO-fed mice.

	Con-Fed	FO-Fed
Glucose (mg/dL)	169.6 ± 15.8	177.1 ± 11.4
NEFA (mEq/L)	0.83 ± 0.07	0.49 ± 0.06 **
TG (mg/dL)	179.9 ± 25.1	70.3 ± 16.4 **
TC (mg/dL)	179.0 ± 13.4	102.3 ± 3.7 ***

Values are mean ± SEM (n = 7). ** $p < 0.01$, *** $p < 0.001$ vs. Con-fed mice. Significant differences between two groups were tested by Student t-test. Con: control; FO: fish oil; NEFA: non-esterified fatty acid; TG: triglyceride; TC: total cholesterol.

2.4. Effects of FO Supplementation on BAT

To confirm the mechanism of increase of DIT in the FO-fed mice, we examined expression profiling of the *Ucp1* gene and UCP1 protein. FO supplementation resulted in a 1.5-fold increase in *Ucp1* mRNA in BAT (Figure 3a). UCP1 protein expression was also analyzed (n = 7 in each group), and representative data (n = 2 in each group) indicating a 1.2-fold increase in expression are shown in Figure 3b. The mRNA expression of *Pparα*, which is one of the nuclear transcription factors whose activation leads to increased fatty acid β-oxidation [39], was significantly increased by FO supplementation (Figure 3a). However, FO supplementation did not affect the mRNA expressions of target genes carnitine palmitoyltransferase I (*Cpt I*), acyl-CoA oxidase (*Aco*) and medium-chain acyl-CoA dehydrogenase (*Mcad*) (Figure 3a). Fibroblast growth factor 21 (*Fgf21*) expression was also not increased by FO administration (Figure 3a). The expression of the mitochondria biogenesis marker peroxisome proliferator-activated receptor gamma coactivator 1-alpha (PGC1α) and that of crucial thermogenesis biomarker type 2 iodothyronine deiodinase (Dio2) in the mice was not different between the two groups (Figure 3a). No difference in β3-adrenergic receptor (β3-AR) mRNA was observed in BAT (Con, 100.0 ± 7.0%; FO, 93.0 ± 11.4%).

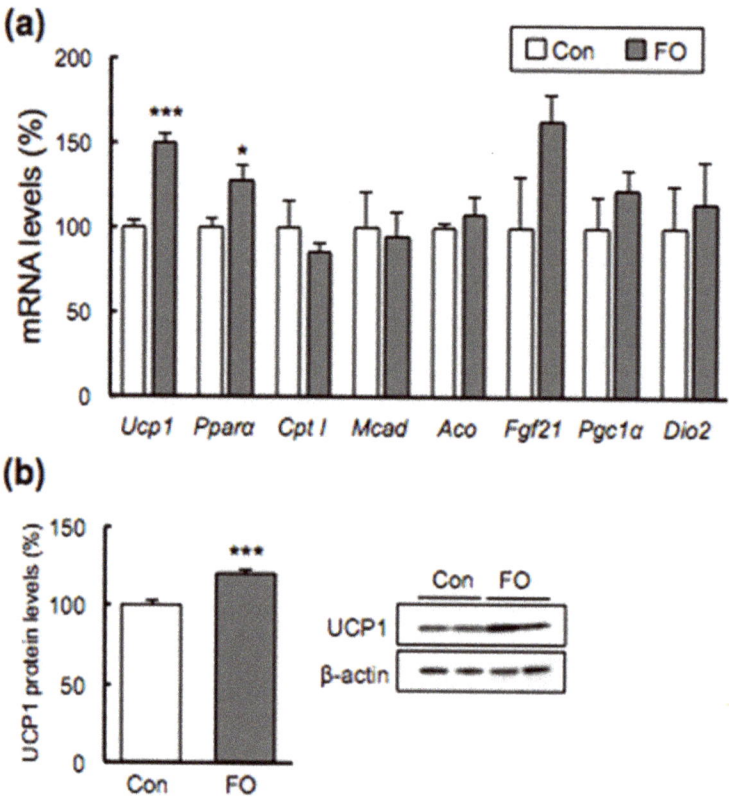

Figure 3. Effect of fish oil (FO) supplementation on gene expression and UCP1 protein levels in brown adipose tissue. mRNA levels of *Ucp1* and *Pparα* and its target genes (**a**) and UCP1 protein (**b**) were assessed by quantitative RT-PCR or western blotting. β-actin was used as the normalization control. The percent of mRNA and protein levels relative to those of Con-fed mice are indicated. White and gray columns represent data from the Con- and FO-fed mice, respectively. Values are mean ± SEM (n = 7). * $p < 0.05$, *** $p < 0.001$ vs. Con-fed mice. Significant differences between two groups were tested by Student *t*-test.

2.5. Effects of FO Supplementation on Gene Expression in subWAT

FO dramatically increased *Ucp1* mRNA expression by 6.3-fold in the subWAT (Figure 4a). UCP1 protein levels were also analyzed (n = 7 in each group), and representative data (n = 2 in each group) indicating a 2.7-fold increase compared with those in the Con-fed mice are shown in Figure 4b. FO supplementation also caused higher expressions of *Pparα* and its target genes of *Cpt I*, *Aco* and *Mcad* in comparison to those in the Con-fed mice (Figure 4a). Fgf21 expression in the FO-fed mice was also increased by 2.3-fold compared with that in the Con-fed mice (Figure 4a). β3-AR mRNA expression was higher in subWAT from the FO-fed mice than that in the Con-fed mice (Con, 100.0 ± 17.9%; FO, 246.1 ± 40.4%, $p < 0.001$).

Among the brown fat-selective genes, expression of cell death-inducing DNA fragmentation factor α-like effector a (Cidea) was significantly increased by 3.9-fold in the FO-fed mice compared with that in the Con-fed mice, whereas that of PR domain containing 16 (Prdm16) mRNA was not different (Figure 4a).

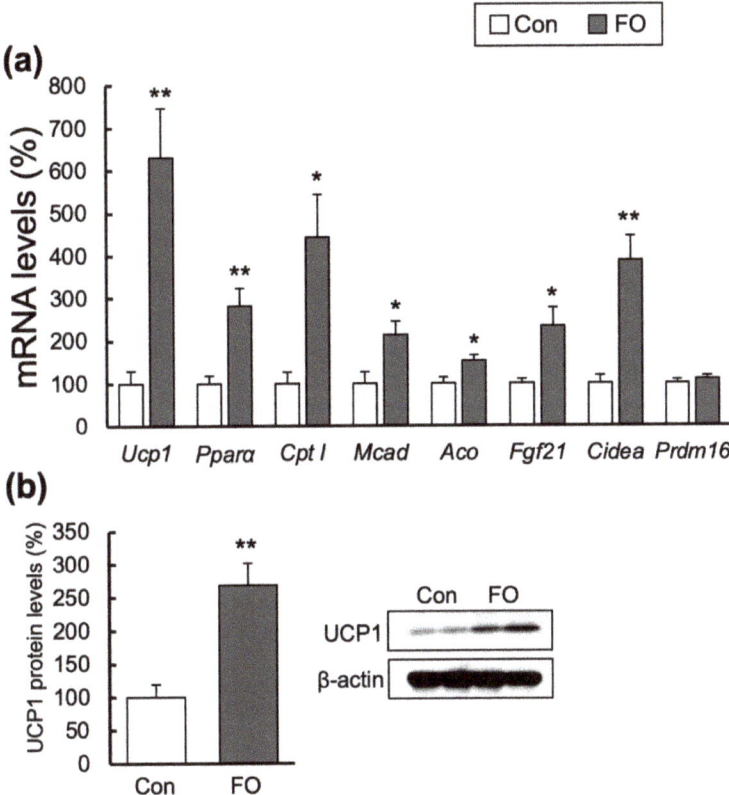

Figure 4. Effect of fish oil (FO) supplementation on gene expression and UCP1 protein levels in subcutaneous white adipose tissue. The mRNA levels of *Ucp1*, *Ppara* and its target genes and beige adipocyte-specific gene (**a**) and UCP1 protein (**b**) were assessed by quantitative RT-PCR or western blotting. β-actin was used as the normalization control. The percent of mRNA and protein levels relative to those of control fat (Con)-fed mice are indicated. White and gray columns represent data from the Con- and the FO-fed mice, respectively. Values are mean ± SEM (n = 7). * $p < 0.05$, ** $p < 0.01$ vs. Con-fed mice. Significant differences between two groups were tested by Student *t*-test.

2.6. Effects of FO Supplementation on Gene Expression in Liver

As the effects of supplementation could also be caused by increased metabolism in the liver, we analyzed gene expressions in the liver related to fatty acid β-oxidation and fatty acid synthesis. As shown in Table S1, fatty acid β-oxidation was induced the FO-fed mice, and fatty acid synthesis was decreased.

3. Discussion

We found that FO increased DIT in mice by 1.2-fold along with the activation of BAT caused by the increased expression of UCP1 and the browning of subWAT. As females are reported to produce less heat than males, we used male mice for our experiment [40]. We observed DIT in both the light period and dark period, although it was higher in the latter because mice eat principally in the dark period. Actually, the Con and FO groups of mice took about 70–80% and 20–30% of their total food intake in the dark and light periods, respectively. It appeared that maintenance of DIT in the light period was caused by feeding in the light period (Figure 1a).

In this study, FO increased the expression of the *Ucp1* gene in BAT by 1.5-fold. Other researchers also reported that FO administration both in vitro and in vivo induced the increased expression of *Ucp1* in BAT. *Ucp1* mRNA expression and UCP1 protein levels were both significantly increased in brown progenitor cells isolated from interscapular BAT supplemented with EPA [35]. EPA also increased mitochondrial content in a dose-dependent manner in HIB 1B brown adipose cells [41]. EPA administration to C57BL/6J mice for 11 weeks, and DHA-enriched FO (DHA 25%, EPA 8%) or EPA-enriched FO (DHA 12%, EPA 28%) administration to mice for 10 weeks, significantly increased UCP1 protein levels and *Ucp1* mRNA expression in BAT [34,42]. UCP1 activity in BAT was significantly increased in rats fed with EPA or a mixture of EPA and DHA for 4 weeks by GDP binding [43]. These reports support our results that UCP1 expression was significantly increased by FO administration in BAT (Figure 3a,b). The nuclear receptor PPARα regulates the expression of *Cpt I*, *Mcad* and *Aco*, which are involved in the fatty acid β-oxidation [41,44,45]. FO administration increased the expression of *Pparα* mRNA by 1.3-fold ($p < 0.05$), but expressions of its target genes *Cpt I*, *Mcad* and *Aco* were not affected in BAT, although that of the other Pparα target gene, *Ucp1*, increased (Figure 3a). Kim et al. reported that the expression of *Cpt I* mRNA in BAT of mice fed EPA-enriched FO increased significantly compared with that of control mice. In contrast, the expression of *Cpt I* mRNA did not increase in mice fed DHA-enriched FO, which has a similar fatty acid ratio as in the present study [34]. The reason why EPA-enriched FO could, but DHA-enriched FO could not, induce *Cpt I* expression in BAT is currently not clear. Further study will be required to reveal the mechanism.

FO also increased the expressions of the *Ucp1* gene and other genes related to the fatty acid β-oxidation in subWAT (Figure 4a). In terms of the marker of browning, *Cidea* mRNA was increased by 3.9-fold, but the expression of *Prdm16* was not increased (Figure 4a). FO enhances fatty acid oxidation through PPARα activation in WAT and causes browning of subWAT [34,46]. When cells derived from subcutaneous adipocytes from overweight females were treated with 200 μM EPA, expressions of *UCP1* and *CIDEA* mRNA increased significantly. The mRNA expression of *PRMD16* increased significantly with 100 μM EPA treatment but not with 200 μM EPA treatment [31]. When the stromal vascular cells isolated from subWAT of C57BL/6J mice were treated with 200 μM EPA during a differentiated process, the expressions of fatty acid β-oxidation-related genes *Ucp1, 2, 3* and *Cpt I*, and *Cidea*, increased significantly, but that of *Prdm16* was still not increased as in our results [32]. The reasons for FO causing different expressions of *Cidea* and *Prdm16* are currently unknown. Due to the increased expressions of *Ucp1* and *Cpt I* mRNA in FO-fed mice, the brown adipocyte-like phenotype was induced in subWAT [33]. The PPARα agonist is known to promote browning in subWAT [47,48] and increase the body temperature [48]. Contrary to these reports, UCP1 protein is reported to be very low or undetectable in subWAT even though mice were fed FO [42]. Our results supported the findings that FO administration markedly increased UCP1 expression in subWAT and induced subWAT browning. Beige adipocytes were shown to have potent thermogenic ability comparable to classical BAT [30], and the thermogenic density and total quantitative contribution in subWAT were maximally one-fifth and one-third of all BAT mitochondria, respectively [49]. Thus, the classical BAT depots would still be predominate in thermogenesis, but the browning of WAT would also contribute to thermogenesis. Sato et al. recently showed that phospholipase A2 group IID, which is expressed in M2-type macrophages in WAT, released n-3 fatty acid and increased energy expenditure and rectal temperature by facilitating subWAT browning, which ameliorated diet-induced obesity [50]. Thus, FO-caused browning of WAT might also contribute to inducing DIT.

FGF21 is reported to have an endocrinological role in BAT and WAT [51,52]. The expression of *Fgf21* mRNA in subWAT increased dramatically in mice after exposure to cold [52]. Moreover, the differentiated primary subWAT treated with β-agonist synthesized and secreted FGF21, suggesting that adipose FGF21 may act mainly in a paracrine/autocrine manner [52]. However, similar to the previous research concerning FO [34], the expression of *Fgf21* did not increase with FO administration in BAT (Figure 3a). However, contrary to that report, *Fgf21* expression in the present study was significantly increased by FO administration in subWAT (Figure 4a). This result leads us to the hypothesis that increased *Fgf21* of subWAT might induce the browning of WAT observed in the present study.

FO is reported to induce UCP1 expression in BAT and WAT via the sympathetic nervous system and transient receptor potential vanilloid 1 [34]. In the present study, β3-AR mRNA expression was higher in subWAT from the FO-fed mice than that in the Con-fed mice. However, no difference in β3-AR mRNA was observed in BAT. Although we did not determine the direct influence of fish oil on sympathetic flow, over the short term of 10 days, FO intake might induce UCP1 expression in subWAT via the sympathetic nervous system at least in part.

G-protein-coupled receptor 120 (GPR120), a receptor for n-3 polyunsaturated fatty acids, was also suggested to contribute to thermogenic activation in BAT and WAT by n-3 fatty acids by suppressing tissue inflammation induced by macrophages, especially in obese mice [53–56]. We used non-obese mice, and the expression of *Gpr120* was not affected in BAT and subWAT by FO supplementation (data not shown).

A systematic review indicated that EPA and DHA lowered serum lipid levels such as TG concentration [57]. Some mechanisms of serum lipid lowering by FO have been reported. EPA increased lipid oxidation in rat liver and reduced serum lipids [58]. FO also lowered serum lipids in adult human subjects [59]. We previously reported that FO administration at the same dose as in the present study decreased fatty acid synthesis genes such as acetyl-CoA carboxylase and increased fatty acid oxidation genes such as *Cpt I*, *Mcad* and *Aco* in mouse liver [60]. The rate limiting step in mitochondrial fatty acid oxidation is mediated by CPT I [61]. Even though CPT I activity in WAT was still low compared with that in liver and BAT in rat [62], activation of CPT I by overexpression of CPT I in 3T3-L1 adipocytes reduced NEFA release [63]. These FO-induced mechanisms in liver and WAT may contribute to lowering of the serum lipid levels. In general, enhanced fatty acid oxidation in the whole body is related to decreased RER. However, in human, RER correlated negatively with plasma palmitate concentrations [64]. In the present study, FO administration caused decreased serum concentrations of NEFA and TG (Table 2). We showed here that the RER of the FO-fed mice was slightly higher than that of the Con-fed mice (Figure 1c), although not significantly so. This was probably due to the reduced serum lipid levels in the FO-fed mice.

The short period of FO administration of 10 days in the present study did not result in weight loss, but weight gain and the weights of epididymal and mesenteric WAT were significantly reduced. Mice fed 21.42 or 42.84 energy% (en%) FO for 6 weeks significantly reduced BW by about 1.5 g or 4 g, respectively [36]. It is likely that mice need to be fed FO for a longer period of time to reduce their weight. BAT-positive subjects would undergo higher DIT than BAT-negative subjects [65]. Thus, BAT activation is expected to have an anti-obesity effect. Interestingly, BAT-positive subjects (young healthy men) showed an increase in EE after oral ingestion of capsinoids (9 mg) [15]. Moreover, capsinoids 6 mg/day taken orally for 12 weeks promoted loss of human abdominal fat [66]. FO supplementation in the present study resulted in a 1.2-fold increase in DIT$_{/intake}$ (Figure 2e). In human, DIT uses 10% of the daily energy intake [67]. The estimated energy requirement for adult men is about 2500 kcal/day [68], and the energy consumed by DIT was calculated to be about 250 kcal/day, and 300 kcal/day if multiplied by 1.2. Thus, a 1.2-fold increase in DIT was estimated to maximally increase energy consumption by 50 kcal/day. Adult human adipose tissue contains 71.6% crude fat [69]. Therefore, an increase in DIT by 1.2-fold was estimated to indicate fat burning of 500 g of adipocytes over about 2 months.

In conclusion, we first showed that FO supplementation significantly increased DIT by 1.2-fold. DIT$_{/intake}$ and DIT$_{/TEE}$ for the FO-fed mice were 11.2% and 22.3%, respectively. The FO-increased DIT was complemented by the increased expression of UCP1, activation of BAT and subWAT browning. FO may be a promising dietary fat for the prevention of overweight and obesity.

4. Materials and Methods

4.1. Animals

Seven-week-old male C57BL/6J mice were obtained from Tokyo Laboratory Animal Science (Tokyo, Japan). They were fed a standard laboratory diet (CE2) from CLEA Japan, Inc, (Tokyo, Japan) for 1 week for stabilization of their metabolism. Mice were maintained under a controlled environment at 22 °C in a 12-h light (0700–1900 h)/12-h dark (1900–0700 h) cycle. They were housed individually and allowed access to the experimental diets and water ad libitum. Care of the mice followed guidelines of the National Institutes of Health's Guide for the Care and Use of Laboratory Animals. The National Institutes of Biomedical Innovation, Health and Nutrition, Japan, reviewed and approved all animal procedures (Approval no. DS27-52R3).

4.2. Diet

Mice received a fat-rich diet (30 en%) containing either mixed fat with safflower oil and butter (control) or FO (n = 7 in each group). Diets were prepared as described previously [60,70], and the composition of the diet is listed in Table 3. Butter and safflower oil were purchased from Snow Brand Milk Corp. (Hokkaido, Japan) and Benibana Food (Tokyo, Japan), respectively. FO (containing 7% EPA and 24% DHA) was kindly provided by the NOF Corporation (Tokyo, Japan). The food was provided to the mice every day. To estimate daily food intake, the food weight of each day was subtracted from the initial food weight of the previous day. Mean food intake over the entire experimental period in the two groups of mice was calculated using these data. The diets were offered for 10 days.

Table 3. Dietary composition.

Dietary Constituents	Con	FO
	g/100 g	
Safflower oil (high oleic)	3.46	0.00
Butter	10.38	0.00
Fish oil	0.00	13.84
Casein	22.2	22.2
α-Starch	52.98	52.98
Vitamin mix (AIN-93)	1.12	1.12
Mineral mix (AIN-93)	3.92	3.92
Cellulose powder	5.60	5.60
L-Cystine	0.34	0.34
	en%	
Fat	30	30
Carbohydrate	50	50
Protein	20	20

Con: control; FO: fish oil; en%: energy %.

4.3. Measurement of O_2 Consumption and CO_2 Production to Calculate DIT and Energy Production

Mice on the 9th day of the experimental diet administration were used for the experiment. The method for calculating DIT was described previously [37]. Briefly, mice were placed in the calorimeter without food 6 days before starting the experiment at 1700 h, and then energy metabolism was measured for the 11-h period from 0000–1100 h. Oxygen consumption (VO_2) and carbon dioxide production (VCO_2) were monitored with a system that measures O_2/CO_2 metabolism in small animals (MK-5000RQ; Muromachi Kikai Co., Ltd., Tokyo, Japan), and their values were used to calculate DIT and EE. The EE was calculated as follows: EE (kcal/min) = 3.9 VO_2 + 1.1 VCO_2 [71]. For the measurements made after feeding, the same mice used in the fasted measurements were placed in the calorimeter at 1600 h. The research diet was provided at 1700 h, and energy metabolism was measured over the 22-h period from 1700–1500 h. VO_2, VCO_2 and activity were monitored by the system at 3-min intervals, and every four data points were averaged. The average value over the 12-min period was considered the mean value. The data were normalized to the square root of the activity count. Under the fasting conditions, 55 (5/h × 11 h) values each for EE and activity were selected from the measurements obtained over the 11-h period; we then plotted EE against the square root of activity and identified a linear regression equation by simple linear regression analysis. Under the fed conditions, 110 (5/h × 22 h) values each for EE and activity were selected from the measurements obtained over the 22-h period, and EE was then plotted against the square root of activity.

4.4. Quantitative Real-Time PCR

On the 10th day of the experimental diet, mice were sacrificed by cervical dislocation, and BAT, subWAT and liver were extracted from the mice. RNA was extracted from these tissues with TRIzol Reagent (Molecular Research Center, Inc., Cincinnati, OH, USA) following manufacturer's instructions. RNA was isolated and quantified with a NanoDrop ND-2000 spectrophotometer (Thermo Fisher Scientific, Waltham, MA, USA). Total RNA isolated from BAT and subWAT was reverse transcribed, and quantitative real-time RT-PCR was performed as described previously [60,72]. The primers for quantitative real-time PCR are listed in Table 4.

Table 4. Primers used for quantitative real-time PCR.

Gene	Forward Primer (5′ to 3′)	Reverse Primer (5′ to 3′)
36b4	GGCCCTGCACTCTCGCTTTC	TGCCAGGACGCGCTTGT
Aco	GCCCAACTGTGACTTCCATT	GGCATGTAACCCGTAGCACT
β3-AR	TCTAGTTCCCAGCGGAGTTTTCATCG	CGCGCACCTTCATAGCCATCAAACC
Cidea	ATCACAACTGGCCTGGTTACG	TACTACCCGGTGTCCATTTCT
Cpt I	GCACTGCAGCTCGCACATTACAA	CTCAGACAGTACCTCCTTCAGGAAA
Dio2	GCACGTCTCCAATCCTGAAT	TGAACCAAAGTTGACCACCA
Fgf21	ATGGAATGGATGAGATCTAGAGTTGG	TCTTGGTCGTCATCTGTGTAGAGG
Mcad	GATCGCAATGGGTGCTTTTGATAGAA	AGCTGATTGGCAATGTCTCCAGCAAA
Pgc1α	AAGTGTGGAACTCTCTGGAACTG	GGGTTATCTTGGTTGGCTTTATG
Pparα	CCTCAGGGTACCACTACGGAGT	GGTCTTCTTCTGAATCTTGCAGCT
Prdm16	GACATTCCAATCCCACCAGA	CACCTCTGTATCCGTCAGCA
Ucp1	GGCCCTTGTAAACAACAAAATAC	GGCAACAAGAGCTGACAGTAAAT

4.5. Serum Chemistry

Blood was obtained from the mice, and serum glucose was measured with an Ascensia autoanalyzer (Bayer Medical, Ltd., Tokyo, Japan). Serum levels of NEFA, TG and TC were measured by enzymatic colorimetry with NEFA C, TG E and TC E test kits (Wako Pure Chemical Industries, Ltd., Osaka, Japan), respectively.

4.6. Western Blotting

To prepare tissue lysates, BAT and subWAT were homogenized on ice in ice-cold lysis buffer consisting of 25 mM Tris-HCl, pH 7.4, 10 mM sodium orthovanadate, 50 mM sodium pyrophosphate, 100 mM sodium fluoride, 10 mM EDTA, 10 mM EGTA, 1 mM phenylmethylsulfonyl fluoride and 1% NP-40 that supplemented with a protease inhibitor cocktail and phosphatase inhibitor cocktail (both, Roche Diagnostics, Mannheim, Germany). After centrifugation of the tissue homogenates at 14,000× g for 10 min at 4 °C, the supernatants were collected for determination of protein concentrations by Bradford protein assay using a Bio-Rad Protein Assay Kit (Bio-Rad Laboratories, Inc., Hercules, CA, USA). Proteins (5 μg for BAT or 25 μg for subWAT) were separated by SDS-PAGE (7.5% gel) and then transferred electrophoretically onto Clear Blot Membrane-P (ATTO, Tokyo, Japan) and immunoblotted with specific primary antibodies: UCP1 (ab10983, 1:2000 dilution; Abcam,) and β-actin (C4) (sc-47778, 1:5000 dilution; Santa Cruz Biotechnology, Inc., Santa Cruz, CA, USA). The secondary antibodies included goat anti-rabbit IgG (sc-2005, 1:8000 dilution) and m-IgGκ BP-HRP (sc-516102, 1:6000 dilution; both from Santa Cruz

Biotechnology, Inc.). ECL detection reagents (Amersham Biosciences, Buckinghamshire, UK) were used to detect the desired proteins, which were then quantified with the NIH Image software program (NIH, Bethesda, MD, USA).

4.7. Statistical Analysis

Values are shown as the mean ± SEM. Significant differences between the mean values of the two groups were evaluated by Student *t*-test with IBM SPSS Statistics 23. Statistical significance was indicated by a p value < 0.05.

Supplementary Materials: The following are available online at https://www.mdpi.com/article/10.3390/md19050278/s1, Table S1: Effect of fish oil (FO) supplementation on gene expression in liver.

Author Contributions: T.Y. designed the research; R.I., D.L. and T.Y. conducted the research, and T.Y. and R.I. analyzed the data. T.Y. and R.I. wrote the manuscript with contributions from D.L. All authors have read and agreed to the published version of the manuscript.

Funding: This work was supported in part by a JSPS Grant-in-Aid for Scientific Research (C) Grant Number 16K01855.

Institutional Review Board Statement: Care of the mice followed guidelines of the National Institutes of Health's Guide for the Care and Use of Laboratory Animals. The National Institutes of Biomedical Innovation, Health and Nutrition, Japan, reviewed and approved all animal procedures (Approval no. DS27-52R3).

Informed Consent Statement: Not applicable.

Data Availability Statement: The data presented in this study are included in the corresponding sections throughout the manuscript.

Conflicts of Interest: The authors declare that they have no conflict of interest.

References

1. Lam, Y.Y.; Ravussin, E. Analysis of energy metabolism in humans: A review of methodologies. *Mol. Metab.* **2016**, *5*, 1057–1071. [CrossRef] [PubMed]
2. Tappy, L. Thermic effect of food and sympathetic nervous system activity in humans. *Reprod. Nutr. Dev.* **1996**, *36*, 391–397. [CrossRef] [PubMed]
3. Diepvens, K.; Westerterp, K.R.; Westerterp-Plantenga, M.S. Obesity and thermogenesis related to the consumption of caffeine, ephedrine, capsaicin, and green tea. *Am. J. Physiol. Regul. Integr. Comp. Physiol.* **2007**, *292*, R77–R85. [CrossRef] [PubMed]
4. Cannon, B.; Nedergaard, J. Brown adipose tissue: Function and physiological significance. *Physiol. Rev.* **2004**, *84*, 277–359. [CrossRef]
5. Heaton, J.M. The distribution of brown adipose tissue in the human. *J. Anat.* **1972**, *112*, 35–39.
6. Van Marken Lichtenbelt, W.D.; Vanhommerig, J.W.; Smulders, N.M.; Drossaerts, J.M.; Kemerink, G.J.; Bouvy, N.D.; Schrauwen, P.; Teule, G.J. Cold-activated brown adipose tissue in healthy men. *N. Engl. J. Med.* **2009**, *360*, 1500–1508. [CrossRef] [PubMed]
7. Virtanen, K.A.; Lidell, M.E.; Orava, J.; Heglind, M.; Westergren, R.; Niemi, T.; Taittonen, M.; Laine, J.; Savisto, N.J.; Enerbäck, S.; et al. Functional brown adipose tissue in healthy adults. *N. Engl. J. Med.* **2009**, *360*, 1518–1525. [CrossRef]
8. Heaton, G.M.; Wagenvoord, R.J.; Kemp, A., Jr.; Nicholls, D.G. Brown-adipose-tissue mitochondria: Photoaffinity labelling of the regulatory site of energy dissipation. *Eur. J. Biochem.* **1978**, *82*, 515–521. [CrossRef]
9. Aquila, H.; Link, T.A.; Klingenberg, M. The uncoupling protein from brown fat mitochondria is related to the mitochondrial ADP/ATP carrier. Analysis of sequence homologies and of folding of the protein in the membrane. *EMBO J.* **1985**, *4*, 2369–2376. [CrossRef]
10. Von Essen, G.; Lindsund, E.; Cannon, B.; Nedergaard, J. Adaptive facultative diet-induced thermogenesis in wild-type but not in UCP1-ablated mice. *Am. J. Physiol. Endocrinol. Metab.* **2017**, *313*, E515–E527. [CrossRef] [PubMed]
11. Kontani, Y.; Wang, Y.; Kimura, K.; Inokuma, K.I.; Saito, M.; Suzuki-Miura, T.; Wang, Z.; Sato, Y.; Mori, N.; Yamashita, H. UCP1 deficiency increases susceptibility to diet-induced obesity with age. *Aging Cell* **2005**, *4*, 147–155. [CrossRef] [PubMed]
12. Nagai, N.; Sakane, N.; Ueno, L.M.; Hamada, T.; Moritani, T. The -3826 A–>G variant of the uncoupling protein-1 gene diminishes postprandial thermogenesis after a high fat meal in healthy boys. *J. Clin. Endocrinol. Metab.* **2003**, *88*, 5661–5667. [CrossRef] [PubMed]
13. Saito, M.; Okamatsu-Ogura, Y.; Matsushita, M.; Watanabe, K.; Yoneshiro, T.; Nio-Kobayashi, J.; Iwanaga, T.; Miyagawa, M.; Kameya, T.; Nakada, K.; et al. High incidence of metabolically active brown adipose tissue in healthy adult humans: Effects of cold exposure and adiposity. *Diabetes* **2009**, *58*, 1526–1531. [CrossRef]

14. Cypess, A.M.; Weiner, L.S.; Roberts-Toler, C.; Elía, E.F.; Kessler, S.H.; Kahn, P.A.; English, J.; Chatman, K.; Trauger, S.A.; Doria, A.; et al. Activation of human brown adipose tissue by a β3-adrenergic receptor agonist. *Cell Metab.* **2015**, *21*, 33–38. [CrossRef] [PubMed]
15. Yoneshiro, T.; Aita, S.; Kawai, Y.; Iwanaga, T.; Saito, M. Nonpungent capsaicin analogs (capsinoids) increase energy expenditure through the activation of brown adipose tissue in humans. *Am. J. Clin. Nutr.* **2012**, *95*, 845–850. [CrossRef]
16. Yoneshiro, T.; Aita, S.; Matsushita, M.; Kayahara, T.; Kameya, T.; Kawai, Y.; Iwanaga, T.; Saito, M. Recruited brown adipose tissue as an antiobesity agent in humans. *J. Clin. Investig.* **2013**, *123*, 3404–3408. [CrossRef]
17. Ramel, A.; Martinéz, A.; Kiely, M.; Morais, G.; Bandarra, N.M.; Thorsdottir, I. Beneficial effects of long-chain n-3 fatty acids included in an energy-restricted diet on insulin resistance in overweight and obese European young adults. *Diabetologia* **2008**, *51*, 1261–1268. [CrossRef]
18. Thorsdottir, I.; Tomasson, H.; Gunnarsdottir, I.; Gisladottir, E.; Kiely, M.; Parra, M.D.; Bandarra, N.M.; Schaafsma, G.; Martinéz, J.A. Randomized trial of weight-loss-diets for young adults varying in fish and fish oil content. *Int. J. Obes.* **2007**, *31*, 1560–1566. [CrossRef] [PubMed]
19. Gunnarsdottir, I.; Tomasson, H.; Kiely, M.; Martinéz, J.A.; Bandarra, N.M.; Morais, M.G.; Thorsdottir, I. Inclusion of fish or fish oil in weight-loss diets for young adults: Effects on blood lipids. *Int. J. Obes.* **2008**, *32*, 1105–1112. [CrossRef] [PubMed]
20. Calder, P.C. Mechanisms of action of (n-3) fatty acids. *J. Nutr.* **2012**, *142*, 592S–599S. [CrossRef]
21. Arterburn, L.M.; Hall, E.B.; Oken, H. Distribution, interconversion, and dose response of n-3 fatty acids in humans. *Am. J. Clin. Nutr.* **2006**, *83*, 1467S–1476S. [CrossRef] [PubMed]
22. Muskiet, F.A.; Fokkema, M.R.; Schaafsma, A.; Boersma, E.R.; Crawford, M.A. Is docosahexaenoic acid (DHA) essential? Lessons from DHA status regulation, our ancient diet, epidemiology and randomized controlled trials. *J. Nutr.* **2004**, *134*, 183–186. [CrossRef] [PubMed]
23. Forman, B.M.; Chen, J.; Evans, R.M. Hypolipidemic drugs, polyunsaturated fatty acids, and eicosanoids are ligands for peroxisome proliferator-activated receptors alpha and delta. *Proc. Natl. Acad. Sci. USA* **1997**, *94*, 4312–4317. [CrossRef] [PubMed]
24. Krey, G.; Braissant, O.; L'Horset, F.; Kalkhoven, E.; Perroud, M.; Parker, M.G.; Wahli, W. Fatty acids, eicosanoids, and hypolipidemic agents identified as ligands of peroxisome proliferator-activated receptors by coactivator-dependent receptor ligand assay. *Mol. Endocrinol.* **1997**, *11*, 779–791. [CrossRef] [PubMed]
25. Escher, P.; Braissant, O.; Basu-Modak, S.; Michalik, L.; Wahli, W.; Desvergne, B. Rat PPARs: Quantitative analysis in adult rat tissues and regulation in fasting and refeeding. *Endocrinology* **2001**, *142*, 4195–4202. [CrossRef] [PubMed]
26. Barbera, M.J.; Schluter, A.; Pedraza, N.; Iglesias, R.; Villarroya, F.; Giralt, M. Peroxisome proliferator-activated receptor alpha activates transcription of the brown fat uncoupling protein-1 gene. A link between regulation of the thermogenic and lipid oxidation pathways in the brown fat cell. *J. Biol. Chem.* **2001**, *276*, 1486–1493. [CrossRef]
27. Ishibashi, J.; Seale, P. Medicine. Beige can be slimming. *Science* **2010**, *328*, 1113–1114. [CrossRef]
28. Seale, P.; Bjork, B.; Yang, W.; Kajimura, S.; Chin, S.; Kuang, S.; Scimè, A.; Devarakonda, S.; Conroe, H.M.; Erdjument-Bromage, H.; et al. PRDM16 controls a brown fat/skeletal muscle switch. *Nature* **2008**, *454*, 961–967. [CrossRef]
29. Wu, J.; Boström, P.; Sparks, L.M.; Ye, L.; Choi, J.H.; Giang, A.H.; Khandekar, M.; Virtanen, K.A.; Nuutila, P.; Schaart, G.; et al. Beige adipocytes are a distinct type of thermogenic fat cell in mouse and human. *Cell* **2012**, *150*, 366–376. [CrossRef]
30. Okamatsu-Ogura, Y.; Fukano, K.; Tsubota, A.; Uozumi, A.; Terao, A.; Kimura, K.; Saito, M. Thermogenic ability of uncoupling protein 1 in beige adipocytes in mice. *PLoS ONE* **2013**, *8*, e84229. [CrossRef]
31. Laiglesia, L.M.; Lorente-Cebrián, S.; Prieto-Hontoria, P.L.; Fernández-Galilea, M.; Ribeiro, S.M.; Sáinz, N.; Martínez, J.A.; Moreno-Aliaga, M.J. Eicosapentaenoic acid promotes mitochondrial biogenesis and beige-like features in subcutaneous adipocytes from overweight subjects. *J. Nutr. Biochem.* **2016**, *37*, 76–82. [CrossRef] [PubMed]
32. Zhao, M.; Chen, X. Eicosapentaenoic acid promotes thermogenic and fatty acid storage capacity in mouse subcutaneous adipocytes. *Biochem. Biophys. Res. Commun.* **2014**, *450*, 1446–1451. [CrossRef] [PubMed]
33. Bargut, T.C.; Souza-Mello, V.; Mandarim-de-Lacerda, C.A.; Aguila, M.B. Fish oil diet modulates epididymal and inguinal adipocyte metabolism in mice. *Food Funct.* **2016**, *7*, 1468–1476. [CrossRef] [PubMed]
34. Kim, M.; Goto, T.; Yu, R.; Uchida, K.; Tominaga, M.; Kano, Y.; Takahashi, N.; Kawada, T. Fish oil intake induces UCP1 upregulation in brown and white adipose tissue via the sympathetic nervous system. *Sci. Rep.* **2015**, *5*, 18013. [CrossRef] [PubMed]
35. Kim, J.; Okla, M.; Erickson, A.; Carr, T.; Natarajan, S.K.; Chung, S. Eicosapentaenoic Acid Potentiates Brown Thermogenesis through FFAR4-dependent Up-regulation of miR-30b and miR-378. *J. Biol. Chem.* **2016**, *291*, 20551–20562. [CrossRef] [PubMed]
36. Bargut, T.C.; Silva-e-Silva, A.C.; Souza-Mello, V.; Mandarim-de-Lacerda, C.A.; Aguila, M.B. Mice fed fish oil diet and upregulation of brown adipose tissue thermogenic markers. *Eur. J. Nutr.* **2016**, *55*, 159–169. [CrossRef]
37. Yamazaki, T.; Ikaga, R.; Li, D.; Nakae, S.; Tanaka, S. A novel method for measuring diet-induced thermogenesis in mice. *MethodsX* **2019**, *6*, 1950–1956. [CrossRef]
38. Hanssen, M.J.; Hoeks, J.; Brans, B.; van der Lans, A.A.; Schaart, G.; van den Driessche, J.J.; Jörgensen, J.A.; Boekschoten, M.V.; Hesselink, M.K.; Havekes, B.; et al. Short-term cold acclimation improves insulin sensitivity in patients with type 2 diabetes mellitus. *Nat. Med.* **2015**, *21*, 863–865. [CrossRef]
39. Lefebvre, P.; Chinetti, G.; Fruchart, J.C.; Staels, B. Sorting out the roles of PPAR alpha in energy metabolism and vascular homeostasis. *J. Clin. Investig.* **2006**, *116*, 571–580. [CrossRef]

40. Leblanc, J.; Dussault, J.; Lupien, D.; Richard, D. Effect of diet and exercise on norepinephrine-induced thermogenesis in male and female rats. *J. Appl. Physiol.* **1982**, *52*, 556–561. [CrossRef]
41. Gulick, T.; Cresci, S.; Caira, T.; Moore, D.D.; Kelly, D.P. The peroxisome proliferator-activated receptor regulates mitochondrial fatty acid oxidative enzyme gene expression. *Proc. Natl. Acad. Sci. USA* **1994**, *91*, 11012–11016. [CrossRef] [PubMed]
42. Pahlavani, M.; Razafimanjato, F.; Ramalingam, L.; Kalupahana, N.S.; Moussa, H.; Scoggin, S.; Moustaid-Moussa, N. Eicosapentaenoic acid regulates brown adipose tissue metabolism in high-fat-fed mice and in clonal brown adipocytes. *J. Nutr. Biochem.* **2017**, *39*, 101–109. [CrossRef] [PubMed]
43. Oudart, H.; Groscolas, R.; Calgari, C.; Nibbelink, M.; Leray, C.; Le Maho, Y.; Malan, A. Brown fat thermogenesis in rats fed high-fat diets enriched with n-3 polyunsaturated fatty acids. *Int. J. Obes. Relat. Metab. Disord.* **1997**, *21*, 955–962. [CrossRef] [PubMed]
44. Mascaró, C.; Acosta, E.; Ortiz, J.A.; Marrero, P.F.; Hegardt, F.G.; Haro, D. Control of human muscle-type carnitine palmitoyltransferase I gene transcription by peroxisome proliferator-activated receptor. *J. Biol. Chem.* **1998**, *273*, 8560–8563. [CrossRef]
45. Leone, T.C.; Weinheimer, C.J.; Kelly, D.P. A critical role for the peroxisome proliferator-activated receptor alpha (PPARalpha) in the cellular fasting response: The PPARalpha-null mouse as a model of fatty acid oxidation disorders. *Proc. Natl. Acad. Sci. USA* **1999**, *96*, 7473–7478. [CrossRef] [PubMed]
46. Goto, T.; Lee, J.Y.; Teraminami, A.; Kim, Y.I.; Hirai, S.; Uemura, T.; Inoue, H.; Takahashi, N.; Kawada, T. Activation of peroxisome proliferator-activated receptor-alpha stimulates both differentiation and fatty acid oxidation in adipocytes. *J. Lipid. Res.* **2011**, *52*, 873–884. [CrossRef]
47. Rachid, T.L.; Penna-de-Carvalho, A.; Bringhenti, I.; Aguila, M.B.; Mandarim-de-Lacerda, C.A.; Souza-Mello, V. Fenofibrate (PPARalpha agonist) induces beige cell formation in subcutaneous white adipose tissue from diet-induced male obese mice. *Mol. Cell. Endocrinol.* **2015**, *402*, 86–94. [CrossRef]
48. Rachid, T.L.; Silva-Veiga, F.M.; Graus-Nunes, F.; Bringhenti, I.; Mandarim-de-Lacerda, C.A.; Souza-Mello, V. Differential actions of PPAR-α and PPAR-β/δ on beige adipocyte formation: A study in the subcutaneous white adipose tissue of obese male mice. *PLoS ONE* **2018**, *13*, e0191365. [CrossRef]
49. Shabalina, I.G.; Petrovic, N.; de Jong, J.M.; Kalinovich, A.V.; Cannon, B.; Nedergaard, J. UCP1 in brite/beige adipose tissue mitochondria is functionally thermogenic. *Cell Rep.* **2013**, *5*, 1196–1203. [CrossRef]
50. Sato, H.; Taketomi, Y.; Miki, Y.; Murase, R.; Yamamoto, K.; Murakami, M. Secreted Phospholipase PLA2G2D Contributes to Metabolic Health by Mobilizing ω3 Polyunsaturated Fatty Acids in WAT. *Cell Rep.* **2020**, *31*, 107579. [CrossRef]
51. Hondares, E.; Iglesias, R.; Giralt, A.; Gonzalez, F.J.; Giralt, M.; Mampel, T.; Villarroya, F. Thermogenic activation induces FGF21 expression and release in brown adipose tissue. *J. Biol. Chem.* **2011**, *286*, 12983–12990. [CrossRef]
52. Fisher, F.M.; Kleiner, S.; Douris, N.; Fox, E.C.; Mepani, R.J.; Verdeguer, F.; Wu, J.; Kharitonenkov, A.; Flier, J.S.; Maratos-Flier, E.; et al. FGF21 regulates PGC-1α and browning of white adipose tissues in adaptive thermogenesis. *Genes Dev.* **2012**, *26*, 271–281. [CrossRef]
53. Quesada-López, T.; Cereijo, R.; Turatsinze, J.V.; Planavila, A.; Cairó, M.; Gavaldà-Navarro, A.; Peyrou, M.; Moure, R.; Iglesias, R.; Giralt, M.; et al. The lipid sensor GPR120 promotes brown fat activation and FGF21 release from adipocytes. *Nat. Commun.* **2016**, *7*, 13479. [CrossRef] [PubMed]
54. Oh, D.Y.; Talukdar, S.; Bae, E.J.; Imamura, T.; Morinaga, H.; Fan, W.; Li, P.; Lu, W.J.; Watkins, S.M.; Olefsky, J.M. GPR120 is an omega-3 fatty acid receptor mediating potent anti-inflammatory and insulin-sensitizing effects. *Cell* **2010**, *142*, 687–698. [CrossRef] [PubMed]
55. Huber, J.; Löffler, M.; Bilban, M.; Reimers, M.; Kadl, A.; Todoric, J.; Zeyda, M.; Geyeregger, R.; Schreiner, M.; Weichhart, T.; et al. Prevention of high-fat diet-induced adipose tissue remodeling in obese diabetic mice by n-3 polyunsaturated fatty acids. *Int. J. Obes.* **2007**, *31*, 1004–1013. [CrossRef] [PubMed]
56. Todoric, J.; Löffler, M.; Huber, J.; Bilban, M.; Reimers, M.; Kadl, A.; Zeyda, M.; Waldhäusl, W.; Stulnig, T.M. Adipose tissue inflammation induced by high-fat diet in obese diabetic mice is prevented by n-3 polyunsaturated fatty acids. *Diabetologia* **2006**, *49*, 2109–2119. [CrossRef]
57. Innes, J.K.; Calder, P.C. The Differential Effects of Eicosapentaenoic Acid and Docosahexaenoic Acid on Cardiometabolic Risk Factors: A Systematic Review. *Int. J. Mol. Sci.* **2018**, *19*, 532. [CrossRef]
58. Madsen, L.; Rustan, A.C.; Vaagenes, H.; Berge, K.; Dyrøy, E.; Berge, R.K. Eicosapentaenoic and docosahexaenoic acid affect mitochondrial and peroxisomal fatty acid oxidation in relation to substrate preference. *Lipids* **1999**, *34*, 951–963. [CrossRef]
59. Buckley, R.; Shewring, B.; Turner, R.; Yaqoob, P.; Minihane, A.M. Circulating triacylglycerol and apoE levels in response to EPA and docosahexaenoic acid supplementation in adult human subjects. *Br. J. Nutr.* **2004**, *92*, 477–483. [CrossRef] [PubMed]
60. Wada, S.; Yamazaki, T.; Kawano, Y.; Miura, S.; Ezaki, O. Fish oil fed prior to ethanol administration prevents acute ethanol-induced fatty liver in mice. *J. Hepatol.* **2008**, *49*, 441–450. [CrossRef] [PubMed]
61. Houten, S.M.; Violante, S.; Ventura, F.V.; Wanders, R.J. The Biochemistry and Physiology of Mitochondrial Fatty Acid β-Oxidation and Its Genetic Disorders. *Annu. Rev. Physiol.* **2016**, *78*, 23–44. [CrossRef]
62. Warfel, J.D.; Vandanmagsar, B.; Dubuisson, O.S.; Hodgeson, S.M.; Elks, C.M.; Ravussin, E.; Mynatt, R.L. Examination of carnitine palmitoyltransferase 1 abundance in white adipose tissue: Implications in obesity research. *Am. J. Physiol. Regul. Integr. Comp. Physiol.* **2017**, *312*, R816–R820. [CrossRef]

63. Gao, X.; Li, K.; Hui, X.; Kong, X.; Sweeney, G.; Wang, Y.; Xu, A.; Teng, M.; Liu, P.; Wu, D. Carnitine palmitoyltransferase 1A prevents fatty acid-induced adipocyte dysfunction through suppression of c-Jun N-terminal kinase. *Biochem. J.* **2011**, *435*, 723–732. [CrossRef] [PubMed]
64. Jensen, M.D.; Bajnárek, J.; Lee, S.Y.; Nielsen, S.; Koutsari, C. Relationship between postabsorptive respiratory exchange ratio and plasma free fatty acid concentrations. *J. Lipid. Res.* **2009**, *50*, 1863–1869. [CrossRef] [PubMed]
65. Hibi, M.; Oishi, S.; Matsushita, M.; Yoneshiro, T.; Yamaguchi, T.; Usui, C.; Yasunaga, K.; Katsuragi, Y.; Kubota, K.; Tanaka, S.; et al. Brown adipose tissue is involved in diet-induced thermogenesis and whole-body fat utilization in healthy humans. *Int. J. Obes.* **2016**, *40*, 1655–1661. [CrossRef] [PubMed]
66. Snitker, S.; Fujishima, Y.; Shen, H.; Ott, S.; Pi-Sunyer, X.; Furuhata, Y.; Sato, H.; Takahashi, M. Effects of novel capsinoid treatment on fatness and energy metabolism in humans: Possible pharmacogenetic implications. *Am. J. Clin. Nutr.* **2009**, *89*, 45–50. [CrossRef] [PubMed]
67. Westerterp, K.R. Diet induced thermogenesis. *Nutr. Metab.* **2004**, *1*, 5. [CrossRef]
68. Trumbo, P.; Schlicker, S.; Yates, A.A.; Poos, M. Dietary reference intakes for energy, carbohydrate, fiber, fat, fatty acids, cholesterol, protein and amino acids. *J. Am. Diet. Assoc.* **2002**, *102*, 1621–1630. [CrossRef]
69. Forbes, R.M.; Cooper, A.R.; Mitchell, H.H. The composition of the adult human body as determined by chemical analysis. *J. Biol. Chem.* **1953**, *203*, 359–366. [CrossRef]
70. Li, D.; Ikaga, R.; Yamazaki, T. Soya protein β-conglycinin ameliorates fatty liver and obesity in diet-induced obese mice through the down-regulation of PPARγ. *Br. J. Nutr.* **2018**, *119*, 1220–1232. [CrossRef]
71. Weir, J.B. New methods for calculating metabolic rate with special reference to protein metabolism. *J. Physiol.* **1949**, *109*, 1–9. [CrossRef] [PubMed]
72. Yamazaki, T.; Okawa, S.; Takahashi, M. The effects on weight loss and gene expression in adipose and hepatic tissues of very-low carbohydrate and low-fat isoenergetic diets in diet-induced obese mice. *Nutr. Metab.* **2016**, *13*, 78. [CrossRef] [PubMed]

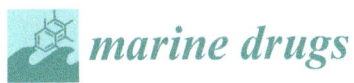

Article

Laminariales Host Does Impact Lipid Temperature Trajectories of the Fungal Endophyte *Paradendryphiella salina* (Sutherland.)

Marine Vallet [1,†,‡], Tarik Meziane [2], Najet Thiney [2], Soizic Prado [1] and Cédric Hubas [3,*,‡]

1. Molécules de Comunications et Adaptation des Microorganismes (MCAM) Muséum National d'Histoire Naturelle, CNRS, 63 Rue Buffon, FR-75005 Paris, France; mvallet@ice.mpg.de (M.V.); soizic.prado@mnhn.fr (S.P.)
2. Laboratoire de Biologie des Organismes et Ecosystèmes Aquatiques (BOREA), Muséum National d'Histoire Naturelle, IRD, SU, CNRS, UA, UCN, 61 Rue Buffon, FR-75005 Paris, France; tarik.meziane@mnhn.fr (T.M.); najet.thiney@mnhn.fr (N.T.)
3. Laboratoire de Biologie des Organismes et Ecosystèmes Aquatiques (BOREA), Muséum National d'Histoire Naturelle, IRD, SU, CNRS, UA, UCN, Station Marine de Concarneau, FR-29900 Concarneau, France
* Correspondence: cedric.hubas@mnhn.fr
† Current address: Max Planck Fellow group Phytoplankton Community Interactions, Max Planck Institute for Chemical Ecology, Hans-Knöll-Straße 8, D-07745 Jena, Germany.
‡ These authors contributed equally to this work.

Received: 4 June 2020; Accepted: 13 July 2020; Published: 22 July 2020

Abstract: Kelps are colonized by a wide range of microbial symbionts. Among them, endophytic fungi remain poorly studied, but recent studies evidenced yet their high diversity and their central role in algal defense against various pathogens. Thus, studying the metabolic expressions of kelp endophytes under different conditions is important to have a better understanding of their impacts on host performance. In this context, fatty acid composition is essential to a given algae fitness and of interest to food web studies either to measure its nutritional quality or to infer about its contribution to consumers diets. In the present study, *Paradendryphiella salina*, a fungal endophyte was isolated from *Saccharina latissima* (L.) and *Laminaria digitata* (Hudson.) and its fatty acid composition was assessed at increasing salinity and temperature conditions. Results showed that fungal composition in terms of fatty acids displayed algal-dependent trajectories in response to temperature increase. This highlights that C18 unsaturated fatty acids are key components in the host-dependant acclimation of *P. salina* to salinity and temperature changes.

Keywords: fatty acids; fungal endophytes; laminariales; *Paradendryphiella salina*

1. Introduction

Kelps are colonized at their surface, but also within their tissues, by a wide range of micro-organisms and thus act as hosts to species-rich assemblages of algae, animals and microbes. The associated microorganisms are responsible for spreading infectious algal diseases, protecting against fouling organisms and pathogens or producing substances that promote algal growth [1]. Among these micro-organisms, endophytic fungi remain poorly documented although recent studies evidenced their high diversity [2] and their key role in algal defence against various pathogens. Their role is still virtually unknown and there is a need to examine how environmental factors influence the relationship between the fungi and their hosts [1].

In that context, isolation of *P. salina* (Ascomycota) strains from several brown algal species has brought new insights into the complex relationships between these macroalgae and their microbiote. The observed association of the fungus to brown algae dates back to 1916 when it was first described as

Cercospora salina [3]. Its ecological mode and habitat were described as saprophytic on seaweeds. It is extremely widespread and has then been found in many ecosystems from the tropics to mid latitudes. It occurs in salt marshes, in sediments, at the surface of living or dead algae thalli [4], sea grasses and woods and has been successfully, isolated from various plant and algal substrates at different geographical locations and climatic zones ([5,6] and references therein).

This fungus was studied for its adaptations to the abiotic and biotic parameters commonly found in its natural marine habitats. All the tested strains grew optimally on culture media with added marine salts, at pH values between 6.5 and 8.0 and at an incubation temperature of 25 °C. It generally exhibits an increased salt optimum with increasing incubation temperature and clearly demonstrate an important phenotypic plasticity and the ability to adapt to diverse biotopes [5]. Recent studies have demonstrated that this common fungal endophyte produce bioactive pyrenocines and pyrenochaceatic acid which may confer protection to the host algae against pathogen infection [2]. Furthermore, bacterial and fungal endophytes associated to four brown algae *Ascophyllum nodosum* (L.), *Pelvetia canaliculata* (L.) *L. digitata*, and *S. latissima* produce metabolites that interfere with bacterial autoinducer-2 quorum sensing (QS), a signalling system involved in virulence and host colonization [7]. Recent results suggest that QS quenching may be linked to a novel α-hydroxy γ-butenolides produced by *P. salina* which interfere with the QS system of the pathogenic bacterial model *Pseudomonas aeruginosa* (Schroeter.) [8]. In addition, a recent study reveals the ability of *P. salina* to degrade alginate of brown algae [9].

Kelps are particularly rich in palmitic acid (16:0), palmitoleic acid (16:1n-7), oleic acid (18:1n-9), linoleic acid (18:2n-6) and arachidonic acid (20:4n-6) but composition may vary according to environmental factors especially temperature and depth [10,11]. A tendency of decreasing unsaturation towards the warmer seasons has been observed and the comparison of fatty acid profiles between *S. latissima* (L.), *Saccorhiza polyschides* (Lightfoot.), and *Laminaria ochroleuca* (Bachelot de la Pylaie.), also indicated species-specific factors [10]. In light of recent evidences of the hitherto unsuspected diversity of fungal endophytes in brown algae, it is not clear whether algal or fungal cells are responsible for previously observed changes in fatty acids composition of kelps (especially in palmitic acid together with oleic, linoleic and linolenic acids 18:3n-3) according to environmental conditions and/or species-specific factors. Most fungi are indeed very rich in C18 fatty acids [12].

These metabolites are important structural components, but also active constituents in several physiological processes. For instance, oxylipins which are key signalling molecules in stress response and immunity [13] and have important implication in fungal development and pathogen/host interactions [14] are produced enzymatically or non-enzymatically as a result of oxygenation of C18 fatty acids by free radicals and reactive oxygen species [15]. The aim of the present study was thus to explore fatty acid synthesis of a common kelp endophyte under different conditions to understand the potential role of *P. salina* on its host metabolism.

2. Results

2.1. Fatty Acid Compositions

Fatty acid compositions of *P. salina* strains LD40H and SL540T are reported in Table 1. A total of 22 fatty acids were detected. Saturated fatty acids (SFA) were lauric acid (12:0), myristic acid (14:0), pentadecylic acid (15:0), palmitic acid (16:0), margaric acid (17:0), stearic acid (18:0), arachidic acid (20:0), and behenic acid (22:0). Altogether, 16:0 and 18:0 were the most abundant SFA and contributed in average 23 $\pm$ 3 and 4 $\pm$ 1% to total fatty acids (TFA), respectively. Mono-unsaturated fatty acids (MUFA) were myristoleic acid (14:1n-5), palmitoleic acid (16:1n-7), hypogeic acid (16:1n-9), 17:1n-7, 17:1n-9, vaccenic acid (18:1n-7), oleic acid (18:1n-9), and 20:1n-9. Across all treatments, 18:1n-9 was the most abundant MUFA (28 $\pm$ 4% of TFA). Measured poly-unsaturated fatty acids (PUFA) were 16:2n-4, 16:2n-6, 17:2n-5, Linoleic acid (18:2n-6), alpha-linolenic acid (18:3n-3), and 20:2n-9. Linoleic acid was the most abundant PUFA as well as the most abundant fatty acid with 40 $\pm$ 3% of TFA.

Table 1. Fatty acids concentrations (μg g^{-1}) in the extracts of endophytic *P. salina* isolated from *L. digitata* (LD) or *S. latissima* (SL) and grown at different salinities (S1, S2 and S3 at 23.5, 50 and 70 PSU respectively) and temperatures (T10, T18 and T25 at 10, 18 and 25 °C respectively). <dl indicates the signal was below detection limit.

Host algae	Temperature	Salinity	12:0 mean	12:0 sd	14:0 mean	14:0 sd	14:1n-5 mean	14:1n-5 sd	15:0 mean	15:0 sd	16:0 mean	16:0 sd	16:1n-7 mean	16:1n-7 sd	16:1n-9 mean	16:1n-9 sd	16:2n-4 mean	16:2n-4 sd
LD	T10	S1	0.02	0.022	0.04	0.007	0.01	0.001	<dl	<dl	4.79	1.069	0.16	0.035	0.03	0.005	0.01	0.003
SL	T10	S1	<dl	<dl	0.03	0.005	<dl	<dl	0.01	0.001	4.55	0.899	0.12	0.045	0.03	0.008	0.01	0.002
LD	T18	S1	0.01	0.010	0.03	0.011	<dl	0.000	0.01	0.002	5.2	1.472	0.25	0.044	0.04	0.008	0.02	0.004
SL	T18	S1	<dl	<dl	0.02	0.003	<dl	<dl	0.01	<dl	3.36	0.810	0.16	0.040	0.03	0.008	0.01	0.001
LD	T25	S1	0.01	0.005	0.03	0.004	0.02	0.015	0.02	0.005	6.24	1.586	0.46	0.126	0.06	0.016	0.03	0.009
SL	T25	S1	<dl	<dl	0.03	0.005	0.01	0.003	0.01	0.003	5.26	1.311	0.34	0.081	0.04	0.008	0.02	0.004
LD	T10	S2	0.01	0.006	0.03	0.007	<dl	<dl	0.01	0.001	3.49	0.741	0.17	0.040	0.02	0.005	0.01	0.002
SL	T10	S2	0.01	0.011	0.02	0.001	<dl	<dl	<dl	<dl	1.87	0.640	0.1	0.044	0.01	0.005	<dl	<dl
LD	T18	S2	0.01	0.017	0.03	0.004	0.01	0.003	0.01	0.003	3.47	1.061	0.27	0.053	0.04	0.008	0.01	0.004
SL	T18	S2	0.01	0.001	0.04	0.009	0.01	0.001	0.02	0.004	4.55	1.194	0.35	0.081	0.04	0.008	0.02	0.005
LD	T25	S2	0.01	0.002	0.08	0.030	0.02	0.010	0.02	0.005	8.5	0.643	0.94	0.088	0.09	0.008	0.07	0.004
SL	T25	S2	<dl	<dl	0.09	0.031	0.02	0.003	0.03	0.007	9.8	3.034	0.95	0.230	0.08	0.014	0.05	0.014
LD	T10	S3	0.01	0.002	0.01	0.004	<dl	<dl	<dl	<dl	0.82	0.373	0.07	0.049	<dl	<dl	<dl	<dl
SL	T10	S3	<dl	<dl	0.01	0.004	<dl	<dl	<dl	<dl	0.62	0.418	0.06	0.051	<dl	<dl	<dl	<dl
LD	T18	S3	<dl	<dl	0.04	0.004	<dl	0.001	0.01	0.001	3.6	0.277	0.38	0.037	0.01	0.003	0.02	0.002
SL	T18	S3	<dl	<dl	0.07	0.044	<dl	<dl	0.02	0.013	5.91	3.655	0.76	0.493	0.03	0.020	0.03	0.017
LD	T25	S3	0.03	0.037	0.07	0.038	<dl	<dl	0.01	0.005	5.19	4.629	0.76	0.937	0.02	0.021	0.06	0.081
SL	T25	S3	<dl	<dl	0.07	0.036	<dl	<dl	0.02	0.008	4.87	1.677	0.78	0.383	0.03	0.008	0.04	0.022

Host algae	Temperature	Salinity	16:2n-6 mean	16:2n-6 sd	17:0 mean	17:0 sd	17:1n-7 mean	17:1n-7 sd	17:1n-9 mean	17:1n-9 sd	17:2n-5 mean	17:2n-5 sd	18:0 mean	18:0 sd	18:1n-7 mean	18:1n-7 sd	18:1n-9 mean	18:1n-9 sd
LD	T10	S1	0.01	0.002	0.03	0.006	0.01	0.003	0.01	0.006	<dl	0.003	<dl	<dl	1.31	0.291	0.1	0.015
SL	T10	S1	0.01	0.010	0.04	0.002	0.01	0.001	0.01	0.002	0.01	0.001	0.01	0.008	1.64	0.251	0.11	0.022
LD	T18	S1	0.02	0.003	0.03	0.006	0.01	<dl	0.01	0.006	<dl	<dl	<dl	<dl	0.97	0.363	0.17	0.090
SL	T18	S1	0.01	0.004	0.03	0.008	0.01	0.001	0.01	0.008	0.01	0.002	<dl	<dl	0.84	0.174	0.11	0.023
LD	T25	S1	0.04	0.014	0.04	0.016	0.01	0.002	0.01	0.016	<dl	0.001	<dl	<dl	0.79	0.161	0.32	0.098
SL	T25	S1	0.02	0.004	0.03	0.007	0.01	0.001	0.01	0.007	<dl	<dl	0.01	0.002	0.93	0.224	0.19	0.034
LD	T10	S2	<dl	<dl	0.01	0.001	<dl	<dl	0.01	0.001	<dl	<dl	<dl	<dl	0.87	0.195	0.06	0.009
SL	T10	S2	<dl	<dl	0.01	0.007	<dl	<dl	0.01	0.007	<dl	<dl	<dl	<dl	0.47	0.135	0.04	0.007

111

Table 1. *Cont.*

Host algae	Temperature	Salinity													
LD	T18	S2	0.02	0.004	0.02	0.004	<dl	<dl	<dl	<dl	0.51	0.203	0.07	0.021	4.21	1.081
SL	T18	S2	0.01	0.004	0.02	0.005	0.01	0.001	<dl	<dl	<dl	<dl	0.71	0.150	0.08	0.019	6.33	1.516
LD	T25	S2	0.05	0.008	0.03	0.008	0.01	0.001	<dl	<dl	<dl	<dl	0.88	0.021	0.27	0.054	9.38	0.268
SL	T25	S2	0.02	0.003	0.02	0.003	0.01	0.001	0.01	0.001	0.01	0.000	1.09	0.341	0.17	0.045	11.85	3.027
LD	T10	S3	<dl	<dl	<dl	<dl	<dl	<dl	<dl	<dl	<dl	<dl	0.11	0.035	0.02	0.011	0.85	0.551
SL	T10	S3	<dl	<dl	<dl	<dl	<dl	<dl	<dl	<dl	<dl	<dl	0.08	0.043	0.03	0.004	0.7	0.599
LD	T18	S3	<dl	<dl	0.01	0.002	<dl	<dl	<dl	<dl	<dl	<dl	0.4	0.056	0.06	0.007	4.53	0.443
SL	T18	S3	<dl	<dl	0.01	0.008	0.01	0.005	<dl	<dl	<dl	<dl	0.6	0.336	0.09	0.054	8.92	5.547
LD	T25	S3	<dl	<dl	0.01	0.002	0.01	0.005	<dl	<dl	<dl	<dl	0.47	0.318	0.1	0.046	5.38	5.823
SL	T25	S3	<dl	<dl	0.01	0.002	0.01	0.002	<dl	<dl	<dl	<dl	0.46	0.096	0.09	0.037	6.37	1.769

Host algae	Temperature	Salinity	18:2n-6		18:3n-3		20:0		20:1n-9		20:2n-9		22:0	
			mean	sd	mean	sd	mean	sd	mean	sd	mean	sd	mean	sd
LD	T10	S1	9.92	1.743	0.97	0.214	0.04	0.009	0.01	0.005	0.03	0.005	0.02	0.003
SL	T10	S1	10.98	1.901	0.92	0.133	0.03	0.006	0.01	0.001	0.04	0.005	0.02	0.002
LD	T18	S1	9.38	2.822	0.16	0.027	0.03	0.015	0.01	0.002	0.04	0.015	0.02	0.005
SL	T18	S1	6.59	1.594	0.16	0.054	0.02	0.003	0.01	0.002	0.02	0.004	0.01	0.001
LD	T25	S1	10.48	2.265	0.07	0.018	0.02	0.004	0.01	0.005	0.07	0.017	0.02	0.002
SL	T25	S1	8.95	1.945	0.11	0.019	0.02	0.005	0.01	0.001	0.04	0.022	0.02	0.004
LD	T10	S2	8.71	2.021	0.66	0.199	0.04	0.008	0.01	0.003	0.05	0.023	0.01	0.005
SL	T10	S2	4.7	1.691	0.37	0.113	0.02	0.007	0.01	0.002	0.03	0.019	0.01	0.008
LD	T18	S2	6.23	1.565	0.08	0.015	0.02	0.008	<dl	<dl	0.05	0.026	0.01	0.003
SL	T18	S2	8.46	1.561	0.12	0.011	0.03	0.007	0.01	0.003	0.03	0.012	0.01	0.003
LD	T25	S2	14.24	0.745	0.07	0.017	0.04	0.005	0.01	0.003	0.05	0.019	0.02	0.002
SL	T25	S2	14.92	3.861	0.09	0.019	0.05	0.017	0.01	0.004	0.05	0.017	0.04	0.011
LD	T10	S3	1.24	0.743	0.07	0.036	<dl	<dl	<dl	<dl	0.01	0.004	<dl	<dl
SL	T10	S3	1.08	0.697	0.08	0.038	<dl	<dl	<dl	<dl	<dl	<dl	<dl	<dl
LD	T18	S3	4.99	0.463	0.05	0.004	0.02	0.003	0.01	0.002	0.02	0.005	0.01	0.002
SL	T18	S3	7.84	4.272	0.09	0.041	0.03	0.015	0.01	0.005	0.02	0.006	0.01	0.005
LD	T25	S3	7.75	8.020	0.03	0.011	0.02	0.020	0.01	0.006	0.03	0.020	0.02	0.009
SL	T25	S3	7.25	2.175	0.04	0.017	0.02	0.004	0.01	0.003	0.02	0.004	0.01	0.002

Concentrations of the most abundant fatty acids were compared according to temperature and salinity treatments. Figure 1 shows the differences between temperatures for each of these fatty acids per salinity treatment and algal host. For both LD and SL temperature changes induced few modifications of fatty acids concentrations at 23.5 practical salinity units (PSU). Significant changes were observed only for minor fatty acids such as 16:1*n*-7 or 18:3*n*-3 whereas most compounds (including major *P. salina* ones) showed significant changes with temperature at 50 and 70 PSU.

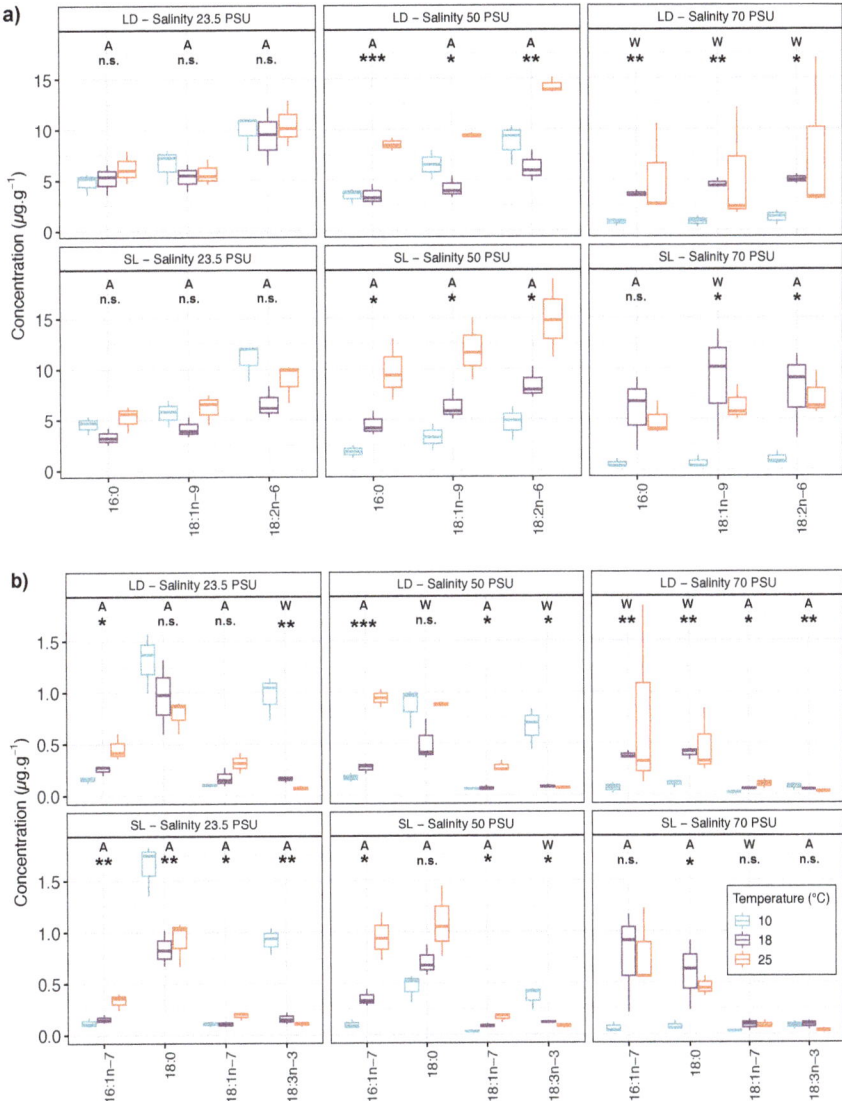

Figure 1. Concentrations ($\mu g\, g^{-1}$) of the 7 most abundant fatty acids. (**a**) Higher concentrations and (**b**) lower concentrations of endophytic *P. salina* isolated from *L. digitata* (LD) or *S. latissima* (SL) and grown at different salinities (23.5, 50 and 70 PSU) and temperatures (10, 18 and 25 °C). One-way Welch ANOVA (W) or One-way ANOVA (A) has been performed depending on the result of Bartlett test: n.s. = not significant, * $p < 0.05$, ** $p < 0.01$, and *** $p < 0.001$.

2.2. Lipid Trajectories

Principal Component Analyses (PCA) were performed using fatty acids relative proportions (in %) for each salinity treatment (Figure 2a–c). The effect of the temperature gradient on fatty acids profiles is displayed for each salinity separately. The PCA allowed to track fatty acids trajectories which corresponded to the path of gradual change in whole fatty acid composition according to T °C. At 70 PSU, no clear trajectories were observed and the PCA ordination explained 55% of the whole inertia in comparison to 61 and 63% for 23.5 and 50 PSU (Figure 2).

Lipid trajectories showed clear opposite directions at 23.5 and 50 PSU between host-algae (LD and SL) meaning that the elevation of temperature induced opposite responses in *P. salina* according to the algal host. Further investigation of lipid trajectories showed an opposition between 18:1*n*-9 and 18:2*n*-6. A fatty acid index (FAI_{18-C}) was calculated using major C18 unsaturated fatty acids relative concentrations (%) :

$$FAI_{18-C} = \frac{[18:2n\text{-}6]}{[18:1n\text{-}9]} \tag{1}$$

FAI_{18-C} was significantly affected by host-algae, temperature and salinity effects (Table 2) but only host-algae:temperature and temperature:salinity interactions were significant.

Table 2. Thee-way analysis of variance (ANOVA) of FAI_{18-C} index as a function of host-algae, temperature and salinity. Normality assumption by group was tested using Shapiro–Wilk. In total, 14 out of 18 groups showed $p > 0.05$. Homogeneity of variance was tested using a Levene's test ($df_1 = 17$, $df_2 = 36$, statistic = 1.19, $p = 0.321$). n.s. = not significant, * $p < 0.05$, and *** $p < 0.001$.

	df	Sum of Square	Mean Squares	F	p-Value	
Host algae (host)	1	0.1020	0.1020	5.661	0.022774	*
Temperature (temp)	2	0.4321	0.2160	11.985	0.000102	***
Salinity (sal)	2	1.2981	0.6491	36.009	2.57×10^{-9}	***
host:temp interaction	2	0.8079	0.4040	22.411	4.76×10^{-7}	***
host:sal interaction	2	0.0098	0.0049	0.272	0.763277	n.s.
temp:sal interaction	4	0.6356	0.1589	8.815	4.55×10^{-5}	***
host:temp:sal interaction	4	0.0804	0.0201	1.115	0.364467	n.s.
Residuals	36	0.6489	0.0180			

It also showed clear opposed linear relationships with temperature according to the algal host (Figure 2d). The index increased with temperature in LD but decreased in SL. At salinities 23.5 and 50 PSU the effect of host algae on FAI_{18-C} was significant as the assumption of homogeneity of slope regression was not met (ANCOVA, interaction host-algae:temperature, $F = 35.509$, $df_n = 1$, $df_d = 14$, $p = 3.49 \times 10^{-5}$ and $F = 34.483$, $df_n = 1$, $df_d = 14$, $p = 4.06 \times 10^{-5}$ respectively). This indicated that slopes of the regression lines were significantly different. At the salinity of 70 PSU, the homogeneity of slope regression was validated (ANCOVA, interaction host-algae:temperature, $F = 2.818$, $p = 0.115$) but the effect of host algae was not significant (ANCOVA–temperature effect: $F = 4.124$, $p = 0.06$, host-algae effect: $F = 0.355$, $p = 0.56$). When regression lines were significantly different, the angle between the two regression lines was calculated (hereafter named α-value). It represented the degree of influence of host-algae in the adaptation of *P. salina* to temperature (Figure 2). This degree of influence was significantly decreasing with salinity (Supplementary Materials Figure S1).

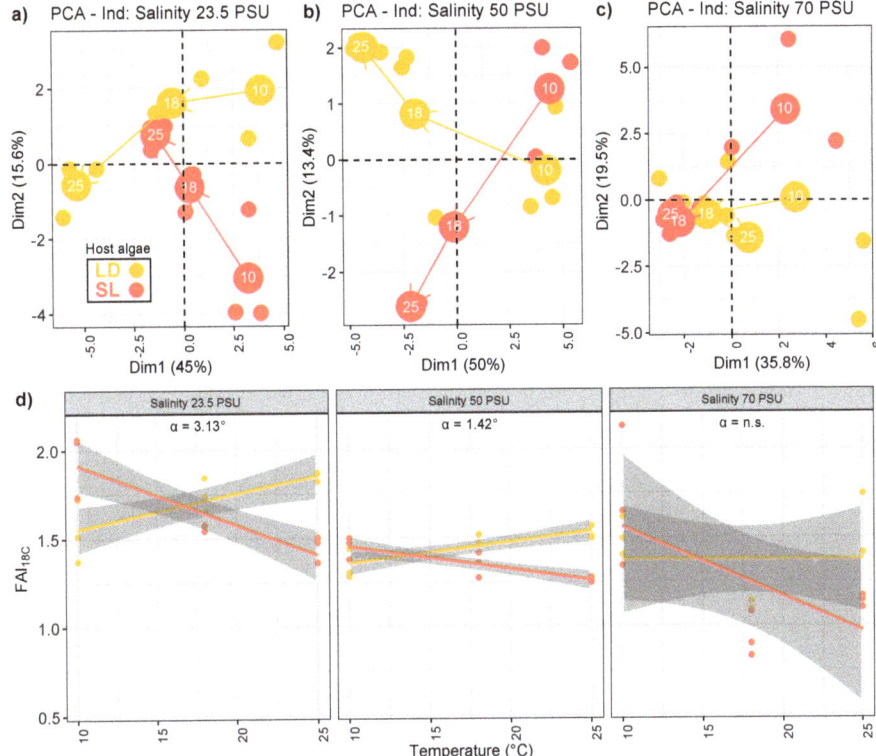

Figure 2. Fatty acid trajectories of endophytic *P. arenaria* isolated from *L. digitata* (LD) or *S. latissima* (SL) grown at different salinities (23.5, 50 and 70 PSU) and different temperatures (10, 18 and 25 °C): (**a**–**c**) PCA scores. (**d**) FAI_{18-C} index calculated with relative contributions (%) of major C18 fatty acids showing opposite trends in the acclimation of *P. salina* to temperature between host algae. α = angle between the two regression lines.

3. Discussion

3.1. Fatty Acid Compositions of P. salina in Relation to Experimental Conditions

The cosmopolitan fungi *P. salina* is widely spread in all type of marine ecosystems, which clearly demonstrate its effective capacity to adapt to diverse temperature and salinity conditions [5,6]. In the present study, salinity levels (including the extreme 70 PSU) did not impact drastically total fatty acid concentrations, except a noticeable decrease at 10 °C and 70 PSU (Supplementary Materials Figure S2), which further illustrate the capacity of the fungi to thrive at salinity conditions well beyond the growth capacity of both host-algae.

Several studies have documented the effect of environmental variables on recruitment, survival, growth, size, biomass and density of kelps, nutrient and light being key factors [16,17]. Along the NE Atlantic (Norwegian) coasts, *L. hyperborea* abundance is, for instance, primarily driven by the interaction between wave exposure and either depth or ocean currents, implying depth-specific effects of wave exposure and wave-specific effects of current speed [18]. In terms of salinity tolerance, *L. digitata* exhibit optimal growth between salinity of 23 and 31 PSU, with a strong reduction of growth at 16 PSU and high mortality below 8 PSU [1]. In a study on Artic kelps, Karsten et al. [19] showed that, on a gradient from 5 to 60 PSU, maximum effective quantum yields (a proxy for photosynthetic efficiency) were measured between 20 and 55 PSU for *L. digitata* and *S. latissima*. Thus, in the present study, while 50 PSU is already a challenging condition; 70 PSU is clearly extreme for these species. Interestingly, despite the recognised phenotypic plasticity of *P. salina* and that the fungi was able to grow at the highest studied salinity without significant loss in total lipid mass, the observed fatty acids trajectories as well as FAI_{18-C} relationships were no longer observed at 70 PSU. This indicated a dynamic relationship of the fatty acid metabolism between *P. salina* and its host-algae and is emphasized by the opposed response to temperature increase between both algal host species.

3.2. Divergent Fatty Acid Trajectories in P. salina Revealed Adaptive Strategies to Temperature Changes

Kelp forests are found on rocky seabeds from temperate to Arctic ecosystems and many species, such as *Laminaria* sp., have an important adaptive capacity to temperature changes [1]. For instance, endemic Arctic *L. solidungula* grow at temperatures between 5 and 16 °C, and cold-temperate NE Pacific species grow between 0 and 18 °C with optima between 5 and 15 °C. The growth range of cold-temperate N Atlantic species extends from 0 to 20 °C with optima between 5 and 15 °C while warm-temperate Atlantic species grow at up to 23–24 °C and have slightly elevated optima [1]. The temperature gradient investigated in the present study is thus within the range of natural temperature conditions.

When submitted to this gradient, endophytic *P. salina* showed divergent fatty acids trajectories as well as FAI_{18-C} relationships depending on the host. At salinities 23.5 and 50 PSU the effect of host algae on FAI_{18-C} was significant. The host effect was more pronounced at 23.5 than at 50 PSU as shown by the α-value and disappeared at the extreme 70 PSU which indicated that the opposition in lipid metabolism and C18 trajectories between LD and SL are conserved throughout the salinity gradient although severe (50 PSU) and extreme (70 PSU) salinities did impact *P. salina* fatty acid metabolism.

In *L. digitata* C18 fatty acids and especially linoleic acid (18:2n-6) are essential in the response of the algae against stressful conditions such as the perception of pathogenic metabolites [20] or against grazing by specialised herbivorous species [21]. The response, in all cases, imply an oxidative stress and the activation of fatty acid oxidation cascades [22]. For instance, early events in the perception of pathogens lipopolysaccharides in this brown alga include the production of 13-hydroxyoctadecadienoic acid (13-HODE) as a result of the oxydation of 18:2n-6 by lipoxygenase activity [20]. A decrease in fatty acid occurs in *S. latissima* during the early development from gametes to gametophytes. The decrease was significant for 18:1n-9, from 45 to 30% of total fatty acids, suggesting that it might be important in the transition from storage lipids to photo-autotrophic strategies [23]. Thus, an increase in FAI_{18-C} in laminariales is likely associated to the redirection of the algal lipid metabolism toward photosynthesis or defence to the detriment of storage lipids.

Homeoviscous and homeophasic adaptations, which is the process of keeping adequate membrane fluidity, as a response to temperature changes are well documented for microorganisms. Degree of unsaturation, variation in chain length, branching and cyclization of fatty acids are known adaptative strategies to enhance membrane fluidity. A considerable decrease in 18:1 and the marked increase in 18:2 or 18:3 with lower temperatures have already been observed in bacteria, fungus and yeast [24]. In the present study, any decrease in temperature is thus expected to induce an increase in FAI_{18-C} as a response. However, this expected relationship was noticed only when the fungal endophyte was isolated from *S. latissima* and, intriguingly, it exhibited an opposite trend when isolated from *L. digitata*.

In absence of dedicated temperature experiments on both *L. digitata* and *S. latissima*, it is difficult to conclude on whether *P. salina* lipid metabolism was fully aligned with its host requirements. However, the observed opposed trend in lipid trajectories between the endophytic fungi of the two hosts revealed a temperature-response that was clearly host dependant.

Host species originated from separate areas (Roscoff-FR and Oban-UK for LD and SL respectively) which, despite being slightly warmer in average (2.6 $\pm$ 0.4) in Roscoff, are relatively similar in terms of sea surface temperature and salinity (SST NOAA). It is thus very likely that the two fungal strains originated from two different populations that were each adapted to their Laminariale host.

Unfortunately, we do not have precise genomics information about the two endophytic strains (other than ITS barcode sequencing) to validate this hypothesis.

However, previous comparative metabolomics on the same endophytic strains, and seven additional *P. salina* isolates from various brown algae, have demonstrated a clearly divergent metabolome between algal species as well as orders (i.e., Fucales vs. Laminariales) [8]. Altogether, the present findings highlight the plasticity of the fungus to adapt to a new environment (i.e., the hosting algae). The fact that the host influenced the expression of *P. salina* metabolome may reflect epigenetic mechanisms as changes in metabolome expression [8] and lipid trajectories (this study) might be conserved across multiple generations.

4. Materials and Methods

4.1. Reagents and Chemicals

Following solvents were used: Sigma-Aldrich methanol ≥ 99.9% Cat No. 34860; ethanol ≥ 99.8% Cat No. 51976; chloroform ≥ 99% Cat No. C7559; hexane ≥ 99% Cat No. 139386. Following reagents were used for fatty acid purification and identification: BF3-methanol (boron-trifluoride methanol, Supelco®, CAS Number: 373-57-9, Cat No. 15716) for derivatization; Sigma-Aldrich tricosanoic acid analytical standards (Sigma-Aldrich–C23–Methyl tricosanoate, CAS Number: 2433-97-8, Cat No. T9900) as internal standard; Supelco® 37 Component FAME Mix, Cat No. CRM47885n, Marine source, Cat No. 47033, and Bacterial Mix, Cat No. 47080-U for fatty acid identification.

4.2. Strain Isolation, Cultivation and Identification

P. salina strains LD40H and SL540T were previously isolated from *L. digitata* (LD) and *S. latissima* (SL) respectively. Complete isolation, cultivation and molecular identification procedures are reported in Vallet et al. [2]. Briefly, three individuals of each species were collected during spring tide and processed within two hours of collection. Algae organs of 5 cm^2 (receptacles, thalli, stipes, fronds and holdfasts) were excised and surface-sterilized by sequential immersion in Ethanol 70% (30 s), in NaCl 0.1% (30 s) and washed three times (30 s) in sterilized sea water [25,26]. Algal segments were plated on solid media (malt extract agar, Millipore) with the internal tissues in contact with the medium and solidified with 20 g·L^{-1} of purified agar. Strains corresponded to *P. salina*, a strictly marine fungus identified with ITS sequencing from all brown algal species investigated [2].

4.3. Experimental Design

Fungal endophytic strains LD40H and SL540T were grown on solid medium Malt Extract Agar for 21 days with 12 h photo-period under both temperature and salinity stress conditions. Several salinity concentrations were tested ranging from low ([NaCl] = 23.5 g·L^{-1}), elevated ([NaCl] = 50 g·L^{-1}) to extreme conditions ([NaCl] = 70 g·L^{-1}). Three incubation temperatures were also tested within the growth range of natural LD and SL population in the temperate Atlantic ocean (10 °C, 18 °C and 25 °C). Experiments were conducted in biological triplicates.

4.4. Fatty Acid Extraction

Fatty acid (FA) analysis was performed following the modified method of Bligh and Dyer [27] as modified by [28,29]. Before extraction, an internal standard (23:0) was added to every sample for quantification purpose (0.5 mg mL^{-1}). Lipids were extracted with a 20 min ultrasonication (sonication bath, 80 kHz, Fisherbrand™) in a mixture of distilled water, chloroform and methanol in ratio 1:1:2 (v:v:v, in mL). Lipids were concentrated under N$_2$ flux, and saponified, in order to separate FA, with a mixture of NaOH (2 mol L^{-1}) and methanol (1:2, v:v, in mL) at 90 °C during 90 min. Saponification was stopped with 500 µL hydrochloric acid. Samples were then incubated with BF3-methanol at 90 °C during 10 min to transform free fatty acids into fatty acids methyl esters (FAME), which were isolated and kept frozen in chloroform. Just before analysis, samples were dried under N$_2$ flux and transferred to hexane. One µL of the mixture was injected in a gas chromatograph (GC, Varian CP-3800 equipped with flame ionization detector), which allowed separation and quantification of FAME. Separation was performed with a Supelco® OMEGAWAX 320 column (30 m × 0.32 mm i.d., 0.25 µm film thickness) with He as carrier gas. The following temperature program was used: 60 °C for 1 min, then raise to 150 °C at 40 °C·min^{-1} (held 3 min), then raise to 240 °C at 3 °C·min^{-1} (held 7 min) at 1 mL min^{-1}. FAME Peaks were identified by comparison of the retention time with analytical standards. Additional identification of the samples was performed using a gas chromatograph coupled to mass spectrometer (GC-MS, Varian 450GC with Varian 220-MS). Compounds annotation was performed by comparing mass spectra with NIST 2017 library. Fatty acids were quantified using the FID detector and the internal standard (C23). Corresponding fatty acids are designated as X:Yn-Z, where X is the number of carbons, Y the number of double bonds and Z the position of the ultimate double bond from the terminal methyl (see [30] for additional information about naming convention).

4.5. Statistics

All statistical analyses were performed using R version 3.5.3 [31] and packages reshape [32], ggplot2 [32], rstatix [33], ade4 [34], factoextra [35] and cowplot [36] for data processing and visualisation. Raw GC-FID text file data together with in-house R script for data processing, univariate and multivariate statistics as well as figures are available at github repository: https://github.com/Hubas-prog/Paradendryphiella_traject.

4.5.1. Univariate

Comparisons in fatty acids concentrations were performed using Analysis of Variances (ANOVA) after prior verification of the normality of the residuals (Shapiro test) and equality of variance (Bartlett test). When Bartlett test indicated that homoscedasticity was not met, one-way Welch's ANOVA (for unequal variances) was performed otherwise, classical one-way ANOVA was used.

Analysis of covariance (ANCOVA) was performed to compare FAI_{18-C} index between temperatures within each salinity treatments. Linearity was inspected visually and homogeneity of regression slopes was checked by testing the interaction between temperature and host-algae. Regression lines were considered different if slopes were different. When slopes were not significantly different, the ANCOVA was performed by checking the presence of outliers and by removing the interaction effect to adjust the ANCOVA model.

4.5.2. Multivariate

Lipid trajectories were calculated using Principal Component Analysis (PCA). PCA allowed to track fatty acids changes in relative proportion in the whole fatty acid profile rather than in a given compound. The aim was to check whether fatty acid trajectories were convergent, divergent or alike in response to temperature increase. Trajectories were studied by comparing PCA scores (i.e., individuals) between host-algae and within each salinity treatment. PCA loadings (i.e., variables) was inspected visually to detect which fatty acids were responsible for lipid trajectories. Univariate staticitics were then performed as described above to validate any changes.

Supplementary Materials: The following are available online at http://www.mdpi.com/1660-3397/18/8/379/s1, Figure S1: α value as a function of salinity; Figure S2: Total fatty acid concentrations of *P. salina*.

Author Contributions: Conceptualization, S.P. and M.V.; Validation, C.H., T.M. and S.P.; Formal analysis, C.H.; Investigation, M.V., S.P., N.T.; Resources, M.V. and S.P.; Data curation, C.H.; Writing–original draft preparation, C.H.; Writing-review and editing, C.H., M.V., T.M., and S.P.; Visualization, C.H.; Supervision, S.P., C.H. and T.M.; Project administration, S.P. and C.H.; Funding acquisition, S.P. and C.H. All authors have read and agreed to the published version of the manuscript.

Funding: This research was funded by the French CNRS-INSU EC2CO program—project "ISLAY".

Acknowledgments: The authors thank the two anonymous reviewers for their constructive comments.

Conflicts of Interest: The authors declare no conflict of interest. The funders had no role in the design of the study; in the collection, analyses, or interpretation of data; in the writing of the manuscript, or in the decision to publish the results.

Abbreviations

The following abbreviations are used in this manuscript:

LD	*Laminaria digitata*
MPB	Microphytobenthos
MUFA	Monounsaturated fatty acid
PUFA	Polyunsaturated fatty acid
QS	Quorum Sensing
SFA	Saturated fatty acid
SL	*Saccharina latissima*
TFA	Total Fatty Acids
PSU	practical salinity units
ANOVA	analysis of variance
PCA	principal component analyses
FAME	Fatty acid methyl esters
NIST	National Institute of Standards and Technology
FID	flame ionization detector

References

1. Bartsch, I.; Wiencke, C.; Bischof, K.; Buchholz, C.M.; Buck, B.H.; Eggert, A.; Feuerpfeil, P.; Hanelt, D.; Jacobsen, S.; Karez, R.; et al. The genus Laminaria sensu lato: Recent insights and developments. *Eur. J. Phycol.* **2008**, *43*, 1–86. [CrossRef]
2. Vallet, M.; Strittmatter, M.; Murúa, P.; Lacoste, S.; Dupont, J.; Hubas, C.; Genta-Jouve, G.; Gachon, C.M.M.; Kim, G.H.; Prado, S. Chemically-Mediated Interactions Between Macroalgae, Their Fungal Endophytes, and Protistan Pathogens. *Front. Microbiol.* **2018**, *9*. [CrossRef] [PubMed]
3. Sutherland, G.K. Marine Fungi Imperfecti. *New Phytol.* **1916**, *15*, 35–48. [CrossRef]
4. Michaelis, K.C.; Gessner, R.V.; Romano, M.A. Population Genetics and Systematics of Marine Species of Dendryphiella. *Mycologia* **1987**, *79*, 514–518. [CrossRef]
5. Dela Cruz, T.E.; Wagner, S.; Schulz, B. Physiological responses of marine Dendryphiella species from different geographical locations. *Mycol. Prog.* **2006**, *5*, 108–119. [CrossRef]
6. Kireev, Y.V.; Konovalova, O.P.; Myuge, N.S.; Shnyreva, A.V.; Bubnova, E.N. Cultural properties and taxonomic position of Helminthosporium-like fungal isolates from the White Sea. *Microbiology* **2015**, *84*, 665–676. [CrossRef]
7. Tourneroche, A.; Lami, R.; Hubas, C.; Blanchet, E.; Vallet, M.; Escoubeyrou, K.; Paris, A.; Prado, S. Bacterial–Fungal Interactions in the Kelp Endomicrobiota Drive Autoinducer-2 Quorum Sensing. *Front. Microbiol.* **2019**, *10*, 1693. [CrossRef]
8. Vallet, M.; Chong, Y.M.; Tourneroche, A.; Genta-Jouve, G.; Hubas, C.; Lami, R.; Gachon, C.; Klochkova, T.; Chan, K.G.; Prado, S. Novel α-hydroxy γ-butenolides of kelp endophytes disrupt bacterial cell-to-cell signaling. *Front. Mar. Sci.* **2020**. [CrossRef]
9. Pilgaard, B.; Wilkens, C.; Herbst, F.A.; Vuillemin, M.; Rhein-Knudsen, N.; Meyer, A.S.; Lange, L. Proteomic enzyme analysis of the marine fungus Paradendryphiella salina reveals alginate lyase as a minimal adaptation strategy for brown algae degradation. *Sci. Rep.* **2019**, *9*, 1–13. [CrossRef]
10. Barbosa, M.; Fernandes, F.; Pereira, D.M.; Azevedo, I.C.; Sousa-Pinto, I.; Andrade, P.B.; Valentão, P. Fatty acid patterns of the kelps Saccharina latissima, Saccorhiza polyschides and Laminaria ochroleuca: Influence of changing environmental conditions. *Arab. J. Chem.* **2020**, *13*, 45–58. [CrossRef]
11. Dawczynski, C.; Schubert, R.; Jahreis, G. Amino acids, fatty acids, and dietary fibre in edible seaweed products. *Food Chem.* **2007**, *103*, 891–899. [CrossRef]
12. Weete, J.D. Fatty Acids. In *Lipid Biochemistry of Fungi and Other Organisms*; Springer: Boston, MA, USA, 1980; pp. 49–95. [CrossRef]

13. Bärenstrauch, M.; Mann, S.; Jacquemin, C.; Bibi, S.; Sylla, O.K.; Baudouin, E.; Buisson, D.; Prado, S.; Kunz, C. Molecular crosstalk between the endophyte Paraconiothyrium variabile and the phytopathogen Fusarium oxysporum—Modulation of lipoxygenase activity and beauvericin production during the interaction. *Fungal Genet. Biol.* **2020**, *139*, 103383. [CrossRef] [PubMed]
14. Fischer, G.J.; Keller, N.P. Production of cross-kingdom oxylipins by pathogenic fungi: An update on their role in development and pathogenicity. *J. Microbiol.* **2016**, *54*, 254–264. [CrossRef] [PubMed]
15. Savchenko, T.V.; Zastrijnaja, O.M.; Klimov, V.V. Oxylipins and plant abiotic stress resistance. *Biochemistry* **2014**, *79*, 362–375. [CrossRef] [PubMed]
16. Hurd, C.L. Water motion, marine macroalgal physiology, and production. *J. Phycol.* **2000**, *36*, 453–472. [CrossRef]
17. Norton, T.; Mathieson, A.; Neushul, M. A Review of Some Aspects of Form and Function in Seaweeds. *Bot. Mar.* **1982**, *25*, 501–510. [CrossRef]
18. Bekkby, T.; Smit, C.; Gundersen, H.; Rinde, E.; Steen, H.; Tveiten, L.; Gitmark, J.K.; Fredriksen, S.; Albretsen, J.; Christie, H.C. The abundance of kelp is modified by the combined impact of depth, waves and currents. *Front. Mar. Sci.* **2019**, *6*. [CrossRef]
19. Karsten, U. Research note: Salinity tolerance of Arctic kelps from Spitsbergen. *Phycol. Res.* **2007**, *55*, 257–262. [CrossRef]
20. Küpper, F.C.; Gaquerel, E.; Boneberg, E.M.; Morath, S.; Salaün, J.P.; Potin, P. Early events in the perception of lipopolysaccharides in the brown alga Laminaria digitata include an oxidative burst and activation of fatty acid oxidation cascades. *J. Exp. Bot.* **2006**, *57*, 1991–1999. [CrossRef]
21. Ritter, A.; Cabioch, L.; Brillet-Guéguen, L.; Corre, E.; Cosse, A.; Dartevelle, L.; Duruflé, H.; Fasshauer, C.; Goulitquer, S.; Thomas, F.; et al. Herbivore-induced chemical and molecular responses of the kelps Laminaria digitata and Lessonia spicata. *PLoS ONE* **2017**, *12*, e0173315. [CrossRef]
22. Küpper, F.C.; Gaquerel, E.; Cosse, A.; Adas, F.; Peters, A.F.; Müller, D.G.; Kloareg, B.; Salaün, J.P.; Potin, P. Free Fatty Acids and Methyl Jasmonate Trigger Defense Reactions in Laminaria digitata. *Plant Cell Physiol.* **2009**, *50*, 789–800. [CrossRef] [PubMed]
23. Steinhoff, F.S.; Graeve, M.; Wiencke, C.; Wulff, A.; Bischof, K. Lipid content and fatty acid consumption in zoospores/developing gametophytes of Saccharina latissima (Laminariales, Phaeophyceae) as potential precursors for secondary metabolites as phlorotannins. *Polar Biol.* **2011**, *34*, 1011–1018. [CrossRef]
24. Neidleman, S.L. Effects of temperature on lipid unsaturation. *Biotechnol. Genet. Eng. Rev.* **1987**, *5*, 245–268. [CrossRef] [PubMed]
25. Kjer, J.; Debbab, A.; Aly, A.H.; Proksch, P. Methods for isolation of marine-derived endophytic fungi and their bioactive secondary products. *Nat. Protoc.* **2010**, *5*, 479–490. [CrossRef]
26. Kientz, B.; Thabard, M.; Cragg, S.M.; Pope, J.; Hellio, C. A new method for removing microflora from macroalgal surfaces: An important step for natural product discovery. *Bot. Mar.* **2011**, *54*, 457–469. [CrossRef]
27. Bligh, E.G.; Dyer, W.J. A Rapid Method of Total Lipid Extraction and Purification. *Can. J. Biochem. Physiol.* **1959**, *37*, 911–917. [CrossRef]
28. Meziane, T.; Tsuchiya, M. Fatty acids as tracers of organic matter in the sediment and food web of a mangrove/intertidal flat ecosystem, Okinawa, Japan. *Mar. Ecol. Prog. Ser.* **2000**, *200*, 49–57. [CrossRef]
29. Passarelli, C.; Meziane, T.; Thiney, N.; Boeuf, D.; Jesus, B.; Ruivo, M.; Jeanthon, C.; Hubas, C. Seasonal variations of the composition of microbial biofilms in sandy tidal flats: Focus of fatty acids, pigments and exopolymers. *Estuarine Coast. Shelf Sci.* **2015**, *153*, 29–37. [CrossRef]
30. Fahy, E.; Subramaniam, S.; Brown, H.A.; Glass, C.K.; Merrill, A.H.; Murphy, R.C.; Raetz, C.R.; Russell, D.W.; Seyama, Y.; Shaw, W.; et al. A comprehensive classification system for lipids. *J. Lipid Res.* **2005**, *46*, 839–861. [CrossRef]
31. R Core Team. *R: A Language and Environment for Statistical Computing*; R Foundation for Statistical Computing: Vienna, Austria, 2019.
32. Wickham, H. *ggplot2: Elegant Graphics for Data Analysis*; Springer: New York, NY, USA, 2016.
33. Kassambara, A. rstatix: Pipe-Friendly Framework for Basic Statistical Tests; 2020. Available online: https://CRAN.R-project.org/package=rstatix (accessed on 21 May 2020).
34. Dray, S.; Dufour, A.B. The ade4 Package: Implementing the Duality Diagram for Ecologists. *J. Stat. Softw.* **2007**, *22*, 1–20. [CrossRef]

35. Kassambara, A.; Mundt, F. *Factoextra: Extract and Visualize the Results of Multivariate Data Analyses*; 2019. Available online: https://CRAN.R-project.org/package=factoextra (accessed on 21 May 2020).
36. Wilke, C.O. cowplot: Streamlined Plot Theme and Plot Annotations for ggplot2; 2019. Available online: https://CRAN.R-project.org/package=cowplot (accessed on 21 May 2020).

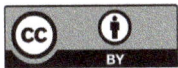 © 2020 by the authors. Licensee MDPI, Basel, Switzerland. This article is an open access article distributed under the terms and conditions of the Creative Commons Attribution (CC BY) license (http://creativecommons.org/licenses/by/4.0/).

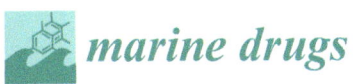

Review

Bioactivities of Lipid Extracts and Complex Lipids from Seaweeds: Current Knowledge and Future Prospects

Diana Lopes [1,2], Felisa Rey [1,2], Miguel C. Leal [3], Ana I. Lillebø [3], Ricardo Calado [3] and Maria Rosário Domingues [1,2,*]

1. Centre for Environmental and Marine Studies, CESAM, Department of Chemistry, Santiago University Campus, University of Aveiro, 3810-193 Aveiro, Portugal; dianasalzedaslopes@ua.pt (D.L.); felisa.rey@ua.pt (F.R.)
2. Mass Spectrometry Centre, LAQV-REQUIMTE, Department of Chemistry, Santiago University Campus, University of Aveiro, 3810-193 Aveiro, Portugal
3. ECOMARE, Centre for Environmental and Marine Studies, CESAM, Department of Biology, Santiago University Campus, University of Aveiro, 3810-193 Aveiro, Portugal; miguelcleal@ua.pt (M.C.L.); lillebo@ua.pt (A.I.L.); rjcalado@ua.pt (R.C.)
* Correspondence: mrd@ua.pt

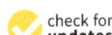

Citation: Lopes, D.; Rey, F.; Leal, M.C.; Lillebø, A.I.; Calado, R.; Domingues, M.R. Bioactivities of Lipid Extracts and Complex Lipids from Seaweeds: Current Knowledge and Future Prospects. *Mar. Drugs* **2021**, *19*, 686. https://doi.org/10.3390/md19120686

Academic Editor: Bill J. Baker

Received: 5 November 2021
Accepted: 28 November 2021
Published: 30 November 2021

Publisher's Note: MDPI stays neutral with regard to jurisdictional claims in published maps and institutional affiliations.

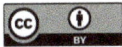

Copyright: © 2021 by the authors. Licensee MDPI, Basel, Switzerland. This article is an open access article distributed under the terms and conditions of the Creative Commons Attribution (CC BY) license (https:// creativecommons.org/licenses/by/ 4.0/).

Abstract: While complex lipids of seaweeds are known to display important phytochemical properties, their full potential is yet to be explored. This review summarizes the findings of a systematic survey of scientific publications spanning over the years 2000 to January 2021 retrieved from Web of Science (WoS) and Scopus databases to map the state of the art and identify knowledge gaps on the relationship between the complex lipids of seaweeds and their reported bioactivities. Eligible publications (270 in total) were classified in five categories according to the type of studies using seaweeds as raw biomass (category 1); studies using organic extracts (category 2); studies using organic extracts with identified complex lipids (category 3); studies of extracts enriched in isolated groups or classes of complex lipids (category 4); and studies of isolated complex lipids molecular species (category 5), organized by seaweed phyla and reported bioactivities. Studies that identified the molecular composition of these bioactive compounds in detail (29 in total) were selected and described according to their bioactivities (antitumor, anti-inflammatory, antimicrobial, and others). Overall, to date, the value for seaweeds in terms of health and wellness effects were found to be mostly based on empirical knowledge. Although lipids from seaweeds are little explored, the published work showed the potential of lipid extracts, fractions, and complex lipids from seaweeds as functional ingredients for the food and feed, cosmeceutical, and pharmaceutical industries. This knowledge will boost the use of the chemical diversity of seaweeds for innovative value-added products and new biotechnological applications.

Keywords: algae; bioactivity; glycolipids; lipidomics; macroalgae; phospholipids; seaweeds

1. Introduction

Marine macroalgae, popularly known as seaweeds, have emerged as one of the contributors to achieve United Nations sustainable development goals (SDG) [1]. Indeed, algae can be used in healthy and sustainable diets, thereby meeting the farm to fork strategy, which is the core of the European Green Deal [2,3]. Moreover, they are a rich source of nutrients and valuable bioactive phytochemicals that act as preventive agents against non-communicable diseases [4] and that can contribute to overcome multiple societal challenges, such as the ongoing fight on obesity [5] and on the issues caused by antimicrobial resistance in microorganisms [6,7]. Additionally, their chemical diversity can also be paramount to fight infectious viral diseases and allow a higher efficiency when tackling future pandemic situations [7,8]. The exploitation of seaweeds as marine resources for new high value-added products thus contributes to increase their economic relevance on multiple niche markets [9].

Seaweeds, have been used since earliest times as a source of food and in traditional medicine in Asian and other seacoast countries around the world [1]. Although their generalized value for human nutrition and health is already recognized, it is mostly based on empirical knowledge. Seaweeds are reservoirs of bioactive compounds [10] yet to be fully used in a plethora of blue biotechnology applications [11], such as functional foods and feeds, pharmaceutical, nutraceutical [12], cosmeceutical [13], and other high-end uses.

Well-known phytochemicals have already been recorded from seaweeds, including polysaccharides, proteins, pigments, and other minor compounds such as phenolics and vitamins [14]. Seaweed lipids are a less abundant fraction of such bioactive phytochemicals that, despite their great value, remain largely over-looked, likely because of their lower content, high structural diversity, and complexity, along with a rather poorly understood biological activity. They are mainly known as reservoirs of omega-3 polyunsaturated fatty acids (PUFA) with well-recognized health benefits [15]. Nevertheless, seaweeds also have complex lipids, such as phospholipids (PLs) and glycolipids (GLs), which display unique features that are not found in terrestrial plants, such as being esterified with omega-3 fatty acids (FA), including eicosapentaenoic acid (EPA) and docosahexaenoic acid (DHA) [16,17]. Marine PLs have better bioavailability, resistance to oxidation, and higher content of omega-3 PUFA than lipids from other sources. Moreover, they are better at delivering dietary omega-3 PUFA than terrestrial PLs, as already demonstrated in several comparative studies [18–21]. On the other hand, and unlike their terrestrial analogues, GLs from seaweeds contain long chain PUFA (20 or more carbon atoms) with potential biotechnological applications [22]. PLs and GLs play a structural role in biological systems, representing the major building blocks of cytoplasmatic and chloroplast membranes [23]. They are also the main carriers of PUFA [24,25].

Recently, complex lipids are being considered, promising phytochemicals with intrinsic bioactive properties, including antioxidant, antitumor, anti-inflammatory, and antimicrobial [7,26,27], fostering potential applications in pharmaceutical, nutraceutical, and cosmeceutical fields (Figure 1) [28]. However, the complexity and structural diversity of complex lipids are hindering their detailed characterization and exploitation. Most published works describing seaweed bioactive lipids refer to assays of total lipid extracts or enriched fractions [29–31], and few studies are focused on the identification and characterization of complex lipids, making it difficult to establish a clear structure–activity relationship. Nevertheless, the rapid development of modern -omics approaches and bioinformatic tools in recent years have been contributing to achieve a detailed mapping of the lipidome of seaweeds from different phyla. Selected species to date include *Ulva rigida* and *Codium tomentosum* from Chlorophyta phylum [32,33]; *Chondrus crispus*, *Palmaria palmata*, *Porphyra dioica*, *Gracilaria* sp. from Rhodophyta phylum [27,34–36]; and *Fucus vesiculosus*, *Saccharina latissima*, *Sargassum muticum*, and *Bifurcaria bifurcata* from Ochrophyta phylum [37–39]. The comparison of seaweeds lipidome revealed unique lipid signatures [40]. While some phylum-specific trends could perceived, lipidomic signatures were rather species-specific [40]. More work is needed to achieve a larger coverage of seaweeds lipidome to fully unravel the specificity of their signatures and support value added uses of these marine bioresources.

Despite its biotechnological potential, our knowledge on naturally occurring bioactive complex lipids from seaweeds is still in its infancy. Only recently sustainably farmed seaweeds have emerged in Europe [41]. The production of seaweeds biomass under controlled conditions has promoted the safeguarding of high food safety standards, and subsequently generated interest in the bioprospecting for new compounds, namely complex lipids, for high-end biotechnological uses. For now, questions such as the relationship between bioactivities already detected and complex lipid structures and their specificity remain to be answered.

The authors have performed a systematic review of scientific literature to establish the state of the art of our knowledge on naturally occurring bioactive complex lipids from seaweeds. The information here assembled provides new insights on how studies are being performed and allows the identification of gaps in knowledge that still need attention in upcoming years.

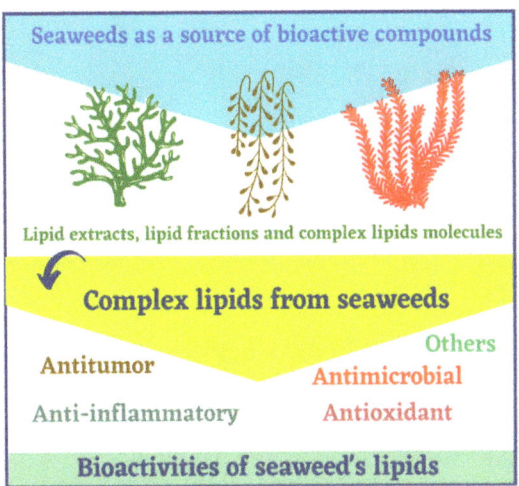

Figure 1. Complex lipids from seaweeds as bioactive compounds with reported bioactivities.

2. Methods

This systematic review followed the Preferred Reporting Items for Systematic Reviews and Meta-Analysis (PRISMA-P) guidelines [42]. We used two databases to retrieve scientific publications: Web of Science (WoS) (www.webofknowledge.com, accessed on 21 January 2021) and Scopus (www.scopus.com, accessed on 25 January 2021). A comprehensive search on the bioactivity of complex lipids from seaweeds was performed based on a query by topic (title, abstract and keywords) of the terms: ((alga* OR seaweed* OR macroalga*) AND ("complex lipid*" OR lipid* OR glycolipid* OR phospholipid*) AND (bioactiv* OR activ*)); spanning over the years 2000 to January 2021. The search query resulted in 3114 papers that were subsequently reviewed by the authors, of which 270 were considered eligible for the present work. From those publications, 29 were included in a more in-depth analysis according to criteria described below (Figure 2).

Selection of Eligibility and Exclusion Criteria

The eligibility and exclusion criteria (Figure 2) were as follows: publication type (1); matrices studied (2); and extraction method using organic solvents (3). In line with the eligibility criteria selected, only journal articles with empirical data were considered (1); only studies reporting bioactivity assays using seaweeds were considered, and studies using seaweeds and mixed were also considered (2); and studies reporting assays with extracts obtained using organic solvents (e.g., n-hexane, diethyl ether, dichloromethane, n-butanol, chloroform, ethyl acetate, acetone, ethanol, and methanol) were considered (3). The following studies were excluded: reviews, book chapters, proceeding papers, conference papers, and notes (1); studies reporting bioactivity from organisms other than seaweeds (2); and studies using water extracts (3). A total of 270 publications were considered eligible, with these subsequently being screened using the following sub-criteria: only studies identifying an isolated complex lipid group, classes, or species, or reaching a molecular structure were considered for a more in-depth analysis to assess a structure–function relationship. After applying these sub criteria, 29 publications were selected, with these being discussed in detail in Section 3.1.

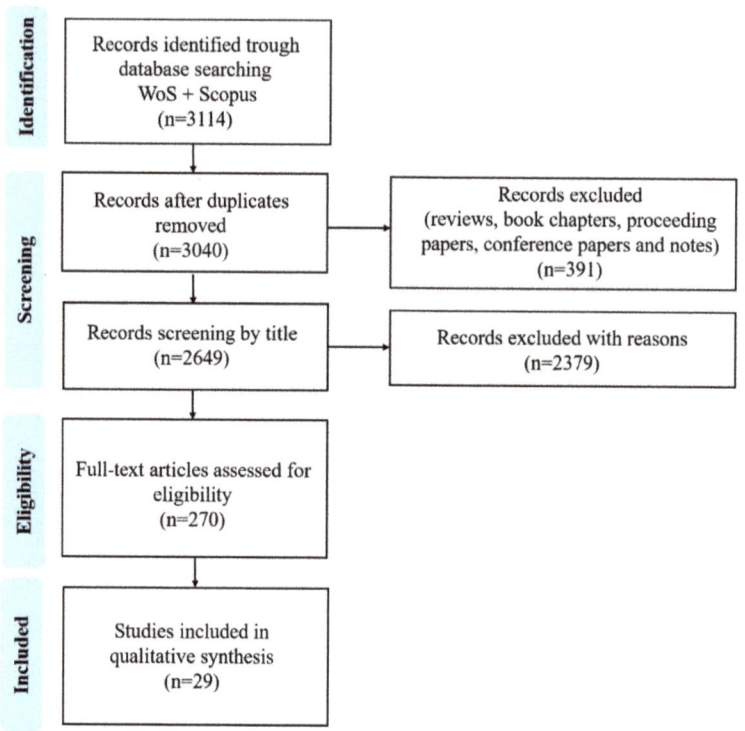

Figure 2. Schematic review selection process performed according to PRISMA 2020 flow diagram [42].

3. Results and Discussion

After applying the eligibility criteria adopted in the present work, 270 publications were considered for further analysis. These publications were evaluated taking in account the methodological approaches employed to perform bioassays, namely in vitro versus in vivo studies. Data analysis revealed that 178 publications referred to in vitro experiments, 73 to in vivo assays, and 19 included both in vitro and in vivo assays (Figure 3). It was also possible to record those in vivo assays included experimental work usually framed within two different approaches: (i) raw seaweed biomass; or (ii) organic extracts administrated intragastrical or in the diet as additives or feed supplements (Figure 3). Papers that described in vitro assays aimed to evaluate bioactive properties of organic extracts, and in some papers, complex lipids were identified or isolated. The papers that describe both in vitro and in vivo results, evaluated bioactive activities of organic extracts using in vitro assays and also the biological effects after oral administration performed mainly in animal models.

Data (270 publications) were plotted in a word cloud (Figure 4) featuring seaweed genus. This representation highlighted genera *Sargassum*, *Fucus*, *Dictyota*, and *Padina* (Ochrophyta; brown seaweeds), genera *Ulva* and *Codium* (Chlorophyta; green seaweeds), and genera *Gracilaria* (Rhodophyta; red seaweeds) as the most reported seaweeds with known bioactivities.

To assess the biological effects reported in eligible studies, data was plotted considering the most frequently prospected bioactivities in the 270 eligible publications (Figure 5). Antioxidant activity (138 studies) was the most reported bioactivity, followed by antimicrobial (61 studies), antitumor (30 studies), anti-inflammatory (19 studies) activities, fat reduction (12 studies), and growth performance (7 studies). Other bioactivities included a wide range of different actions, which was not possible to group within a specific classification. It was also possible to record that most bioactivities reported were related to antioxidant or anti-inflammatory activities; the accurate bioactivity or bioactivities reported on each of these studies are summarized in Table S1.

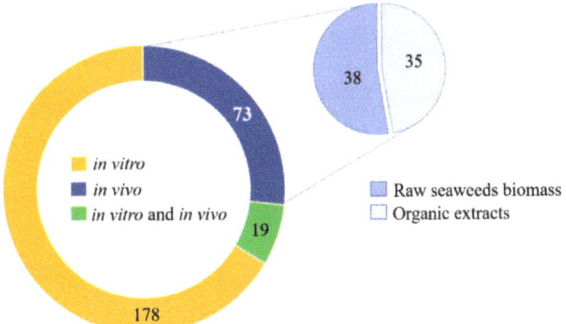

Figure 3. Number of eligible studies that recorded bioactivity on raw seaweed biomass or seaweeds organic extracts, distributed by type of performed assays (in vitro, in vivo and both in vitro and in vivo).

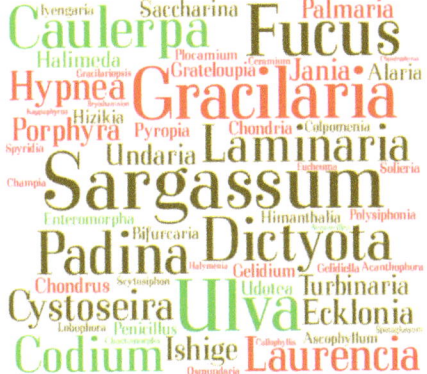

Figure 4. Word cloud assembled using the genera of seaweed species reported in the 270 eligible publications that reported bioactivity on raw seaweed biomass or seaweeds organic extracts. Genera featured with a larger size in the word cloud indicate that species within those genera were the ones mostly reported. Words in brown, green and red refer to genus within phylum Ochrophyta, Chlorophyta, and Rhodophyta, respectively (brown, green, and red seaweeds, respectively).

Data (270 publications) was also ranked based on biomass of various seaweeds, or their extracts used in the bioassays performed, being grouped in five categories: studies using seaweed as raw seaweed biomass (category 1); studies using organic extracts (category 2); studies using organic extracts with identified complex lipids (category 3); studies of extracts enriched in isolated groups or classes of complex lipids (category 4); and studies of isolated complex lipid molecular species (category 5).

In some of the selected categories (e.g., category 1 and 2) most studies did not highlight the identification of lipids, neither attributed the bioactivity reported to lipids. However, to our knowledge, the role of complex lipids in the observed bioactivity cannot be excluded. The distribution of eligible studies by category 1-5 and bioactivity assayed is summarized in Figure 6. Most studies were classified according to category 2 (177 studies), followed by category 1 (39 studies) and 3 (25 studies). Category 4 and 5 displayed a smaller number of studies (18 and 11, respectively). Category 1 included studies addressing the improvement of growth and/or immune system/health status, fat reduction, including reduction in hyperlipidemia/cholesterolemia/triglycerides, anti-obesity/anti-adipogenic effects; antioxidant and other activities (Table S1). Studies related with categories 2 to 5 pinpoint antioxidant, antitumor, anti-inflammatory, and antimicrobial (including antibacterial, antiviral, anti-protozoal, anti-microalgal, and anti-fouling) bioactivities. It is important to highlight that several studies reported more than one single bioactivity.

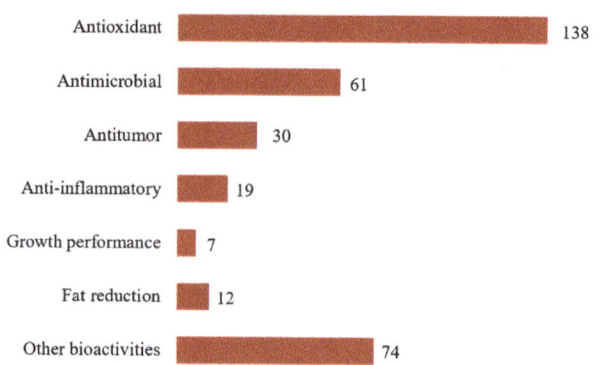

Figure 5. Number of eligible publications that reported bioactivity on raw seaweed biomass or seaweeds organic extracts.

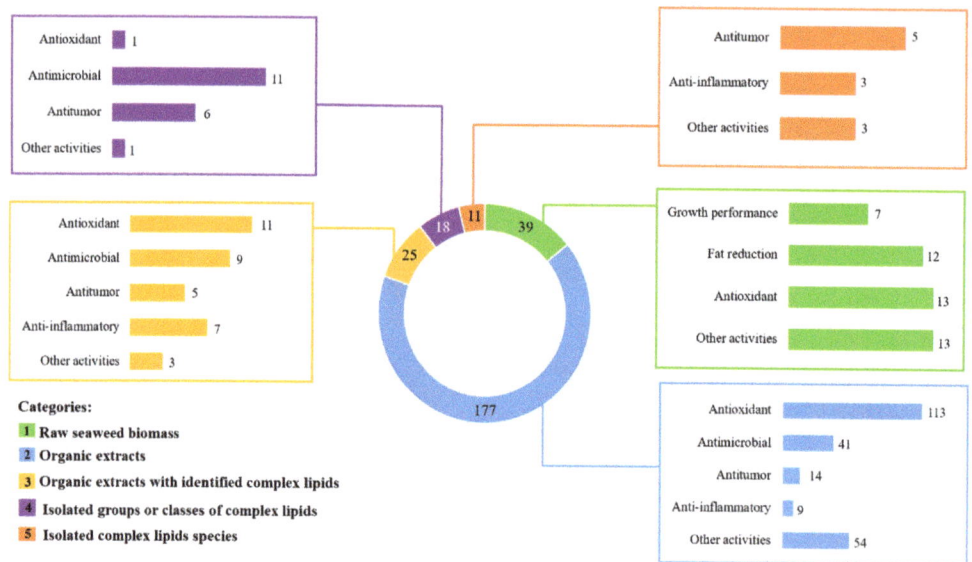

Figure 6. Ranking of eligible studies that reported bioactivity of raw seaweed or seaweeds organic extracts distributed by distinct categories.

Antioxidant activity was most studied in categories 1 (13 studies out of 39), 2 (113 studies out of 177), and 3 (11 studies out of 25). In category 1, most studies that evaluated the antioxidant activity tested the inclusion of the raw seaweed biomass on diet, with no specification of the bioactive compound. In category 2, most studies tested organic extracts and were oriented towards phenolic compounds, which were recognized by their antioxidant properties. In category 3, the antioxidant activity was evaluated testing organic extracts with identified complex lipids, assigning the bioactivity to the whole extract and the synergic effect between molecules. The in vitro assays of antioxidant evaluation using free radical scavenging activities were one of the bioactivities more intensively investigated, likely because of well-established and easy-to-use methodologies. However, these *in chemico* assays have limited biological relevance considering the effect in the modulation of redox homeostasis of in vivo organisms. Therefore, additional studies are still needed using in vivo models, and measuring biologically relevant biomarkers of redox homeostasis, such as catalase, and superoxide dismutase enzymes, or addressing the proper value of seaweeds lipid antioxidant bioactivities.

Antimicrobial and antitumor activities were mostly studied on categories 4 (11 studies out of 18) and 5 (5 studies out of 11), respectively. Several studies reported the antimicrobial properties of lipid extracts from seaweeds. However, the majority of the studies reported only the estimation of inhibition of bacterial growth, lacking information on the identification of the bioactive lipids promoting such response and/or elucidating the mechanism of antimicrobial action. Interestingly, some studies reported antibacterial and antiviral activity of lipid extract from specific seaweeds and activities seem to be dependent on their origin. As society urgently needs new antibiotics to overcome the current scenario of antibiotic resistance, along with powerful new antiviral drugs to face future pandemics [7], it is urgent to further explore these bioactivities in seaweeds. Concerning antitumor activity, information is also scarce and lacks key information on putative structure function relationship.

To unravel the most studied phyla of seaweeds, data (270 publications) were ranked considering how reported bioactivities were distributed over the phyla Ochrophyta, Chlorophyta, and Rhodophyta (Figure 7). Seaweed species belonging to the Ochrophyta were the most reported on antioxidant, antimicrobial, antitumor, and anti-inflammatory activities, followed by species within the Rhodophyta. Species within the Chlorophyta were the less studied.

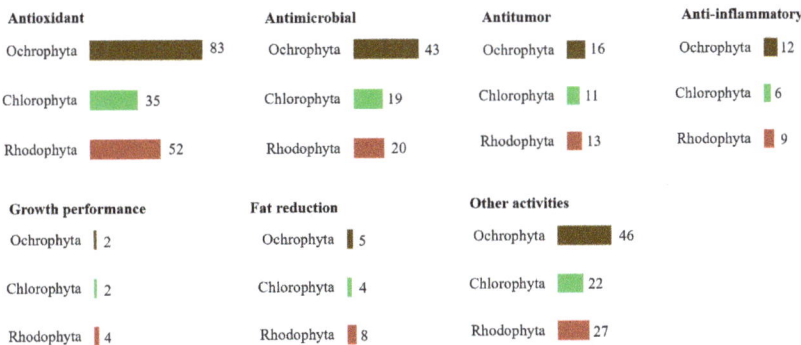

Figure 7. Number of eligible studies that reported bioactivity on raw seaweed biomass or seaweeds organic extracts distributed by bioactivities and seaweed phyla.

Bioactivity distributed by phylum combined with the five categories selected in the present study is plotted in Figure 8. Seaweeds within the Ochrophyta were the most screened to evaluate antioxidant, antimicrobial, antitumor, and anti-inflammatory bioactivities on category 2–4. On the other hand, seaweeds from the Rhodophyta were the most investigated to screen for growth performance, fat reduction, and antioxidant activity over criteria 1. Although with a lower number of studies on category 5, seaweed species within the Chlorophyta and Ochrophyta appeared as the most screened for antitumor activity. Seaweed species within the Rhodophyta were the most studied for anti-inflammatory activity under category 5.

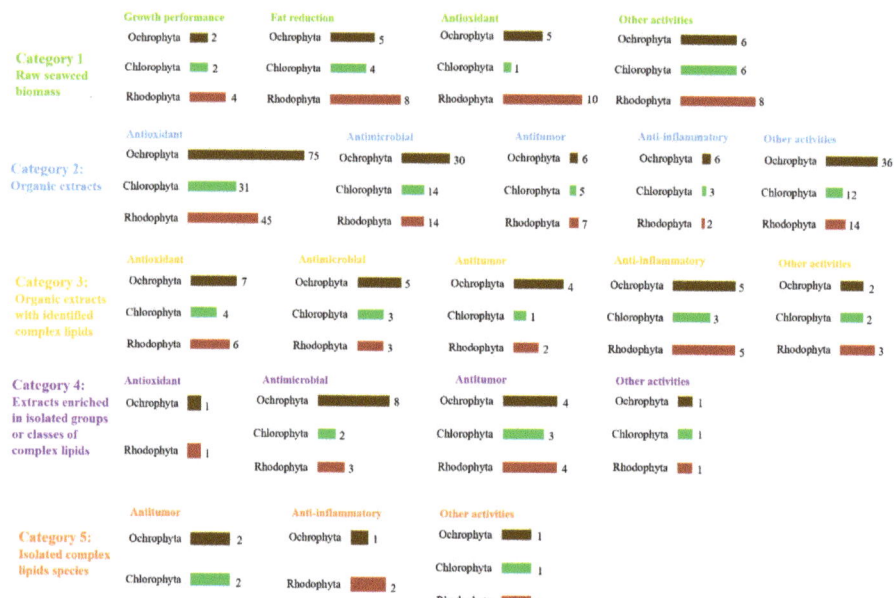

Figure 8. Number of eligible studies that reported bioactivity distributed over the five categories and seaweed phyla.

In most studies (Table S1), the bioactivity reported for seaweed lipids was often associated with the most abundant molecules identified in organic extracts, or with other molecules detected by the methodology used for structural characterization (e.g., fatty acid identification by Gas Chromatography–Mass Spectrometry (GC-MS)). PUFA have been frequently identified as bioactive lipids in many studies because FA identification was the only approach used for extract characterization on those publications [31,43–46]. Nevertheless, this is an inadequate approach since FA commonly exist in low amounts as free FA and they are mostly esterified in complex lipids. Other studies tested extracts obtained with organic solvents, which also extract complex lipids. However, these studies only focused on the identification of well-known phytochemicals, which are present at a lower abundance in seaweeds, such as phenolic compounds, excluding the putative role of lipids and/or the synergic effect of other lipid-soluble compounds [47–49].

Knowledge progression of natural bioactive products and their application depends on the isolation of pure molecules to achieve a possible structure–function relationship [50,51]. While this is a very laborious and time-consuming task, it is also essential to understand specific biological effects of these biomolecules. Moreover, this task will also provide a new perspective to plan chemical synthesis and subsequent applications on different fields, such as in the pharmaceutical industry, aiming to add-value to seaweeds as natural sources of bioactive compounds. To date, few studies have tried to overcome this drawback. New studies being performed on bioassays using specific groups or class of seaweed lipids are scarce; although, they are paramount to isolate molecules to address a proper clarification of structure–bioactivity relationship. These studies are detailed bellow.

3.1. The Complex Lipids of Seaweeds as Derived Bioactive Phytochemicals

Studies addressing extracts enriched in isolated groups or classes of complexes lipids (category 4) and studies of isolated complex lipid species (category 5) are a minority. However, they provide a greater level of confidence concerning the bioactivity reported on complex lipids. These studies were selected for inclusion criteria following PRISMA-P workflow. Herein, they were ranked based on the bioactivities they evaluated.

3.1.1. Antitumor Activity

Naturally occurring compounds have been tested for antiproliferative/cytotoxic, pro-apoptotic, anti-metastatic, and anti-neoplastic activities, among others [52–54].

Screening of antiproliferative activity is the most common approach to evaluate antitumor potential of complex lipids. Several cancer cell lines have been used including hepato [55,56], cervix [57], breast [56,58], leukemia [58,59], colon [58,60], lung [58,61], melanoma [62], and prostate and ovarian cancer [58]. The majority of these studies used lipid fractions enriched in a specific lipid group or class, obtained by using silica gel columns and solvents with different polarities. This approach was performed, for example, to evaluate the PLs fraction of the brown seaweed *Sargassum marginatum* inhibiting promyelocytic cells (HL-60) [59]. There is a huge variety of classes within PLs group that can contribute for bioactivity of these fractions; thus, the analysis of enriched lipid fractions solely provides a partial interpretation of results. Fractions enriched in GLs classes were isolated, allowing the identification of inhibitory activity against several cancer cells lines in digalactosyldiacylglycerol (DGDG) [60] and sulfoquinovosyldiacylglycero (SQDG) [55–57,60] enriched fractions (Table 1).

Few works have evaluated bioactivities of isolated lipid classes. The monogalactosyldiacylglycerol (MGDG) (MGDG 14:0_16:1) from the red seaweed *Solieria chordalis* and DGDG (14:0_18:3) from the green seaweed *Ulva armoricana* were found to have activity against NSCLC-N6 cancer cells [61]. However, to the best of our knowledge, the authors only identified the most abundant lipid species in the fraction, undervaluing other unidentified lipid species. Therefore, the antiproliferative activity of previous GLs molecular species could be incorrectly attributed.

There are very few studies that achieved the isolation and identification of pure compounds, such as 1-*O*-(5Z, 8Z, 11Z, 14Z, 17Z-eicosapentanoyl)-2-*O*-(6Z,9Z,12Z,15Z-octadecatetraenoyl)-3-*O*-β-D-galactopiranosyl-*sn*-glycerol, (MGDG (20:5/18:4)) (Figure 9A) from the brown seaweed *Fucus evanescence* [62] with activity against malignant melanoma (SK-MEL-28), and 1-*O*-(palmitoyl)-2-*O*-(5Z, 8Z, 11Z, 14Z-eicosatetraenoyl)-3-*O*-β-D-galactopyranosylglycerol, (MGDG 20:4/16:0) (Figure 9B) from the red seaweed *Hydrolithon reinboldii*, which demonstrated inhibitory activity against a range of 12 cancer cell lines [58].

Along with the assessment of cell viability and the antiproliferative effect of lipid extracts, several biochemical approaches have also been developed in order to interrupt the cancer cells progression, including the inhibition of enzymes and disruption of mitotic process. The inhibition of DNA polymerases α was achieved by GLs species identified as galactosyldiacylglycerol esterified with the FAs C18:1 and C16:0 (GDG(18:1/16:0)) (Figure 9C) isolated from the brown seaweed *Petalonia bingbamiae* [63]. Likewise, the inhibition of MYT1 kinase by two GLs lipid species from unknown seaweed species were reported and these bioactive GLs species were identified as *sn*-1,2-dipalmitoyl-3-(*N*-palmitoyl-6-deoxy-6-amino-α-D-glucosyl)-glycerol and *sn*-1-palmitoyl-2-myristoyl-3-(*N*-stearyl-6-deoxy-6-aminoglucosyl)-glycerol (Figure 9D) [64]. The total synthesis of 1,2-dipalmitoyl-3-(*N*-palmitoyl-6′-amino-6′-deoxy-α-D-glucosyl)-*sn*-glycerol based on previous study [64], was achieved by Göllner and co-authors that confirmed those GLs lipids species as bioactive [65].

The species of GL isolated from the green seaweed *Avrainvillea nigricans*, named Nigricanoside A (Figure 9E), showed the capacity to arrest MCF-7 cells in mitosis, stimulating the polymerization of pure tubulin in vitro and thus inhibiting the proliferation of MCF-7 and HCT-116 cells [66]. The potent antimitotic activity of Nigricanoside A was seen without precedent among previously known GL.

3.1.2. Anti-Inflammatory Activity

Inflammation is a multifactorial condition ubiquitously present in most diseases and particularly in non-communicable diseases. It involves a large number of identified mediators, comprising leukocyte cells that release specialized substances such as pro-inflammatory cytokines [67] and high levels of nitric oxide (NO) in response to the inflammatory process [68].

NO is a potent pro-inflammatory mediator in over inflammation conditions [69]. On a small scale, and for research purposes, inhibition of NO, represents a protective effect of several anti-inflammatory compounds. The reduction in NO production from immune cells is assessed as a first step in the anti-inflammatory potential of natural products. Using this approach, several studies evaluated the anti-inflammatory activity of isolated and characterized seaweed lipid molecules (Table 2) including (2S)-1-O-eicosapentaenoyl-2-O-myristoyl-3-O-(6-sulfo-α-D-quinovopyranosyl)-glycerol SQDG (20:5/14:0), (2S)-1-O-eicosapentaenoyl-2-O-palmitoyl-3-O-(6-sulfo-α-D-quinovopyranosyl)-glycerol SQDG(20:5/16:0), 1-O-eicosapentaenoyl-2-O-trans-3-hexadecanoyl-3-phospho-(1′-glycerol)-glycerol PG(20:5/trans-16:1), 1-O-eicosapentaenoyl-2-O-palmitoyl-3-phospho-(1′-glycerol)-glycerol PG(20:5/16:1), and 1,2-bis-O-eicosapentanoylglycero-3-phosphocholine PC(20:5/20:5) (Figure 10(A1–A3)) from the red seaweed *Palmaria palmata* [70]; and isolated galactolipid species from the red seaweed *Chondrus crispus*, such as (2S)-1,2-bis-O-eicosapentaenoyl-3-O-β-D-galactopyranosylglycerol MGD(20:5/20:5), (2S)-1-O-eicosapentaenoyl-2-O-arachidonoyl-3-O-β-D-galactopyranosylglycerol MGDG(20:5/20:4), (2S)-1-O-eicosapentaenoyl-2-O-palmitoyl-3-O-β-D-galactopyranosylglycerol MGDG(20:5/16:0), (2S)-1-O-eicosapentaenoyl-2-O-palmitoyl-3-O-(β-D-galactopyranosyl-6-1-α-D-galactopyranosyl)-glycerol DGDG(20:5/16:0), (2S)-1,2-bis-O-arachidonoyl-3-O-β-D-galactopyranosylglycerol MGDG(20:4/20:4), (2S)-1-O-arachidonoyl-2-O-palmitoyl-3-O-β-D-galactopyranosylglycerol MGDG(20:4/16:0), (2S)-1-O-arachidonoyl-2-O-palmitoyl-3-O-(β-D-galactopyranosyl-6-1α-D-galactopyranosyl)-glycerol DGDG(20:4/16:0), and (2S)-1-O-(6Z,9Z,12Z,15Z-octadecatetranoyl)-2-O-palmitoyl-3-O-β-D-galactopyranosylglycerol MGDG(18:4/16:0) (Figure 10(B1–B3)) [71], which showed significant NO inhibition through down-regulation of inducible Nitric Oxide Synthase (iNOS). PUFA side chains, mainly EPA and arachidonic acid (AA), esterified to polar lipid structure seem to be relevant for their potent NO inhibition. Curiously, isolated PUFA, such as EPA, AA, and DHA, showed less NO inhibitory activity when compared to their esterified forms in polar lipid [70,71].

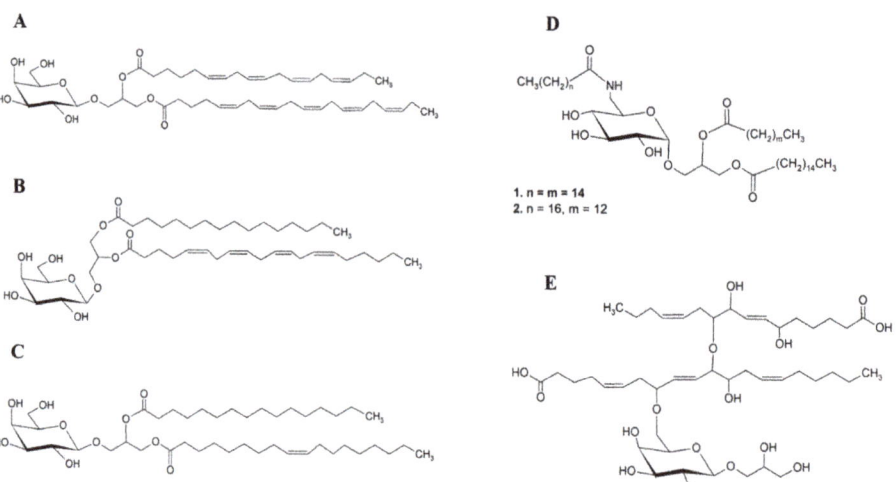

Figure 9. Chemical structures of bioactive complex lipids reported with antitumor activity. (**A**) 1-O-(5Z, 8Z, 11Z, 14Z, 17Z-eicosapentanoyl)-2-O-(6Z,9Z,12Z,15Z-octadecatetraenoyl)-3-O-β-D-galactopiranosyl-sn-glycerol MGDG (20:5/18:4) (brown seaweed *Fucus evanescence*); (**B**) 1-O-(palmitoyl)-2-O-(5Z, 8Z, 11Z, 14Z eicosatetraenoyl)-3-O-β-D-galactopyranosyl-glycerol MGDG (20:4/16:0) (red seaweed *Hydrolithon reinboldii*); (**C**) GDG (16:0, 18:1) (brown seaweed *Petalonia bingbamiae*) [63]; (**D**) sn-1,2-dipalmitoyl-3-(N-palmitoyl-6-deoxy-6-amino-α-D-glucosyl)-glycerol (1) and sn-1-palmitoyl-2-myristoyl-3-(N-stearyl-6-deoxy-6-aminoglucosyl)-glycerol (2); (**E**) Nigricanoside A (green seaweed *Avrainvillea nigricans*).

Table 1. Lipid species extracted from seaweeds with antitumor activities. Extraction and characterization methodologies and cell lines used in in vitro assays are reported. Data is reported by phylum (Ochrophyta, Rhodophyta, Chlorophyta, or mixed phyla) and ranked by alphabetical order of seaweed species name within each phylum (or mixed phyla).

Study Category	Seaweed Species	Phylum	Lipid Species	Model and Obtained Results	Extraction Procedure	Identification/Characterization	Ref.
Category 5	*Fucus evanescens*	Ochrophyta	MGDG (20:5/18:4)	Melanoma (SK-MEL-28), IC$_{50}$ of 104 µM, (MTS assay)	Extraction solvents: ethanol (40 °C); deionized water, aqueous ethanol (70%), chloroform. Fractionation/isolation: silica gel, Sephadex LH-20 column chromatography	TLC, ESI-MS; ^{1}H-, ^{13}C-NMR; GC-FID, GC-MS	[62]
Category 5	*Petalonia binghamiae*	Ochrophyta	GDG (16:0/18:1)	Inhibition of DNA polymerase α, IC$_{50}$ of 54 µM, (WST-1 assay)	Extraction solvents: acetone; ethyl acetate and water. Fractionation/isolation: silica gel, Sephadex LH-20 column chromatography	GC-FID; EI mass; FABHR mass; ^{1}H-, ^{13}C- and DEPT-NMR	[63]
Category 4	*Sargassum horneri*	Ochrophyta	DGDD, SQDG,	Colon carcinoma (Caco-2), inhibition effect at 100 µM, (action improved with 1.0 mM NaBT)	Extraction solvents: chloroform, methanol, water (Bligh and Dyer). Fractionation: silica gel column chromatography	TLC, GC-FID	[64]
Category 4	*Sargassum marginatum*	Ochrophyta	PL	Human pro-myelocytic leukemia (HL-60), inhibition >70% at 40 µg mL^{-1} (trypan blue dye exclusion assay)	Extraction solvents: methanol, chloroform: methanol (1:1), water. Fractionation: silica gel column chromatography	GC-FID; GC-MS	[59]
Category 4	*Gracilaria corticata*	Rhodophyta	SQDG	Epithelioid cervix carcinoma (HeLa), IC$_{50}$ of 106.88 µg mL^{-1} (MTT assay)	Extraction solvents: ethyl acetate/methanol (1:1), *n*-hexane, dichloromethane, butanol, water. Fractionation: silica gel column chromatography	GC-MS, TLC, ^{1}H-^{13}C-NMR (1H-1H COSY, DEPT, HSQC, HMBC spectra), HPLC	[57]
Category 5	*Hydrolithon reinboldii*	Rhodophyta	MGDG (20:4/16:0) (designated as Lithonoside)	Colon cancer (HCT116), prostate cancer (PC-3, LNcap-FGC, Du145), ovarian cancer (A2780/DDP-S), lung cancer (NCI-H446, SHP-77), leukemia (CCRF-CEM), breast cancer (BT-549, DU4475, MDA-MB-468, MDA-MB-231), average IC$_{50}$ of 19.8 µM (MTS assay)	Extraction solvents: methanol, methanol: dichloromethane (1:1), methanol: water (9:1), hexane, ethyl acetate, butanol. Fractionation/isolation: semi-preparative reversed-phase HPLC, C18 HPLC	HPLC(C18)-Q-TOF-MS; ^{1}H-, ^{13}C-NMR (DEPT, COSY, HSQC, HMBC spectra)	[58]
Category 4	*Porphyra crispata*	Rhodophyta	SQDG	Liver carcinoma (HepG2), IC$_{50}$ of 126 µg mL^{-1} (MTT assay)	Extraction solvents: ethanol. Fractionation: HP-20 column, DEAE-cellulose acetate column, TLC	GC-FID; TLC, normal-phase HPLC-ELSD	[35]
Category 5	*Avrainvillea nigricans*	Chlorophyta	Nigricanoside A	Breast adenocarcinoma (MCF-7) colon cancer (HCT-116) antimitotic activity, IC$_{50}$ of 3 nM	Extraction solvents: methanol, water, ethyl acetate, hexane, dichloromethane. Fractionation/isolation: normal phase flash, Sephadex LH-20, reversed-phase flash column chromatographies, reversed-phase HPLC	HRESIMS; ^{1}H-, ^{13}C-NMR (DEPT, COSY, HSQC, HMBC spectra)	[66]
Category 4	*Solieria chordalis*; *Ulva armoricana*	Rhodophyta Chlorophyta	MGDG (14:0_16:1) DGDG (14:0_18:3)	Bronchopulmonary carcinoma (NSCLC-N6), IC$_{50}$ of 23.5 µg mL^{-1} for MGDG (14:0_16:1) and IC50 of 24.0 µg mL^{-1} for DGDG (14:0_18:3) (MTT assay)	Extraction solvents: chloroform/methanol (1:1), water, dichloromethane, acetone, methanol. Fractionation: flash column chromatography	GC-MS; TLC; LC-MS	[61]

Table 1. Cont.

Study Category	Seaweed Species	Phylum	Lipid Species	Model and Obtained Results	Extraction Procedure	Identification/ Characterization	Ref.
Category 4	Dilophus fasciola; Galaxaura cylindrica; Laurencia papillosa; Taonia atomaria; Ulva fasciata.	Rhodophyta Chlorophyta	Sulfolipid class	Hepato cellular carcinoma (Hep G2), IC_{50} in a range of 0.60 to 2.75 µg mL^{-1}, Breast adenocarcinoma (MCF-7), IC_{50} in a range of 0.40 to 0.67 µg mL^{-1} (SRB assay)	Extraction solvents: methanol/chloroform (2:1). Fractionation: DEAE-cellulose column chromatography	IR; GC-FID; GC-MS; LC-MS/MS	[56]
Category 5	Unknown algal species			sn-1,2-dipalmitoyl-3-(N-palmitoyl-6-deoxy-6-amino-α-D-glucosyl)-glycerol; sn-1-palmitoyl-2-myristoyl-3-(N-stearyl-6-deoxy-6-aminoglucosyl)-glycerol	Inhibition of MYT1 kinase, IC_{50} of 0.12 and 0.43 µg mL^{-1}	Extraction solvents: methanol, water, n-hexane, dichloromethane, butanol. Fractionation/isolation: Sephadex LH-20; RP-18 reverse phase silica gel;	^{1}H, ^{13}C-NMR; MALDI-TOF-MS	[64]

The capacity to inhibit phospholipase A2 (PLA2) has been linked to the efficacy for the treatment of inflammatory processes, since PLA2 hydrolyze membrane phospholipids releasing AA, the precursor of the pro-inflammatory mediators prostaglandins, thromboxanes, and leukotrienes [72,73]. Inhibition of PLA2 is the pharmacological mechanism of action of corticosteroids, a group of drugs with potent anti-inflammatory properties. The 7-methoxy-9-methylhexadeca-4,8-dienoic acid (MMHDA) (Figure 10C) isolated from the brown seaweed *Ishige okamurae* was tested in vitro for inhibition of PLA2 activity, and in vivo on edema and erythema induced in rat models. In both models, it demonstrated potent inhibitor of PLA2 activity and inflammation, with IC_{50} concentrations lower than the ones reported for rutin, a flavonoid model [74].

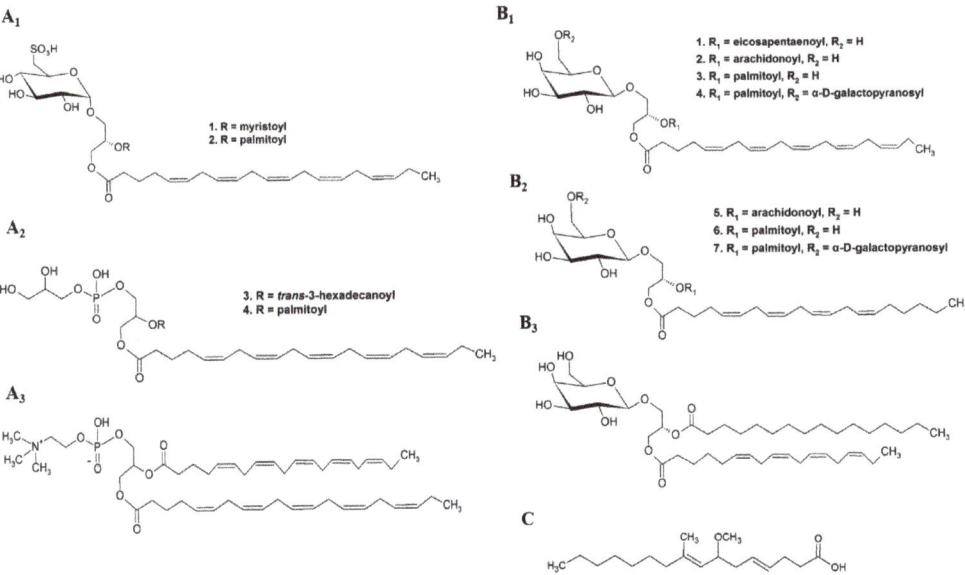

Figure 10. Chemical structures of bioactive complex lipids reported with anti-inflammatory activity: (**A1**) (2S)-1-*O*-eicosapentaenoyl-2-*O*-myristoyl-3-*O*-(6-sulfo-α-D-quinovopyranosyl)-glycerol SQDG (20:5/14:0) (1); (2S)-1-*O*-eicosapentaenoyl-2-*O*-palmitoyl-3-*O*-(6-sulfo-α-D-quinovopyranosyl)-glycerol SQDG(20:5/16:0) (2); (**A2**) 1-*O*-eicosapentaenoyl-2-*O*-trans-3-hexadecanoyl-3-phospho-(1′-glycerol)-glycerol PG(20:5/*trans*-16:1) (3); 1-*O*-eicosapentaenoyl-2-*O*-palmitoyl-3-phospho-(1′-glycerol)-glycerol PG(20:5/16:1) (4); (**A3**) 1,2-*bis*-*O*-eicosapentanoylglycero-3-phosphocholine PC(20:5/20:5) (red seaweed *Palmaria palmata*); (**B1**) (2S)-1,2-*bis*-*O*-eicosapentaenoyl-3-*O*-β-D-galactopyranosylglycerol MGDG(20:5/20:5) (1); (2S)-1-*O*-eicosapentaenoyl-2-*O*-arachidonoyl-3-*O*-β-D-galactopyranosylglycerol MGDG(20:5/20:4) (2); (2S)-1-*O*-eicosapentaenoyl-2-*O*-palmitoyl-3-*O*-β-D-galactopyranosylglycerol MGDG(20:5/16:0) (3); (2S)-1-*O*-eicosapentaenoyl-2-*O*-palmitoyl-3-*O*-(β-D-galactopyranosyl-6-1-α-D-galactopyranosyl)-glycerol DGDG (20:5/16:0)(4); (**B2**) (2S)-1,2-*bis*-*O*-arachidonoyl-3-*O*-β-D-galactopyranosylglycerol MGDG(20:4/20:4) (5); (2S)-1-*O*-arachidonoyl-2-*O*-palmitoyl-3-*O*-β-D-galactopyranosylglycerol MGDG(20:4/16:0) (6); (2S)-1-*O*-arachidonoyl-2-*O*-palmitoyl-3-*O*-(β-D-galactopyranosyl-6-1-α-D-galactopyranosyl)-glycerol DGDG(20:4/16:0) (7); (**B3**) (2S)-1-*O*-(6Z,9Z,12Z,15Z-octadecatetranoyl)-2-*O*-palmitoyl-3-*O*-β-D-galactopyranosylglycerol MGDG (18:4/16:0) (red seaweed *Chondrus crispus*); (**C**) 7-methoxy-9-methylhexadeca-4,8-dienoic acid (MMHDA) (brown seaweed *Ishige okamurae*).

Table 2. Lipid species extracted from seaweeds with anti-inflammatory activities. Extraction and characterization methodologies and cell lines used in bioassays are reported. Data is reported by phylum (Ochrophyta, Rhodophyta, Chlorophyta, or mixed phyla) and ranked by alphabetical order of seaweed species name within each phylum (or mixed phyla).

Study Category	Seaweed Species	Phylum	Lipid Species	Model and Obtained Results	Compounds Extraction	Identification/Characterization	Ref.
Category 5	*Chondrus crispus*	Rhodophyta	MGDG(20:5/20:5) MGDG(20:5/20:4) MGDG(18:4/16:0) MGDG(20:5/16:0) MGDG(20:4/20:4) MGDG(20:4/16:0) DGDG(20:5/16:0) DGDG(20:4/16:0)	Raw 264.7 cells NO inhibition at 100 µM	Extraction solvents: methanol, water, ethyl acetate. Fractionation/isolation: SPE, HPLC (synergy MAX-RP column), semi-preparative HPLC	LC/MS; ^{1}H, ^{13}C-NMR; GC; HRMS	[71]
	Ishige okamurae	Ochrophyta	MMHDA	*in vitro* inhibition of PLA2, IC$_{50}$ of 1.9 µg mL^{-1} *in vivo* inhibition of oedema, IC$_{50}$ of 3.5 mg mL^{-1} *in vivo* inhibition of erythema, IC$_{50}$ of 4.6 mg mL^{-1}	Extraction solvents: methanol, chloroform. Fractionation/isolation: Sephadex LH-20 column, silica gel column, reverse-phase HPLC, µBondapak C-18 column	HPLC (C18); GC-MS-QP5050A; EIMS;	[74]
	Palmaria palmata	Rhodophyta	SQDG(20:5/14:0) SQDG(20:5/16:0) PG(20:5/*trans*-16:1) PG(20:5/16:1) PC(20:5/20:5)	Raw 264.7 cells NO inhibition SQDG(20:5/14:0), IC$_{50}$ of 36.5 µM SQDG(20:5/16:0), IC$_{50}$ of 11.0 µM PG(20:5/*trans*-16:1), IC$_{50}$ of 16.7 µM PG(20:5/16:0), IC$_{50}$ of 42.9 µM PC(20:5/20:5), IC$_{50}$ of 43.5 µM All species reduced iNOS expression >85% at 100 µM	Extraction solvents: methanol: chloroform (1:1), water, ethyl acetate. Fractionation/isolation: silica gel column chromatography; semi-preparative HPLC	ESI-MS; ^{1}H, ^{13}C-NMR (COSY, HSQC HMBC spectra)	[70]

3.1.3. Antimicrobial Activity

The emergence of antibiotic resistance of human pathogenic microorganisms and the need for new antiviral drugs has been a key driver for searching new antimicrobial compounds [75]. Complex lipids from seaweeds could play an active role in this field. In this section we describe the lipids from seaweeds with reported antibacterial, antiviral, anti-algal, anti-fouling, antifungal and anti-protozoal activities (Table 3). In spite of the range of antimicrobial activities tested, there is still opportunity to gain a more in-depth knowledge on this bioactive property of seaweed lipids, namely by testing against other strains of bacteria and virus that are major drivers of infection diseases

The GLs classes MGDG, DGDG, and SQDG from some species of *Laminaria* genus [76,77]; the brown seaweeds *Fucus evanescens* [78], *Alaria fistulosa* [76], *Saccharina cichorioides* [79]; and the red seaweed *Chondria armata* [80], demonstrated activity against a range of bacteria, yeast, and fungus. Likewise, sulfolipids classes from several seaweed species proved antibacterial activity [56]. In addition to antibacterial and antifungal activity, an isolated mixture of SQDG species from the brown seaweed *Lobophora variegata* showed anti-protozoal activity [81]. Isolated sub-fractions enriched in GL from the green seaweed *Ulva prolifera* [82] and the brown seaweed *Sargassum vulgare* [83] showed anti-algal and anti-fouling activities, respectively.

The studies surveyed pinpoint the evaluation of the complex lipid antiviral activity on Herpes simplex virus (HSV). The SQDG class from the red seaweed *Osmundaria obtusiloba*, the brown seaweed *Sargassum vulgare* and several species within genus *Laminaria* (brown seaweeds), were highlighted by its antiviral activity against HSV-1 [56,84,85] and HSV-2 [84,85]. The role of palmitic acid and sulfonate group on SQDG molecular structure was considered as relevant on activity against HSV virus and on cellular receptors [85].

Prospecting new antimicrobial compounds should follow a systemic protocol once the goal is to design solutions for human protection. Tested compounds must also show low toxicity against erythrocytes, which was evaluated in parallel in some studies that revealed hemolytic activity [76–78].

Table 3. Lipid species extracted from seaweeds with antimicrobial activities. Extraction and characterization methodologies and cell lines used in bioassays are reported. Data is reported by phylum (Ochrophyta, Rhodophyta, Chlorophyta, or mixed phyla) and ranked by alphabetical order of seaweed species name within each phylum (or mixed phyla).

Study Category	Seaweed Species	Phylum	Lipid Species	Activity (Microorganisms) and Obtained Results	Extraction	Identification/ Characterization	Ref.
	Fucus evanescens	Ochrophyta	MGDG, DGDG, SQDG classes	Antibacterial and antifungal (*Candida albicans*, *Fusarium oxysporum*, *Staphylococcus aureus*, *Escherichia coli*) Paper disk assay Unknown concentration	Extraction solvents: ethanol; ethanol:acetone (1:1); chloroform:ethanol (1:1); chloroform; water. Fractionation: silica gel column chromatography	TLC; GC-MS	[78]
	Laminaria cichorioides	Ochrophyta	MGDG, DGDG, SQDG classes	Antibacterial and antifungal (Safale S04, *Candida albicans*, *Fusarium oxysporum*, *Aspergillus niger*, *Staphylococcus aureus*, *Escherichia coli*) Paper disk assay 3 mg mL^{-1}	Extraction solvents: 96% ethanol, chloroform, water. Fractionation: silica gel column chromatography	TSC	[77]
	Lobophora variegata	Ochrophyta	Mixture of SQDG(16:0/14:0), SQDG(16:0/16:0) and SQDG(16:0/18:1) species	Antiprotozoal (*Giardia intestinalis*, *Entamoeba histolytica* (Eh), *Trichomonas vaginalis*) Susceptibility assays IC$_{50}$ of 3.9 μg mL^{-1} for *E. histolytica*, IC$_{50}$ of 8.0 μg mL^{-1} for *T. vaginalis*, IC$_{50}$ of 20.9 μg mL^{-1} for *G. intestinalis*	Extraction solvents: dichloromethane/methanol (7:3), methanol/water (9:1), hexane, chloroform, ethyl acetate and n-butanol. Fractionation: Sephadex LH20 column chromatograph	FAB-MS; ^{1}H-13C-NMR (COSY, TOCSY, DEPT, HSQC and HMQC spectra)	[81]
	Saccharina cichorioides	Ochrophyta	Glycolipids (GL) group MGDG class	Antibacterial GL group: activity against *Staphylococcus aureus*, *Escherichia coli*, *Fusarium oxysporum*, and *Aspergillus niger* MGDG class: activity against *S. aureus* and oxysporum Paper disk assay Unknown concentration	Extraction solvents: ethanol: acetone (1:1, v/v), chloroform:ethanol (1:1, v/v). Fractionation: silica gel column	TLC	[79]
	Sargassum vulgare	Ochrophyta	Isolated SQDG fraction, identified SQDG(14:0/16:0), SQDG(16:0/16:0), SQDG(17:0/16:0), SQDG(18:1/16:0), SQDG(19:0/16:0), SQDG(23:0/17:0) species	Antiviral Inhibition HSV-1 and HSV-2 with maximum non-toxic concentrations (MNTC) of 50 μg mL^{-1} and viral inhibition index (VII) in a range of 96 (minimum) to 99.9% (maximum) Titer reduction assay	Extraction solvents: chloroform/methanol (2:1 and 1:2). Fractionation: silica column chromatography.	TLC; ESI-MS; ^{1}H, ^{13}C-NMR	[85]
Category 4	*Sargassum vulgare*	Ochrophyta	Fraction enriched in MGDG (16:0/19:1) DGDG (16:0/16:1) SQDG (16:0/19:0) species	Antifouling Biofilm-forming marine bacteria (*Pseudoalteromonas elyakovii*, *Halomonas marina*, *Shewanella putrefaciens* and *Polaribacter irgensii*) and marine microalgae (*Chlorarachnion reptans*, *Pleurochrysis roscoffensis*, *Exanthemachrysis gayraliae*, *Cylindrotheca closterium*, and *Navicula jeffreyi*) MIC in a range of 0.01 to >10 μg/mL	Extraction solvents: chloroform/methanol (2:1 and 1:2), water. Fractionation: silica gel column chromatography.	HPTLC silica gel; TLC; LC-MS	[83]

Table 3. *Cont.*

Study Category	Seaweed Species	Phylum	Lipid Species	Activity (Microorganisms) and Obtained Results	Extraction	Identification/ Characterization	Ref.
	Alaria fistulosa, Laminaria bongardiana, Laminaria longipes, Laminaria yezoensis	Ochrophyta	MGDG, DGDG, SQDG classes	Antibacterial (Staphylococcus aureus, Escherichia coli) and antifungal (Candida albicans, Fusarium oxysporum) Paper disk assay Unknown concentration	Extraction solvents: ethanol; ethanol:acetone (1:1); chloroform:ethanol (1:1); chloroform; water. Fractionation: silica gel column chromatography.	TLC; GC-MS	[76]
	Chondria armata	Rhodophyta	Glycolipids (GL) group, identified the species 1-oleoyl-2-palmitoyl-3-O-(linolenyl-6′-galactosyl)-glycerol, 2-O-palmitoyl-3-O-(6′-sulfoquinovopyranosyl)-glycerol and 3-digalactosyl-2-palmitoyl glycerol	Antibacterial (Klebsiella sp., Shigella flexineri, Vibrio cholerae) and antifungal (Candida albicans, Cryptococcus neoformans, Aspergillus fumigatus) Paper disk assay impregnated with extract in a range of 65–130 µg/disk	Extraction solvents: methanol, chloroform, n-butanol and water. Fractionation: Sephadex LH20 for gel filtration, silica gel column chromatography, RP-18 column	TLC; QSTARXL MS/MS; ^{1}H-, ^{13}C-NMR (COSY, HMQC, and HMBC spectra)	[80]
	Osmundaria obtusiloba	Rhodophyta	SQDG class	Antiviral Inhibition HSV-1 and HSV-2 with 50% of effective concentration (EC$_{50}$) values of 42 µg mL^{-1} to HSV-1 and 12 µg mL^{-1} to HSV-2 Titer reduction assay	Extraction solvents: acetone, chloroform/methanol (2:1 and 1:2). Fractionation: silica gel column chromatography, preparative TLC.	TLC; ESI-MS; ^{1}H-, ^{13}C-NMR (HSQC, COSY and TOCSY spectra)	[84]
	Ulva prolifera	Chlorophyta	Enriched subfraction on MGMG(18:0) MGMG(16:0) MGDG(16:0/18:1)	Antialgal: Inhibition > 50% of red tide microalgae (Karenia mikimitoi, Skeletonema costatum, Alexandrium tamarense, Heterosigma akashivo, Prorocentrum donghaiense) at concentration of 28.8 µg mL^{-1}	Extraction solvents: methanol, water, ethyl acetate Fractionation: silica gel column, Sephadex LH-20, preparative TLC.	TLC	[82]
	Dilophys fasciola, Galaxoura cylindrica, Laurencia papillosa, Taonia atomaria, Ulva fasciata	Ochrophyta Rhodophyta Chlorophyta	Sulfolipids classes	Antiviral: Inhibition HSV-1, IC$_{50}$ ranged from 15 to 25 µg mL^{-1} (plaque reduction assay) Antibacterial (Bacillus subtilis, Escherichia coli) with MIC in a range of 40 to 80 µg mL^{-1} for G. cylindrica, U. fasciata, and T. atomaria (agar diffusion assay)	Extraction solvents: methanol:chloroform (2:1, v/v) Fractionation: DEAE-cellulose column chromatography.	IR, GC MS/MS, LC-MS/MS.	[56]

3.1.4. Other Bioactivities Attribute to Seaweed Lipids

Complex lipids from seaweeds have showed a broad spectrum of bioactivates (Table 4), including antioxidant activity associated with GL and PL groups from the red seaweed *Solieria chordalis* and the brown seaweed *Sargassum muticum*, and evidenced through in vitro free radical scavenging activity [86]. However, the study did not characterize the compounds in the isolated fractions, which raises doubts about their purity and possible interference of other compounds.

Fractionated lipid classes, such as MGDG, were suggested to play an important role in the design of optimized nanoparticulate tubular immune-stimulating complexes. Sanina et al. (2021) found different degrees of effectiveness on anti-porin response, porin conformation, and cytokine profile of MGDG from different phyla with different FA composition [87].

A study that bio-prospected and isolated bioactive molecular species from the green seaweed *Capsosiphon fulvescens* highlighted two GL species: (2S)-l-O-(6Z,9Z,12Z,15Z-octadecatetraenoyl)-2-O-(4Z,10Z,13Z-hexadecatetraenoyl)-3-O-β-D-galactopyranosylglycerol and (2S)-l-O-(9Z,12Z,15Z-octadecatrienoyl)-2-O-(10Z,13Z-hexadecadienoyl)-3-O-β-D-galactopyranosylglycerol (designated by capsofulvesin A and B, respectively) (Figure 11A) that showed capacity to inhibit rat lens aldose reductase (RLAR), thus showing potential for application as anti-diabetic agents [88]. The inhibitory effect on lipid accumulation of (2S)-1-O-myristoyl-2-O-linoleyl-3-O-β-D-galactopyranosyl-sn-glycerol MGDG (14:0/18:2) and (2S)-1-O-palmitoyl-2-O-linoleyl-3-O-β-D-galactopyranosyl-sn-glycerol MGDG (16:0/18:2) glycolipids species (Figure 11B) from the brown seaweed *Sargassum horneri* was also reported in 3T3-L1 adipocytes [89]. These two MGDG species have in common the presence of linoleic acid (LA) (18:2 *n*-6) on *sn*-2 FA chain position, and when compared to other isolated MGDG species they were the most effective. Thus, this study suggested that LA on the *sn*-2 position of MGDG species played an important role on the inhibition of triglyceride accumulation in this biological model.

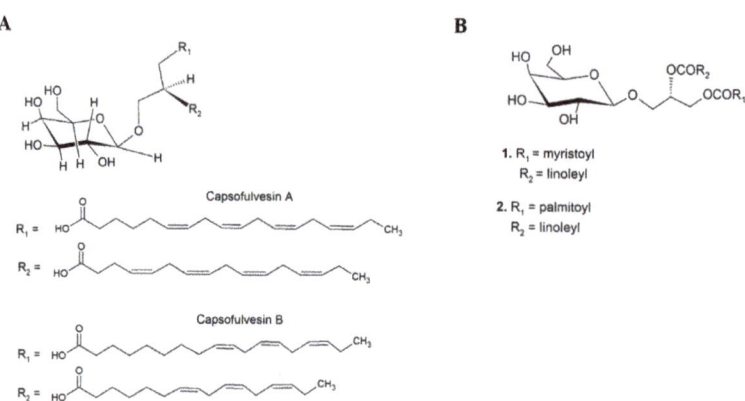

Figure 11. Chemical structures of bioactive complex lipids reported with anti-diabetic and anti-obesity activities. (**A**) (2S)-l-O-(6Z,9Z,12Z,15Z-octadecatetraenoyl)-2-O-(4Z,10Z,13Z-hexadecatetraenoyl)-3-O-β-D-galactopyranosylglycerol and (2S)-l-O-(9Z,12Z,15Z-octadecatrienoyl)-2-O-(10Z,13Z-hexadecadienoyl)-3-O-β-D-galactopyranosylglycerol capsofulvesin A and B (green seaweed *Capsosiphon fulvescens*); (**B**) (2S)-1-O-myristoyl-2-O-linoleyl-3-O-β-D-galactopyranosyl-*sn*-glycerol MGDG(14:0/18:2) (1) and (2S)-1-O-palmitoyl-2-O-linoleyl-3-O-β-D-galactopyranosyl-*sn*-glycerol MGDG(16:0/18:2) (2) (brown seaweed *Sargassum horneri*).

A human sperm motility stimulating activity was achieved by an isolated sulfonoglycolipid (named by S-ACT-1) from the red seaweed *Gelidiella acerosa*, whose molecular structure was not evidenced [90].

Table 4. Lipid species extracted from seaweeds with other activities. Extraction and characterization methodologies and tested bioactivities are reported. Data is reported by phylum (Ochrophyta, Rhodophyta, Chlorophyta, or mixed phyla) and ranked by alphabetical order of seaweed species name within each phylum (or mixed phyla).

Study Category	Seaweed Species	Phylum	Lipid Species	Activity and Action	Extraction	Identification/Characterization	Ref.
Category 4	*Solieria chordalis*, *Sargassum muticum*	Rhodophyta Ochrophyta	Glycolipids (GLs) and Phospholipids (PLs) groups	Antioxidant through DPPH free radical scavenging activity *Solieria chordalis*: GL with EC_{50} in a range of 0.9 to >5 mg mL^{-1} PL with EC_{50} in a range of 1.1 to >5 mg mL^{-1} *Sargassum muticum* GL with EC_{50} in a range of 0.9 to 4.1 mg mL^{-1} PL with EC_{50} in a range of 1 to 4.8 mg mL^{-1}	Extraction solvents: chloroform/methanol (1/1) or supercritical carbon dioxide pure or with 2% or 8% of ethanol. Fractionation: silica gel column chromatography.	No characterization	[86]
	Ahnfeltia tobuchiensis, *Laminaria japonica*, *Sargassum pallidum*, *Ulva fenestrata*	Rhodophyta Ochrophyta Chlorophyta	MGDG class	Regulation of the immunogenicity of protein antigen in the content of TI-complexes	Extraction solvents: chloroform, methanol. Fractionation: silica gel column chromatography, purified by preparative silica TLC.	GC-FID	[87]
	Capsosiphon fulvescens	Chlorophyta	Capsofulvesin A and B	Anti-diabetic Rat lens aldose reductase (RLAR) inhibitory assay capsofulvesin A: IC_{50} of 52.53 µM capsofulvesin B: IC_{50} of 101.92 µM	Extraction solvents: 95% ethanol at 80 °C, water, partitioned dichloromethane, ethyl acetate, and n-butanol. Fractionation/isolation: silica gel column chromatography, reversed-phase (RP-C18) chromatography.	^{1}H, ^{13}C-NMR	[88]
Category 5	*Sargassum horneri*	Ochrophyta	MGDG(14:0/18:2) MGDG(16:0/18:2)	Inhibitory effects on triglyceride and free fatty acids accumulation in 3T3-L1 adipocytes at concentration of 10 µM	Extraction: 70% alcohol, ethyl acetate. Fractionation/isolation: vacuum liquid chromatography (VLC) over silica gel, Sephadex LH-20, flash silica gel column chromatography	TLC; ^{1}H, ^{13}C-NMR; GC-FID; HPLC–MS/MS	[89]
	Gelidiella acerosa	Rhodophyta	SQDG (S-ACT-1)	Human sperm motility stimulating activity	Extraction: dichloromethane: methanol (1:1). Fractionation/isolation: Sephadex LH-20	TLC; ^{1}H, ^{13}C-NMR, IR	[90]

4. Concluding Remarks and Future Prospects

Seaweeds remain largely untapped reservoirs of natural bioactive molecules [10]. In fact, more than 11,300 species of seaweeds are reported on Algabase, of which only 42 species were surveyed on category 4 (studies of extracts enriched in isolated groups or classes of complex lipids) and category 5 (studies of isolated complex lipid molecular species), most of them within the Ochrophyta phylum. This reveals that the bioprospecting potential of seaweed lipids remains largely untapped.

Complex lipids from seaweeds are emerging as bioactive molecules with hidden potential; however, their exploitation is far from being optimized and their action mechanisms are still poorly understood. This figure is likely to change as more seaweeds have their bioactive complex lipids characterized and more mechanism-oriented studies are performed.

To date, not only do most studies lack a systematic research approach, but most of the lipid bioactivities already identified refer to total lipid extracts. Indeed, only a few studies have achieved molecular isolation and characterization of bioactive lipids. Interestingly, complex lipids isolated from seaweed species with reported bioactivity have been classified mainly as GLs species. This systematic analysis pinpoints the promising results of naturally occurring GLs in seaweeds, with emphasis to their antitumor and anti-inflammatory potential. The advances of emerging food/feed, nutraceutical, cosmeceutical, pharmaceutical, and complementary medicine research fields [91–93], as well as biological and experimental sciences, will contribute to boost structural characterization of complex lipids and to link lipid structure and bioactivity through different mechanisms of action.

Regardless of their polyphyletic nature, it is unquestionable that seaweeds as a whole, remain an important reservoir of lipid phytochemicals. Despite the low abundance of these biomolecules in seaweeds, they remain largely uncharacterized and unexplored. Complex lipids from seaweeds offer an unmatched chemical diversity and structural complexity when compared to terrestrial phytochemicals. It seems that seaweeds species or genera feature unique lipidomes, which likely enhances the potential number of target applications. Lipidomic characterization strategies using high-resolution apparatus, such as mass spectrometry, can be paramount to unleash the true potential of these biomolecules. The species-specific lipidome for each seaweed could be applied to the production of target bioactive lipids. Otherwise, isolated bioactive complex lipids can be used as a large-scale synthesis model. While some of their natural chemotherapy diversity has already been studied, resulting in open access and proprietary compound libraries, there is still a multitude of lipids from algal origin that have hardly been characterized. The potential of these biomolecules to develop new products and processes is certainly far from being exhausted. It is expected that the bioprospecting of seaweed extracts enriched in active lipids for the formulation of high-end products can foster the added value of seaweed biomass production.

Under this scope it will be possible to put forward innovative processes for the production of farmed seaweeds biomass under controlled conditions, as these will allow to target new markets and consumers under a circular and sustainable blue bioeconomy framework.

Supplementary Materials: The following are available online at https://www.mdpi.com/article/10.3390/md19120686/s1, Table S1: Eligible studies distributed by title, published year, doi (when applicable), seaweeds species, genus, phylum, bioactivity reported, and category where they were inserted.

Author Contributions: Conceptualization, D.L. and M.R.D.; methodology, D.L.; validation, M.R.D., F.R., M.C.L., A.I.L., R.C. and M.R.D.; formal analysis, D.L.; data curation, D.L. and F.R.; writing—original draft preparation, D.L.; writing—review and editing, F.R., M.C.L., A.I.L., R.C. and M.R.D.; supervision, A.I.L., R.C. and M.R.D. All authors have read and agreed to the published version of the manuscript.

Funding: The authors are grateful to Fundação para a Ciência e a Tecnologia (FCT, Portugal), European Union, QREN, POPH, FEDER, and COMPETE by funding CESAM (UIDP/50017/2020 + UIDB/50017/2020), and LAQV/REQUIMTE (UIDP/50006/2020 + UIDB/50006/2020). Thanks to the project Omics 4 Algae: Lipidomic tools for chemical phenotyping, traceability, and valorization of seaweeds from aquaculture as a sustainable source of high added-value compounds (POCI-01-0145-FEDER-030962), funded by Centro2020, through FEDER and PT2020.Diana Lopes (SFRH/BD/119027/2016) is grateful to FCT, Programa Operacional do Capital Humano (POCH) and European Union through European Social Fund (FSE) for her grant. FCT is also thanked for the Scientific Employment Stimulus 2017, with a Junior Researcher contract to Felisa Rey (CEECIND/00580/2017), and an Assistant Researcher contract to Miguel Leal (CEECIND/01618/2020). This is a contribution of the Marine Lipidomics Laboratory.

Conflicts of Interest: The authors declare no conflict of interest.

References

1. Mahadevan, K. *Chapter 13—Seaweeds: A Sustainable Food Source*; Tiwari, B.K., Troy, D.J.B.T.-S.S., Eds.; Academic Press: San Diego, CA, USA, 2015; pp. 347–364.
2. European Union. *Farm to Fork Strategy: For a Fair, Healthy and Environmentally-Friendly Food System*; EU: Maastricht, The Netherlands, 2020.
3. WHO. *Sustainable Healthy Diets: Guiding Principles*; Food and Agriculture Organization of the United Nations: Rome, Italy, 2019; p. 37.
4. Collins, K.G.; Fitzgerald, G.F.; Stanton, C.; Ross, R.P. Looking beyond the terrestrial: The potential of seaweed derived bioactives to treat non-communicable diseases. *Mar. Drugs* **2016**, *14*, 60. [CrossRef]
5. Wan-Loy, C.; Siew-Moi, P. Marine algae as a potential source for anti-obesity agents. *Mar. Drugs* **2016**, *14*, 222. [CrossRef] [PubMed]
6. Shannon, E.; Abu-Ghannam, N. Antibacterial Derivatives of Marine Algae: An Overview of Pharmacological Mechanisms and Applications. *Mar. Drugs* **2016**, *14*, 81. [CrossRef] [PubMed]
7. Alves, E.; Dias, M.; Lopes, D.; Almeida, A.; Domingues, M.D.R.; Rey, F. Antimicrobial lipids from plants and marine organisms: An overview of the current state-of-the-art and future prospects. *Antibiotics* **2020**, *9*, 441. [CrossRef] [PubMed]
8. Pereira, L.; Critchley, A.T. The COVID 19 novel coronavirus pandemic 2020: Seaweeds to the rescue? Why does substantial, supporting research about the antiviral properties of seaweed polysaccharides seem to go unrecognized by the pharmaceutical community in these desperate times? *J. Appl. Phycol.* **2020**, *32*, 1875–1877. [CrossRef] [PubMed]
9. Vincent, A.; Stanley, A.; Ring, J. *Hidden Champion of the Ocean: Seaweed as a Growth Engine for a Sustainable European Future*. 2020. Available online: https://www.seaweedeurope.com/wp-content/uploads/2020/10/Seaweed_for_Europe-Hidden_Champion_of_the_ocean-Report.pdf (accessed on 5 November 2021).
10. Leal, M.C.; Munro, M.H.G.; Blunt, J.W.; Puga, J.; Jesus, B.; Calado, R.; Rosa, R.; Madeira, C. Biogeography and biodiscovery hotspots of macroalgal marine natural products. *Nat. Prod. Rep.* **2013**, *30*, 1380–1390. [CrossRef]
11. Vieira, H.; Leal, M.C.; Calado, R. Fifty Shades of Blue: How Blue Biotechnology is Shaping the Bioeconomy. *Trends Biotechnol.* **2020**, *38*, 940–943. [CrossRef]
12. Gomez-Zavaglia, A.; Prieto Lage, M.A.; Jimenez-Lopez, C.; Mejuto, J.C.; Simal-Gandara, J. The Potential of Seaweeds as a Source of Functional Ingredients of Prebiotic and Antioxidant Value. *Antioxidants* **2019**, *8*, 406. [CrossRef]
13. Pereira, L. Seaweeds as Source of Bioactive Substances and Skin Care Therapy—Cosmeceuticals, Algotheraphy, and Thalassotherapy. *Cosmetics* **2018**, *5*, 68. [CrossRef]
14. Rengasamy, K.R.R.; Mahomoodally, M.F.; Aumeeruddy, M.Z.; Zengin, G.; Xiao, J.; Kim, D.H. Bioactive compounds in seaweeds: An overview of their biological properties and safety. *Food Chem. Toxicol.* **2020**, *135*, 111013. [CrossRef]
15. van Ginneken, V.J.; Helsper, J.P.; de Visser, W.; van Keulen, H.; Brandenburg, W.A. Polyunsaturated fatty acids in various macroalgal species from north Atlantic and tropical seas. *Lipids Health Dis.* **2011**, *10*, 1–8. [CrossRef]
16. Cyberlipid. Available online: http://cyberlipid.gerli.com/description/complex-lipids/ (accessed on 5 November 2021).
17. Kagan, M.L.; Levy, A.; Leikin-Frenkel, A. Comparative study of tissue deposition of omega-3 fatty acids from polar-lipid rich oil of the microalgae *Nannochloropsis oculata* with krill oil in rats. *Food Funct.* **2015**, *6*, 185–191. [CrossRef] [PubMed]
18. Che, H.; Zhou, M.; Zhang, T.; Zhang, L.; Ding, L.; Yanagita, T.; Xu, J.; Xue, C.; Wang, Y. EPA enriched ethanolamine plasmalogens significantly improve cognition of Alzheimer's disease mouse model by suppressing β-amyloid generation. *J. Funct. Foods* **2018**, *41*, 9–18. [CrossRef]
19. Drouin, G.; Catheline, D.; Guillocheau, E.; Gueret, P.; Baudry, C.; Le Ruyet, P.; Rioux, V.; Legrand, P. Comparative effects of dietary n-3 docosapentaenoic acid (DPA), DHA and EPA on plasma lipid parameters, oxidative status and fatty acid tissue composition. *J. Nutr. Biochem.* **2019**, *63*, 186–196. [CrossRef] [PubMed]
20. Lordan, R.; Tsoupras, A.; Zabetakis, I. Phospholipids of animal and marine origin: Structure, function, and anti-inflammatory properties. *Molecules* **2017**, *22*, 1964. [CrossRef] [PubMed]
21. Haq, M.; Suraiya, S.; Ahmed, S.; Chun, B.-S. Phospholipids from marine source: Extractions and forthcoming industrial applications. *J. Funct. Foods* **2021**, *80*, 104388. [CrossRef]
22. Kalisch, B.; Dörmann, P.; Hölzl, G. *DGDG and Glycolipids in Plants and Algae BT—Lipids in Plant and Algae Development*; Nakamura, Y., Li-Beisson, Y., Eds.; Springer International Publishing: Cham, Switzerland, 2016; pp. 51–83.

23. Kumari, P.; Kumar, M.; Reddy, C.R.K.; Jha, B. Algal lipids, fatty acids and sterols. In *Functional Ingredients from Algae for Foods and Nutraceuticals*; Woodhead Publishing: Sawston, UK, 2013; pp. 87–134.
24. Shen, L.; Yang, Y.; Ou, T.; Key, C.-C.C.; Tong, S.H.; Sequeira, R.C.; Nelson, J.M.; Nie, Y.; Wang, Z.; Boudyguina, E.; et al. Dietary PUFAs attenuate NLRP3 inflammasome activation via enhancing macrophage autophagy. *J. Lipid Res.* **2017**, *58*, 1808–1821. [CrossRef]
25. Barros, R.; Moreira, A.; Fonseca, J.; Delgado, L.; Graça Castel-Branco, M.; Haahtela, T.; Lopes, C.; Moreira, P. Dietary intake of α-linolenic acid and low ratio of n-6: N-3 PUFA are associated with decreased exhaled NO and improved asthma control. *Br. J. Nutr.* **2011**, *106*, 441–450. [CrossRef]
26. Lopes, D.; Melo, T.; Rey, F.; Meneses, J.; Monteiro, F.L.; Helguero, L.A.; Abreu, M.H.; Lillebø, A.I.; Calado, R.; Domingues, M.R. Valuing bioactive lipids from green, red and brown macroalgae from aquaculture, to foster functionality and biotechnological applications. *Molecules* **2020**, *25*, 3883. [CrossRef]
27. Lopes, D.; Melo, T.; Meneses, J.; Abreu, M.H.; Pereira, R.; Domingues, P.; Lillebø, A.I.; Calado, R.; Rosário Domingues, M. A new look for the red macroalga *Palmaria palmata*: A seafood with polar lipids rich in EPA and with antioxidant properties. *Mar. Drugs* **2019**, *17*, 533. [CrossRef]
28. Plouguerné, E.; da Gama, B.A.P.; Pereira, R.C.; Barreto-Bergter, E. Glycolipids from seaweeds and their potential biotechnological applications. *Front. Cell. Infect. Microbiol.* **2014**, *4*, 1–5. [CrossRef] [PubMed]
29. Yuan, S.; Wang, P.; Xiao, L.; Liang, Y.; Huang, Y.; Ye, H.; Wu, K.; Lu, Y. Enrichment of lipids from agar production wastes of *Gracilaria lemaneiformis* by ultrasonication: A green sustainable process. *Biomass Convers. Biorefinery* **2020**, *11*, 2899–2908. [CrossRef]
30. do-Amaral, C.C.F.; Pacheco, B.S.; Segatto, N.V.; Paschoal, J.D.F.; Santos, M.A.Z.; Seixas, F.K.; Pereira, C.M.P.; Astorga-España, M.S.; Mansilla, A.; Collares, T. Lipidic profile of sub-Antarctic seaweed *Mazzaella laminarioides* (Gigartinales, Rhodophyta) in distinct developmental phases and cell cytotoxicity in bladder cancer. *Algal Res.* **2020**, *48*, 101936. [CrossRef]
31. Pacheco, B.S.; dos Santos, M.A.Z.; Schultze, E.; Martins, R.M.; Lund, R.G.; Seixas, F.K.; Colepicolo, P.; Collares, T.; Paula, F.R.; De Pereira, C.M.P. Cytotoxic activity of fatty acids from Antarctic macroalgae on the growth of human breast cancer cells. *Front. Bioeng. Biotechnol.* **2018**, *6*, 185. [CrossRef] [PubMed]
32. Lopes, D.; Moreira, A.S.P.; Rey, F.; da Costa, E.; Melo, T.; Maciel, E.; Rego, A.; Abreu, M.H.; Domingues, P.; Calado, R.; et al. Lipidomic signature of the green macroalgae *Ulva rigida* farmed in a sustainable integrated multi-trophic aquaculture. *J. Appl. Phycol.* **2019**, *31*, 1369–1381. [CrossRef]
33. Rey, F.; Cartaxana, P.; Melo, T.; Calado, R.; Pereira, R.; Abreu, H.; Domingues, P.; Cruz, S.; Rosário Domingues, M. Domesticated populations of *Codium tomentosum* display lipid extracts with lower seasonal shifts than conspecifics from the wild-relevance for biotechnological applications of this green seaweed. *Mar. Drugs* **2020**, *18*, 188. [CrossRef] [PubMed]
34. Melo, T.; Alves, E.; Azevedo, V.; Martins, A.S.; Neves, B.; Domingues, P.; Calado, R.; Abreu, M.H.; Domingues, M.R. Lipidomics as a new approach for the bioprospecting of marine macroalgae—Unraveling the polar lipid and fatty acid composition of chondrus crispus. *Algal Res.* **2015**, *8*, 181–191. [CrossRef]
35. da Costa, E.; Azevedo, V.; Melo, T.; Rego, A.M.; Evtuguin, D.V.; Domingues, P.; Calado, R.; Pereira, R.; Abreu, M.H.; Domingues, M.R. High-resolution lipidomics of the early life stages of the red seaweed *Porphyra dioica*. *Molecules* **2018**, *23*, 187. [CrossRef]
36. Da Costa, E.; Melo, T.; Moreira, A.S.P.; Bernardo, C.; Helguero, L.; Ferreira, I.; Cruz, M.T.; Rego, A.M.; Domingues, P.; Calado, R.; et al. Valorization of lipids from *Gracilaria* sp. through lipidomics and decoding of antiproliferative and anti-inflammatory activity. *Mar. Drugs* **2017**, *15*, 62. [CrossRef]
37. da Costa, E.; Domingues, P.; Melo, T.; Coelho, E.; Pereira, R.; Calado, R.; Abreu, H.M.; Domingues, R.M. Lipidomic signatures reveal seasonal shifts on the relative abundance of high-valued lipids from the brown algae *Fucus vesiculosus*. *Mar. Drugs* **2019**, *17*, 335. [CrossRef]
38. Rey, F.; Lopes, D.; Maciel, E.; Monteiro, J.; Skjermo, J.; Funderud, J.; Raposo, D.; Domingues, P.; Calado, R.; Domingues, M.R. Polar lipid profile of *Saccharina latissima*, a functional food from the sea. *Algal Res.* **2019**, *39*, 101473. [CrossRef]
39. Santos, F.; Monteiro, J.P.; Duarte, D.; Melo, T.; Lopes, D.; da Costa, E.; Domingues, M.R. Unraveling the Lipidome and Antioxidant Activity of Native *Bifurcaria bifurcata* and Invasive *Sargassum muticum* Seaweeds: A Lipid Perspective on How Systemic Intrusion May Present an Opportunity. *Antioxidants* **2020**, *9*, 642. [CrossRef] [PubMed]
40. Lopes, D.; Melo, T.; Rey, F.; Costa, E.; Moreira, A.S.P.; Abreu, M.H.; Domingues, P.; Lillebø, A.I.; Calado, R.; Rosário Domingues, M. Insights of species-specific polar lipidome signatures of seaweeds fostering their valorization in the blue bioeconomy. *Algal Res.* **2021**, *55*, 102242. [CrossRef]
41. Araújo, R.; Vázquez Calderón, F.; Sánchez López, J.; Azevedo, I.C.; Bruhn, A.; Fluch, S.; Garcia Tasende, M.; Ghaderiardakani, F.; Ilmjärv, T.; Laurans, M. Current status of the algae production industry in Europe: An emerging sector of the Blue Bioeconomy. *Front. Mar. Sci.* **2021**, *7*, 1247. [CrossRef]
42. Moher, D.; Liberati, A.; Tetzlaff, J.; Altman, D.G.; Prisma Group. Preferred reporting items for systematic reviews and meta-analyses: The PRISMA statement. *PLoS Med.* **2009**, *6*, e1000097. [CrossRef]
43. Kindleysides, S.; Quek, S.-Y.; Miller, M.R. Inhibition of fish oil oxidation and the radical scavenging activity of New Zealand seaweed extracts. *Food Chem.* **2012**, *133*, 1624–1631. [CrossRef]
44. Francavilla, M.; Franchi, M.; Monteleone, M.; Caroppo, C. The red seaweed *Gracilaria gracilis* as a multi products source. *Mar. Drugs* **2013**, *11*, 3754–3776. [CrossRef] [PubMed]

45. Nagappan, T.; Vairappan, C.S. Nutritional and bioactive properties of three edible species of green algae, genus *Caulerpa* (Caulerpaceae). *J. Appl. Phycol.* **2014**, *26*, 1019–1027. [CrossRef]
46. Rodeiro, I.; Olguín, S.; Santes, R.; Herrera, J.A.; Pérez, C.L.; Mangas, R.; Hernández, Y.; Fernández, G.; Hernández, I.; Hernández-Ojeda, S.; et al. Gas Chromatography-Mass Spectrometry Analysis of *Ulva fasciata* (Green Seaweed) Extract and Evaluation of Its Cytoprotective and Antigenotoxic Effects. *Evid.-Based Complement. Altern. Med.* **2015**, *2015*, 520598. [CrossRef]
47. Farvin, K.H.S.; Jacobsen, C. Antioxidant activity of seaweed extracts: In vitro assays, evaluation in 5% fish oil-in-water emulsions and characterization. *J. Am. Oil Chem. Soc.* **2015**, *92*, 571–587. [CrossRef]
48. Honold, P.J.; Jacobsen, C.; Jónsdóttir, R.; Kristinsson, H.G.; Hermund, D.B. Potential seaweed-based food ingredients to inhibit lipid oxidation in fish-oil-enriched mayonnaise. *Eur. Food Res. Technol.* **2016**, *242*, 571–584. [CrossRef]
49. Trigui, M.; Gasmi, L.; Zouari, I.; Tounsi, S. Seasonal variation in phenolic composition, antibacterial and antioxidant activities of *Ulva rigida* (Chlorophyta) and assessment of antiacetylcholinesterase potential. *J. Appl. Phycol.* **2013**, *25*, 319–328. [CrossRef]
50. Newman, D.J.; Cragg, G.M. Marine Natural Products and Related Compounds in Clinical and Advanced Preclinical Trials. *J. Nat. Prod.* **2004**, *67*, 1216–1238. [CrossRef]
51. Cragg, G.M.; Newman, D.J. Natural products: A continuing source of novel drug leads. *Biochim. Biophys. Acta (BBA)-Gen. Subj.* **2013**, *1830*, 3670–3695. [CrossRef] [PubMed]
52. Luo, H.; Vong, C.T.; Chen, H.; Gao, Y.; Lyu, P.; Qiu, L.; Zhao, M.; Liu, Q.; Cheng, Z.; Zou, J.; et al. Naturally occurring anti-cancer compounds: Shining from Chinese herbal medicine. *Chin. Med.* **2019**, *14*, 48. [CrossRef]
53. Cragg, G.M.; Kingston, D.G.I.; Newman, D.J. *Anticancer Agents from Natural Products*; CRC Press: Boca Raton, FL, USA; Taylor & Francis: Abingdon, UK, 2005.
54. Newman, D.J.; Cragg, G.M.; Snader, K.M. Natural Products as Sources of New Drugs over the Period 1981–2002. *J. Nat. Prod.* **2003**, *66*, 1022–1037. [CrossRef]
55. Tsai, C.-J.; Sun Pan, B. Identification of sulfoglycolipid bioactivities and characteristic fatty acids of marine macroalgae. *J. Agric. Food Chem.* **2012**, *60*, 8404–8410. [CrossRef]
56. El Baz, F.K.; El Baroty, G.S.; Abd El Baky, H.H.; Abd El-Salam, O.I.; Ibrahim, E.A. Structural characterization and biological activity of sulfolipids from selected marine algae. *Grasas Aceites* **2013**, *64*, 561–571.
57. Akbari, V.; Abedi, B.; Yegdaneh, A. Bioassay-guided isolation of glycolipids from the seaweed *Gracilaria corticata*. *Res. Pharm. Sci.* **2020**, *15*, 473–480. [CrossRef]
58. Jiang, R.-W.; Hay, M.E.; Fairchild, C.R.; Prudhomme, J.; Le Roch, K.; Aalbersberg, W.; Kubanek, J. Antineoplastic unsaturated fatty acids from Fijian macroalgae. *Phytochemistry* **2008**, *69*, 2495–2500. [CrossRef]
59. Bhaskar, N.; Hosakawa, M.; Miyashita, K. Growth inhibition of human pro-myelocytic leukemia (HL-60) cells by lipid extracts of marine alga *Sargassum marginatum* (Fucales, Phaeophyta) harvested of Goa (west coast of India) with special reference to fatty acid composition. *Indian J. Mar. Sci.* **2004**, *33*, 355–360.
60. Hossain, Z.; Kurihara, H.; Hosokawa, M.; Takahashi, K. Growth inhibition and induction of differentiation and apoptosis mediated by sodium butyrate in Caco-2 cells with algal glycolipids. *Vitr. Cell. Dev. Biol.-Anim.* **2005**, *41*, 154–159. [CrossRef] [PubMed]
61. Kendel, M.; Wielgosz-collin, G.; Bertrand, S.; Roussakis, C.; Bourgougnon, N.; Bedoux, G. Lipid Composition, Fatty Acids and Sterols in the Seaweeds *Ulva armoricana*, and *Solieria chordalis* from Brittany (France): An Analysis from Nutritional, Chemotaxonomic, and Antiproliferative Activity Perspectives. *Mar. Drugs* **2015**, *13*, 5606–5628. [CrossRef] [PubMed]
62. Imbs, T.I.; Ermakova, S.P.; Fedoreyev, S.A.; Anastyuk, S.D.; Zvyagintseva, T.N. Isolation of Fucoxanthin and Highly Unsaturated Monogalactosyldiacylglycerol from Brown Alga *Fucus evanescens* C Agardh and in vitro Investigation of Their Antitumor Activity. *Mar. Biotechnol.* **2013**, *15*, 606–612. [CrossRef] [PubMed]
63. Mizushina, Y.; Sugiyama, Y.; Yoshida, H.; Hanashima, S.; Yamazaki, T.; Kamisuki, S.; Ohta, K.; Takemura, M.; Yamaguchi, T.; Matsukage, A.; et al. Galactosyldiacylglycerol, a Mammalian DNA Polymerase Alpha-Specific Inhibitor from a Sea Alga, *Petalonia bingbamiae*. *Biol. Pharm. Bull.* **2001**, *24*, 982–987. [CrossRef]
64. Zhou, B.-N.; Tang, S.; Johnson, R.K.; Mattern, M.P.; Lazo, J.S.; Sharlow, E.R.; Harich, K.; Kingston, D.G.I. New glycolipid inhibitors of Myt1 kinase. *Tetrahedron* **2005**, *61*, 883–887. [CrossRef]
65. Göllner, C.; Philipp, C.; Dobner, B.; Sippl, W.; Schmidt, M. First total synthesis of 1,2-dipalmitoyl-3-(N-palmitoyl-6′-amino-6′-deoxy-α-d-glucosyl)-sn-glycerol—A glycoglycerolipid of a marine alga with a high inhibitor activity against human Myt1-kinase. *Carbohydr. Res.* **2009**, *344*, 1628–1631. [CrossRef]
66. Williams, D.E.; Sturgeon, C.M.; Roberge, M.; Andersen, R.J. Nigricanosides A and B, antimitotic glycolipids isolated from the green alga *Avrainvillea nigricans* collected in Dominica. *J. Am. Chem. Soc.* **2007**, *129*, 5822–5823. [CrossRef]
67. Abdulkhaleq, L.A.; Assi, M.A.; Abdullah, R.; Zamri-Saad, M.; Taufiq-Yap, Y.H.; Hezmee, M.N.M. The crucial roles of inflammatory mediators in inflammation: A review. *Vet. World* **2018**, *11*, 627. [CrossRef]
68. Kamali, A.N.; Noorbakhsh, S.M.; Hamedifar, H.; Jadidi-Niaragh, F.; Yazdani, R.; Bautista, J.M.; Azizi, G. A role for Th1-like Th17 cells in the pathogenesis of inflammatory and autoimmune disorders. *Mol. Immunol.* **2019**, *105*, 107–115. [CrossRef]
69. Sharma, J.N.; Al-Omran, A.; Parvathy, S.S. Role of nitric oxide in inflammatory diseases. *Inflammopharmacology* **2007**, *15*, 252–259. [CrossRef]

70. Banskota, A.H.; Stefanova, R.; Sperker, S.; Lall, S.P.; Craigie, J.S.; Hafting, J.T.; Critchley, A.T. Polar lipids from the marine macroalga *Palmaria palmata* inhibit lipopolysaccharide-induced nitric oxide production in RAW264.7 macrophage cells. *Phytochemistry* **2014**, *101*, 101–108. [CrossRef]
71. Banskota, A.H.; Stefanova, R.; Sperker, S.; Lall, S.; Craigie, J.S.; Hafting, J.T. Lipids isolated from the cultivated red alga *Chondrus crispus* inhibit nitric oxide production. *J. Appl. Phycol.* **2014**, *26*, 1565–1571. [CrossRef]
72. Jang, Y.; Kim, M.; Hwang, S.W. Molecular mechanisms underlying the actions of arachidonic acid-derived prostaglandins on peripheral nociception. *J. Neuroinflammation* **2020**, *17*, 30. [CrossRef]
73. Burke, J.E.; Dennis, E.A. Phospholipase A2 structure/function, mechanism, and signaling. *J. Lipid Res.* **2009**, *50*, S237–S242. [CrossRef]
74. Cho, J.Y.; Gyawali, Y.P.; Ahn, S.H.; Khan, M.N.A.; Kong, I.S.; Hong, Y.K. A methoxylated fatty acid isolated from the brown seaweed *Ishige okamurae* inhibits bacterial phospholipase A2. *Phyther. Res.* **2008**, *22*, 1070–1074. [CrossRef] [PubMed]
75. Cos, P.; Vlietinck, A.J.; Berghe, D.V.; Maes, L. Anti-infective potential of natural products: How to develop a stronger in vitro 'proof-of-concept'. *J. Ethnopharmacol.* **2006**, *106*, 290–302. [CrossRef] [PubMed]
76. Gerasimenko, N.I.; Martyyas, E.A.; Busarova, N.G. Composition of lipids and biological activity of lipids and photosynthetic pigments from algae of the families Laminariaceae and Alariaceae. *Chem. Nat. Compd.* **2012**, *48*, 737–741. [CrossRef]
77. Gerasimenko, N.I.; Chaykina, E.L.; Busarova, N.G.; Anisimov, M.M. Antimicrobic and hemolytic activity of low-molecular metabolits of brown seaweed *Laminaria cichorioides* (Miyabe). *Appl. Biochem. Microbiol.* **2010**, *46*, 426–430. [CrossRef]
78. Gerasimenko, N.I.; Busarova, N.G.; Martyyas, E.A. Composition of lipids from *Fucus evanescens* (Seas of Okhotsk and Japan) and biological activity of lipids and photosynthetic pigments. *Chem. Nat. Compd.* **2012**, *48*, 742–747. [CrossRef]
79. Martyyas, E.A.; Gerasimenko, N.I.; Busarova, N.G.; Yurchenko, E.A.; Skriptsova, A.V.; Anisimov, M.M. Seasonal changes in biological activity of lipids and photosynthetic pigments of *Saccharina cichorioides* (Miyabe) (Laminariaceae Family). *Russ. J. Bioorganic Chem.* **2013**, *39*, 720–727. [CrossRef]
80. Al-Fadhli, A.; Wahidulla, S.; D'Souza, L. Glycolipids from the red alga *Chondria armata* (Kütz.) Okamura. *Glycobiology* **2006**, *16*, 902–915. [CrossRef]
81. Cantillo-Ciau, Z.; Moo-Puc, R.; Quijano, L.; Freile-Pelegrín, Y. The tropical brown alga *Lobophora variegata*: A source of antiprotozoal compounds. *Mar. Drugs* **2010**, *8*, 1292–1304. [CrossRef] [PubMed]
82. Sun, Y.Y.; Wang, H.; Guo, G.L.; Pu, Y.F.; Yan, B.L.; Wang, C.H. Isolation, purification, and identification of antialgal substances in green alga *Ulva prolifera* for antialgal activity against the common harmful red tide microalgae. *Environ. Sci. Pollut. Res.* **2016**, *23*, 1449–1459. [CrossRef] [PubMed]
83. Plouguerné, E.; de Souza, L.M.; Sassaki, G.L.; Hellio, C.; Trepos, R.; da Gama, B.A.P.; Pereira, R.C.; Barreto-Bergter, E. Glycoglycerolipids From *Sargassum vulgare* as Potential Antifouling Agents. *Front. Mar. Sci.* **2020**, *7*, 116. [CrossRef]
84. De Souza, L.M.; Sassaki, G.L.; Romanos, M.T.V.; Barreto-Bergter, E. Structural characterization and anti-HSV-1 and HSV-2 activity of glycolipids from the marine algae *Osmundaria obtusiloba* isolated from Southeastern Brazilian coast. *Mar. Drugs* **2012**, *10*, 918–931. [CrossRef]
85. Plouguerné, E.; De Souza, L.M.; Sassaki, G.L.; Cavalcanti, J.F.; Romanos, M.T.V.; Da Gama, B.A.P.; Pereira, R.C.; Barreto-Bergter, E. Antiviral sulfoquinovosyldiacylglycerols (SQDGs) from the Brazilian brown seaweed *Sargassum vulgare*. *Mar. Drugs* **2013**, *11*, 4628–4640. [CrossRef] [PubMed]
86. Terme, N.; Boulho, R.; Kucma, J.-P.; Bourgougnon, N.; Bedoux, G. Radical scavenging activity of lipids from seaweeds isolated by solid-liquid extraction and supercritical fluids. *OCL* **2018**, *25*, D505. [CrossRef]
87. Sanina, N.M.; Kostetsky, E.Y.; Shnyrov, V.L.; Tsybulsky, A.V.; Novikova, O.D.; Portniagina, O.Y.; Vorobieva, N.S.; Mazeika, A.N.; Bogdanov, M. V The influence of monogalactosyldiacylglycerols from different marine macrophytes on immunogenicity and conformation of protein antigen of tubular immunostimulating complex. *Biochimie* **2012**, *94*, 1048–1056. [CrossRef] [PubMed]
88. Islam, M.N.; Choi, S.H.; Moon, H.E.; Park, J.J.; Jung, H.A.; Woo, M.H.; Woo, H.C.; Choi, J.S. The inhibitory activities of the edible green alga *Capsosiphon fulvescens* on rat lens aldose reductase and advanced glycation end products formation. *Eur. J. Nutr.* **2014**, *53*, 233–242. [CrossRef]
89. Ma, A.-C.; Chen, Z.; Wang, T.; Song, N.; Yan, Q.; Fang, Y.-C.; Guan, H.-S.; Liu, H.-B. Isolation of the Molecular Species of Monogalactosyldiacylglycerols from Brown Edible Seaweed *Sargassum horneri* and Their Inhibitory Effects on Triglyceride Accumulation in 3T3-L1 Adipocytes. *J. Agric. Food Chem.* **2014**, *62*, 11157–11162. [CrossRef] [PubMed]
90. Premakumara, G.A.; Ratnasooriya, W.D.; Tillekeratne, L.M.; Amarasekare, A.S. Human sperm motility stimulating activity of a sulfono glycolipid isolated from Sri Lankan marine red alga *Gelidiella acerosa*. *Asian J. Androl.* **2001**, *3*, 27–31. [PubMed]
91. Holdt, S.L.; Kraan, S. Bioactive compounds in seaweed: Functional food applications and legislation. *J. Appl. Phycol.* **2011**, *23*, 543–597. [CrossRef]
92. Mohamed, S.; Hashim, S.N.; Rahman, H.A. Seaweeds: A sustainable functional food for complementary and alternative therapy. *Trends Food Sci. Technol.* **2012**, *23*, 83–96. [CrossRef]
93. Wijesinghe, W.A.J.P.; Jeon, Y.-J. Biological activities and potential cosmeceutical applications of bioactive components from brown seaweeds: A review. *Phytochem. Rev.* **2011**, *10*, 431–443. [CrossRef]

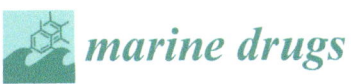

Review

Advances in Technologies for Highly Active Omega-3 Fatty Acids from Krill Oil: Clinical Applications

Alessandro Colletti [1], Giancarlo Cravotto [1,2], Valentina Citi [3,4,5], Alma Martelli [3,4,5], Lara Testai [3,4,5] and Arrigo F. G. Cicero [6,7,*]

1. Department of Drug Science and Technology, University of Turin, Via P. Giuria 9, 10125 Turin, Italy; Alessandro.colletti@unito.it (A.C.); giancarlo.cravotto@unito.it (G.C.)
2. World-Class Research Center "Digital Biodesign and Personalized Healthcare", Sechenov First Moscow State Medical University, 8 Trubetskaya ul, 101000 Moscow, Russia
3. Department of Pharmacy, University of Pisa, 56121 Pisa, Italy; valentina.citi@unipi.it (V.C.); alma.martelli@unipi.it (A.M.); lara.testai@unipi.it (L.T.)
4. Interdepartmental Research Centre "Nutraceuticals and Food for Health (NUTRAFOOD)", University of Pisa, 56121 Pisa, Italy
5. Interdepartmental Research Centre of Ageing, Biology and Pathology, University of Pisa, 56121 Pisa, Italy
6. Medical and Surgical Sciences Department, Alma Mater Studiorum University of Bologna, 40138 Bologna, Italy
7. IRCCS Policlinico S. Orsola-Malpighi, 40138 Bologna, Italy
* Correspondence: arrigo.cicero@unibo.it

Abstract: *Euphausia superba*, commonly known as krill, is a small marine crustacean from the Antarctic Ocean that plays an important role in the marine ecosystem, serving as feed for most fish. It is a known source of highly bioavailable omega-3 polyunsaturated fatty acids (eicosapentaenoic acid and docosahexaenoic acid). In preclinical studies, krill oil showed metabolic, anti-inflammatory, neuroprotective and chemo preventive effects, while in clinical trials it showed significant metabolic, vascular and ergogenic actions. Solvent extraction is the most conventional method to obtain krill oil. However, different solvents must be used to extract all lipids from krill because of the diversity of the polarities of the lipid compounds in the biomass. This review aims to provide an overview of the chemical composition, bioavailability and bioaccessibility of krill oil, as well as the mechanisms of action, classic and non-conventional extraction techniques, health benefits and current applications of this marine crustacean.

Keywords: krill oil; omega-3 polyunsaturated fatty acids; bioavailability; nutraceuticals; dietary supplements

1. Introduction

Euphausia superba, commonly known as krill, is a small marine crustacean from the Antarctic Ocean that plays an important role in the marine ecosystem, serving as feed for most fish [1]. Although measuring krill biomass is difficult, it has been estimated at approximately 379 million metric tons. The Commission for the Conservation of Antarctic Marine Living Resources (CCAMLR) has set a catch limit of 620,000 tons per year to protect the marine ecosystem [2]. Nevertheless, the annual catch is around 250,000 tons, indicating use below the established limits, which is probably due to the difficulty in conserving krill and its fragility [3].

In fact, krill is commonly used in the sport fishing market as well as in the aquaculture industry. However, in recent years, krill has been successfully investigated for its role as a nutritional supplement to improve human health. This is because krill is rich in nutrients, including vitamins A and E, minerals, n-3 polyunsaturated fatty acids (n-3 PUFAs), phospholipids (PLs), astaxanthin and flavonoids [4].

Particular attention has been paid to lipid content (0.5% to 3.6%) [5], including phospholipids (30–65%) and triglycerides, while fish oil is only comprised of triglycerides. The main phospholipid in krill oil is phosphatidylcholine, with 40% of the total fatty acids bound to phosphatidylcholine being eicosapentaenoic acid (EPA) and docosahexaenoic acid (DHA) [6]. The EPA and DHA omega-3 fatty acids found in krill oil have shown several useful pharmacological properties in the management of numerous chronic dysfunctions, including cardiovascular, neurological and inflammatory diseases, as well as the prevention of cancer and promoting gut microbiota health [7–10]. In this regard, supplementation with krill polyunsaturated fatty acids may be a natural way to relieve the symptoms of these conditions, potentially in combination with conventional therapies [11]. EPA and DHA from krill oil have also shown higher bioaccessibility than other forms of n-3 PUFAs (ethyl-ester and re-esterified omega 3), demonstrating similar benefits, but at smaller dosages [12].

Krill oil was authorized in 2008 by the U.S. Food and Drug Administration (FDA) as GRAS (Generally Recognized as Safe), was approved in Europe by EFSA as a novel food in 2009 and was also approved in China in 2014. Finally, krill oil was authorized by EFSA for pregnant and lactating women in 2014.

This review aims to provide an overview of the chemical composition, bioavailability and bioaccessibility, mechanism of actions, classic and non-conventional extraction techniques, health benefits and current applications of krill oil underlying the future perspectives of this nutraceutical.

2. Krill Oil Composition

Krill oil composition provides a large variety of substances beneficial to health which justifies its use as a novel food ingredient for pharmacological and nutraceutical applications in different pathological conditions, such as cardiometabolic and neurodegenerative diseases. Generally, although the content of the different classes of nutritional components is influenced by the extraction technologies, krill oil contains a high level of n-3 PUFAs and phospholipids (PLs), and minor components such as vitamins, minerals, astaxanthin and flavonoids [13,14].

2.1. Lipid Fraction

The analysis of the lipid component of krill oil revealed a very complex composition which is characterized by the presence of polar lipids representing the major lipid class in krill oil, followed by triacylglycerols (TAG) [15,16]. Many factors have been reported to influence the specific composition of the lipid fraction, for example interannual environmental changes, seasonal variation, krill sample variety and sexual maturity of krill samples as well as transportation process, storage conditions and pretreatment methods [17]. For example, larger amounts of FFAs have been obtained by dehydrating krill through hot air [18]. Many studies have analyzed krill oil composition through different methods of analysis [19,20]. The range of krill oil PLs ranges between 39.9% found in gravid females of *Euphausia superba* in South Georgia and 80.7% in krill oil found in Aker BioMarine (Table 1). This content varies depending on analysis methods and sample variety. Other differences in krill oil composition have been found considering feeding behavior, krill age and regions. Higher PL levels have been found in ovarian tissues and in gravid females compared to muscle tissues. Another important factor leading to variation in krill composition is extraction methods. A larger amount of PL can be obtained by using ethanol and isopropanol rather than acetone and hexane. PE and phosphatidylcholine (PC) results in the most abundant types of phospholipids ranging from 44.58–99.80%, with the low end of this range reported by Araujo and colleagues using HPTLC as the analysis method and the high end of the range described by Castro-Gomez and coworkers in 2015 using HPLC-ELSD as the analysis method. Phosphatidylethanolamine (PE), even if less abundant, has been found as 0.20% to 24.74% of total PLs [21]. Interestingly, in studies that reported a minor presence of PC, a higher amount of lysophosphatidylcholine (LPC) has been described ranging from 43.3–44.4%, probably due to PC hydrolysis caused by inappropriate storage or inadequate treatment of krill samples [22]. Other important components have been described sometimes in small amounts (less than 10% of total PLs) including phosphatidylglycerol, sphingomyelin, cardiolipin phosphatidylserine and phosphatidic acid. Due to the high content of PC, krill oil is now considered a very promising marine supply of PLs and an alternative to PLs deriving from vegetable oils, egg yolk and dairy products [23].

It is worth noting that the PL fraction obtained from the krill lipid had much higher percentages of PUFA and n-3 PUFA [24,25]. In particular, 31.13% of EPA and 14.87% of DHA were measured in the PL fraction, while only 3.17% of EPA and 1.5% of DHA were found in the TAG fraction. However, as reported by Paluchová and colleagues, the TAG lipid class containing esterified DHA proved to be the best substrate for a better bioavailability of DHA for polyunsaturated fatty acid esters of hydroxy fatty acids (FAHFA) synthesis. This is crucial for selection of novel food sources, which could stimulate endogenous synthesis of functional lipids from a nutritional point of view [26].

Table 1. The different content of polar lipids, monoacylglycerols, diacylglycerols, sterols, free fatty acids and triacylglycerols that have been found in different krill samples expressed as percent of total lipids.

Krill Sample	Polar Lipids	Monoacylglycerols	Diacylglycerols	Sterols	Free Fatty Acids	Triacyl Glycerols	Ref.
Euphausia superba in South Georgia	41.25	1.4	0.43	16.17	14.36	21.50	[19]
Euphausia superba in Gerlache Strait	44	0.9	3.6	1.4	8.5	40.4	[16]
Euphausia superba in Scotia Sea	45.7	0.4	1.3	1.7	16.1	33.3	[27]
Euphausia superba US AMLR Elephant Islands	ND	66–72	ND	4–6	1.1–1.8	22–38.4	[16]
Euphausia superba US AMLR Elephant Islands Extracted with ethanol	69.8	ND	ND	1.1	28.5	0.6	[28]
Euphausia superba US AMLR Elephant Islands Extracted with hexane	48.6	ND	ND	0.6	13.5	37.6	[29]
Krill oil from *Aker BioMarine*	80.7	ND	0.93	2.8	3.46	11.85	[30]

2.2. Fatty Acid Composition

As reported by the Codex Alimentarius Commission (STANDARD FOR FISH OILS CXS 32 9-2017 Adopted in 2017), the most abundant fatty acids in krill oil that have been described are C14:0 myristic acid (5.0–13.0), C16:0 palmitic acid (17.0–24.6), C16:1 (n-7) palmitoleic acid (2.5–9.0), C18:1 (n-7) vaccenic acid (4.7–8.1), C18:1 (n-9) oleic acid (6.0–14.5), C20:5 (n-3) eicosapentaenoic acid (14.3–28.0) and C22:6 (n-3) docosahexaenoic acid (7.1–15.7) (Table 2). DHA and EPA are known as n-3 PUFAs and play a fundamental role in mediating beneficial effects in different mammalian systems [29]. In general, consuming fish oil represents a daily practice for increasing EPA and DHA intake. Since EPA and DHA krill oil content are similar to other common fish oils (anchovy, tuna or salmon), consuming krill oil may represent a potential alternative for a nutritional approach as a dietary supplement [31]. Interestingly, krill lipid fraction is characterized by a higher amount of n-3 PUFA and very low levels of saturated fatty acid (SFA) and monounsaturated fatty acid (MUFA) than TAG in fish oil [32]. Indeed, EPA and DHA (respectively 31.13% and 14.87%) have been mainly found in PLs fraction, while only 3.17% of EPA and 1.5% of DHA were present in the TAG fraction [33]. This composition has been confirmed by many studies, which demonstrated that n-3 PUFAs in the PLs fraction are characterized by a higher quantity of EPA and DHA, significantly improving the bioavailability of these two pharmacological and nutraceutical components, compared to EPA and DHA contained in TAG fraction [34,35].

Table 2. The table reports the fractions expressed as % of total fatty acid characterized in krill samples.

Fatty Acid	Krill
C14:0 Myristic acid	5.0–13.0
C16:0 Palmitic acid	17.0–24.6
C16:1 (n-7) Palmitoleic acid	2.5–9.0
C18:1 (n-7) Cis-11-octadecenoic acid	4.7–8.1
C18:1 (n-9) Elaidic acid	6.0–14.5
C18:2 (n-6) Linoleic acid	ND–3.0
C18:3 (n-3) Alpha linolenic acid	0.1–4.7
C20:5 (n-3) Eicosapentaenoic acid	14.3–28.0
C22:5 (n-3) Docosapentaenoic Acid	ND–0.07
C22:6 (n-3) Docosahexaenoic acid (DHA)	7.1–15.7

2.3. Astaxanthin

One of the most important minor components of krill oil is represented by astaxanthin, a carotenoid that has been characterized in different algae and marine animals [36]. This compound is responsible for the typical dark red color of krill oil and is endowed with potent antioxidant properties, even more than other carotenoids such as zeaxanthin, lutein, canthaxanthin, β-carotene and α-tocopherol [37]. Generally, the amount of astaxanthin in krill oil ranges from 40 to 5000 mg/kg and depends on intrinsic features of krill (for example raw material, krill species) or can vary due to extraction and analysis methods [38]. Indeed, as reported in the below section, a high concentration of astaxanthin can be achieved by using acetone as the extraction solvent [39]. Chemically, astaxanthin can be found in krill oil as a fatty acid ester. In particular, 51% of total astaxanthin is present as diester, 43% as monoesters and only 6% as free astaxanthin [40]. The main fatty acids that are conjugated with astaxanthin are myristic acid, palmitic acid, palmitoleic acid, vaccenic acid, arachidic acid, eicosapentaenoic acid and docosahexaenoic acid [41]. Furthermore, three different isomers of astaxanthin have been identified by Grynbaum and colleagues, such as (all-trans) astaxanthin, which represents the most abundant isomers, (13-cis) astaxanthin, and (9-cis) astaxanthin [41].

2.4. Sterols

Krill oil also contains an important fraction of sterols that range between 2.3–3.9% of total lipids [42]. Desmosterol and cholesterol represent the most abundant sterols of the total sterols [30]. Desmosterol is the precursor of cholesterol and represents 1.70–18.63% of total sterols [17]. The component variation is due to the different food intake of krill since crustaceans are not able to endogenously synthetize sterols but are supplied by diet and phytosterol dealkylation. Cholesterol has been reported as 81.33–82.34% of total sterols with a concentration of 18.95 to 31.96 mg/g of oil [43]. Compared to other fish oil, cholesterol amount in krill oil is even higher than hoki oil, which contains 5.15 mg/g of oil, 2.04 mg/g of tuna oil and 11.81 mg/g of egg yolk oil [17]. Considering the potential nutraceutical application of krill oil, a higher content of cholesterol may represent a matter of concern due to the onset of cardiovascular diseases, for example atherosclerosis, in a cholesterol rich diet. However, extraction methods could limit the content of total cholesterol in krill oil as reported by Bruheim and Cameron who demonstrated that using pure ethanol instead of ethanol mixed with water significantly reduced the cholesterol concentration. Minor percentages are represented by other sterols found in krill samples in 1977, such as

24-nordehydrocholesterol (0.1–1.7%), trans-dehydrocholesterol (1.1–1.5%), brassicasterol (0.5–1.7%), 24-methylenecholesterol (0.1–0.4%), and two stanols (0.1–0.2%) [44].

2.5. Vitamins

Krill oil contains a high amount of α-tocopherol (Vitamin E) which is characterized by a potent antioxidant effect. The concentration of this isoform ranges between 14.74 to 63.0 mg/100 g of oil and represents 90% of total tocopherols, while the other homologues of tocopherols (β-, γ-, δ-) are present only in traces (γ (0.25 to 3.67 mg/100 g of oil) and δ-tocopherol (0 to 0.65 mg/100 g of oil)) [45]. Besides vitamin E, vitamin A has also been found in frozen krill (about 0.11 mg/100 g of wet weight) [21]. The presence of vitamin A in krill samples represents an important feature contributing to making krill oil a very promising food supplement for the regulation of human immune function and for counteracting some infectious diseases. Depending on extraction methods, the vitamin A content of krill oil ranges between 16.4 to 28.5 mg per 100 g of krill oil, a concentration which is significantly higher than tuna oil (11.1 mg/100 g of oil) [45].

2.6. Flavonoids

In general, flavonoids represent a large variety of compounds with a similar chemical structure and are endowed with antioxidant activities, antibacterial and immunomodulatory effects. They also exert cardio protection and reduce the production of proinflammatory mediators. Krill oil has been reported to contain a particular flavonoid whose chemical structure is similar to 6,8-di-C-glucosyl luteolin. As reported by Sampalis and colleagues, by using specific extraction methods, a krill extract containing a significative level of flavonoid (7 mg/100 mL) can be obtained and used for protecting the skin from ultraviolet B (UVB) radiation [46]. Although some studies report that the C-glycosylation of flavonoids in krill oil could improve their antioxidant and anti-diabetic effects, there are no direct data on the use of krill oil for this purpose.

2.7. Minerals

Other than the organic compounds responsible for the pharmacological activity of krill oil, there is also a large quantity of minerals that have been characterized in some krill samples. Indeed, one of the most abundant minerals contained in krill is calcium (1322 mg/100 g) which can be exploited for bone health, phosphorus (1140 mg/100 g), and magnesium (360 mg/100 g) [30]. Other minerals are contained in minor quantities such as zinc, selenium and potassium. Besides these essential elements, krill is characterized by a large quantity of fluoride (2400 mg/kg dry matter) which may cause skeletal fluorosis if its intake is high. However, the major quantity of fluoride is contained in the krill exoskeleton which could be removed during krill oil extraction to avoid excessive fluoride content reaching low fluoride levels (<0.5 ppm) [47].

3. Mechanism of Action

Due to the complex composition of krill oil, which contains structurally different chemical compounds such as PUFAs, flavonoids, astaxanthin and vitamins, the pharmacological effects that have been described are ascribable to multiple mechanisms of action. Krill oil is characterized by a high quantity of (n-3) PUFA (mainly EPA and DHA) which are natural PPAR's ligands responsible for the activation of PPAR [33]. These transcription factors play a fundamental role in regulating cell and tissue behavior to different stimuli. Generally, PPAR forms a heterodimer with the retinoic-X-receptor whose ligand is represented by cis-9-retinoic acid [48]. PPARα and PPARγ are the most investigated isoforms of PPAR. PPARα is mainly expressed in hepatic cells and regulates lipid accumulation [49], while PPARγ has been mainly described in adipose tissues where it promotes insulin sensitivity, adipocyte differentiation and regulates metabolic responses, fat storage and energy homeostasis [50]. Furthermore, PPARγ has also been described in inflammatory cells, where it controls the release of proinflammatory mediators and promotes anti-inflammatory effects [51]. The PPARγ activation occurs in the cells and the uptake of EPA and DHA seems to be due to the expression of FAT/CD36 (a transmembrane fatty acid transporter) [52]. Intriguingly, PPARγ also regulates the expression of FAT/CD36 itself, indicating that n3-PUFA can increase their own uptake inside the adipocytes, promoting the production of adiponectin [53]. The involvement of PPARγ have been demonstrated using PPARγ antagonists (e.g., bisphenol-A-diglycidyl ether or GW9662) that suppressed the secretion of adiponectin [54]. Furthermore, n-3 PUFA are able to activate PPAR through a non-covalent interaction, promoting the reduction of inflammatory responses with a consequent reduction of the release of TNFα and IL-6 after LPS stimulation [55].

Another important target mediating the pharmacological effects of krill oil is represented by G protein-coupled transmembrane receptors (GPCRs) which are involved in the regulation of many metabolic processes. In particular, EPA and DHA activate GPR120 (also known as FFA receptor 4; FFAR4) leading to the increase of intracellular cAMP level and Ca2+ concentrations, consequently promoting the phosphorylation of extracellular signal-regulated kinases 1/2 (ERK1/2) [56]. Since EPA and DHA are involved in the regulation of inflammatory processes mainly in adipose tissue, the involvement of GPR120 has been investigated. In particular, DHA inhibited the IKK (Inhibitor of κB kinase) complex activation and JNK phosphorylation resulting in a reduction of TNF-α release in macrophages treated with LPS [57]. The involvement of GPR120 has been confirmed by GPR120 knockdown. In addition, DHA has been reported to facilitate the formation of GPR120 and β-arrestin2 complex (GPR120-βarr2) that blocks the pro-inflammatory stimulus due to LPS exposure [58]. The GPR120-mediated anti-inflammatory effects of DHA and EPA have also been confirmed in 3T3-L1 adipocytes, resulting in a significant reduction in MCP-1, IL-1β and TNF-α gene expression [58].

The inflammatory process is mainly regulated by NF-κB. Once this transcription factor is activated after IκB phosphorylation due to external stimuli such as UV radiation, endotoxins, oxidative stress, saturated fatty acids, it is able to translocate into the nucleus. It can then promote the production of several pro-inflammatory mediators, adhesion molecules, COX-2, and inducible NO synthase [59]. EPA and DHA, as reported above, reduce the production of a variety of pro inflammatory molecules, such as TNFα, IL-1, IL-6, IL-8, and IL-12 and limit the transcription of those enzymes involved in the inflammatory process including inducible NO synthase and COX-2 in different cell lines (for example endothelial cells, macrophages and monocytes) [60]. This effect seems to involve the reduction of IκB phosphorylation and consequently the reduction of the activation of NF-κB in a GPR120 and PPARγ dependent manner. Indeed, PPAR physically interacts with NF-κB, avoiding its translocation into the nucleus. Furthermore, NF-κB activity is also related to GPR120 since DHA strongly inhibited IKK activity via GPR120 in both stimulated macrophages and adipocytes [61].

In addition, treatment with n3-PUFA limited NF-κB DNA binding activity in adipocytes, macrophages and THP-1 monocytes stimulated with LPS, which prevents the production of IL-6, IL-1β and TNF-α [62]. Intriguingly, as along with NF-κB DNA binding activity being reduced, the authors demonstrated that PPARγ DNA binding activity was also significantly abolished, providing evidence of the tight connection between PPARγ and NF-κB activity in regulating the inflammatory processes. Alongside the reduction of pro inflammatory mediators, treatment with EPA and DHA promoted the release of IL10 in 3T3-L1 adipocytes [63]. IL10 is an important interleukin that is involved in the anti-inflammatory response and inhibits IKK, preventing NF-κB DNA binding activity and PPARγ binding motif. This demonstrates that n3-PUFA may regulate NF-κB activity by inducing IL-10 expression in a PPARγ dependent manner [64].

Besides the high content of EPA and DHA, krill oil also contains potent antioxidant molecules. In particular, many studies have demonstrated that the presence of astaxanthin is responsible for the potent antioxidant effect and potentially the well-known anti-inflammatory properties of EPA and DHA. Oxidative stress is the leading cause of many pathological conditions by triggering the activation of important proinflammatory intracellular pathways which feed a vicious circle. This is especially true in neurodegenerative processes and in cardiovascular diseases characterized by endothelial dysfunction. Preventing the excessive production of reactive oxygen species (ROS) through a nutraceutical approach may be a promising strategy to manage several pathological conditions. In this context, Nrf-2 is one of the main transcriptional factors controlling antioxidant machinery. Indeed, its activation is reported to exert beneficial effects through the increased production of direct antioxidant molecules as well as the hyper activation of antioxidant enzymes SOD, CAT, and GPX [65]. Nrf-2 is one of the main targets of the antioxidant effect of astaxanthin, which induces Nrf2–ARE-mediated antioxidant enzymes in different in vitro models. Astaxanthin reduced oxidative stress in neuronal cells exposed to doxorubicin results in an increase in cell viability and reduction of pro inflammatory mediators [66]. Similarly, astaxanthin protected human mesangial cells exposed to high glucose exert an anti-inflammatory and anti-oxidant effect [67].

Oxidative stress, beyond promoting the inflammatory response, is also responsible for insulin resistance due to the activation of several kinases, among which JNK promotes the phosphorylation of IRS-1, inhibiting its activity and preventing its interaction with the insulin receptor. In addition, elevated levels of ROS cause the degradation of the GLUT4 vesicle, dramatically decreasing glucose uptake [68]. The potent antioxidant effect of astaxanthin facilitates insulin secretion, accelerates glucose metabolism and improves insulin sensitivity, IRS-1 activation, Akt phosphorylation, and GLUT4 translocation in skeletal muscle. This leads to increased insulin sensitivity and a decrease in blood glucose level, which in turn paves the way for using the astaxanthin nutraceutical supply for the management of type 2 diabetes [69] (Table 3).

4. Krill Oil Extraction Technologies

Krill oil can be extracted from different biomasses of fresh krill and dried krill [70,71]. However, fresh krill contains high levels of proteolytic enzymes that induce the rapid autolysis of the crustacean. For this reason, it is necessary to process krill immediately after it is caught [72]. The extraction techniques (Figure 1) can be divided into classic and non-conventional methods. Conventional techniques include several solvent extractions, while the innovative methods include non-solvent extractions, super- and sub-critical fluid extractions and enzyme-assisted extractions.

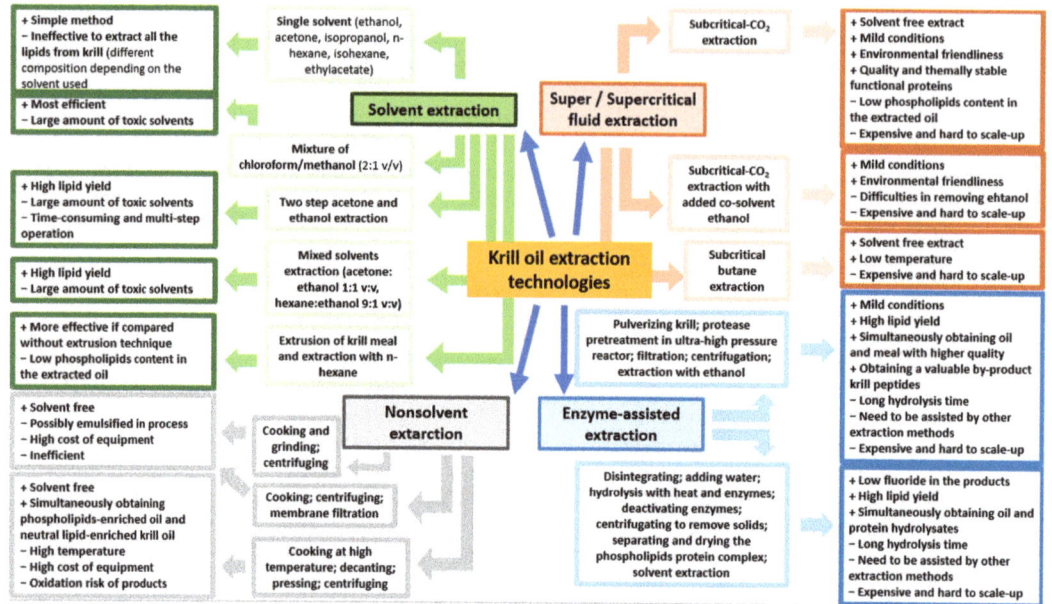

Figure 1. The advantages and disadvantages of krill oil extraction technologies.

4.1. Conventional Extraction Techniques

Solvent extraction is the most conventional method to obtain krill oil. However, different solvents must be used to extract all the lipids from krill because of the diversity of the polarities of the lipid compounds in the biomass. As reported in a study by Xie et al., ethanol and isopropanol can extract most of the phospholipids, although the obtained krill oil is lacking in other lipid components [21]. Hexane is the most common solvent for vegetable oil production due to its low cost, high extraction efficiency and because it is easily eliminated and leaves few traces of residues in food sources. Nevertheless, data on the use of hexane for krill oil production has demonstrated that this solvent only has moderate PL-extracting ability [28,73].

Acetone has proven to be effective for the extraction of minor molecules from krill, but not for PLs. In this regard, a combination of nonpolar and polar solvents is a good compromise for the extraction of both the PLs and other molecules from krill [74]. Two-step acetone and ethanol extraction techniques are the most common methods used for krill [71], as other methods, including the Folch method (which is popular for lipid extraction from animal tissues), are not commercially feasible because of the toxicity of the solvents used (e.g., chloroform and methanol) [75]. Similar results have been obtained using a single-step extraction method with a mixture of acetone and ethanol as the solvents (1:1, v/v) [76]. Moreover, lipid efficiency can be improved by combining the extrusion pre-treatment of krill meal with the solvent extraction technique [77].

Environmental concerns, which have a real impact even in krill oil production, are one of the main limitations with the use of solvents. In addition, this technique is time-consuming and labor intensive because of the multiple extraction and evaporation steps. However, it remains the most economical and easily scalable.

Krill oil can also be extracted using non-solvent techniques including mechanical pressing, which is commonly used for oilseed extraction, such as in sesame oil and sunflower oil [78]. However, this method is inefficient compared to solvent extraction, for two reasons in particular: the low lipid content present in fresh krill (0.5–3.6%) and the difficulty of the mechanical processing used for krill [77].

Non-solvent sequential procedures, such as cooking, decanting, pressing and centrifuging, are able to successfully separate krill oil from the mixture (Figure 2). In fact, the release of PLs from the lipid fraction of fresh or defrosted krill—after conventional grinding into a slurry which involves mechanical disruption procedures and centrifugation—does not facilitate the complete separation of the oil fraction due to the amphipathic nature of PLs, which act as emulsifying agents in the formed slurry [79]. Katevas et al., have developed a method that can extract both the PL fraction and the neutral lipid-enriched krill oil. In this method, the first cooking step is conducted at 90° C without grinding and agitation, thus avoiding the emulsification process. The same authors concluded that fresh krill is a better option than defrosted krill as it was able to avoid or reduce the emulsification process, which may occur in defrosted krill due to the formation of ice crystals (after freezing) and the consequent disruption of krill tissue [70].

Although the non-solvent extraction technique avoids the use of solvents, making it safer and more eco-friendly than solvent-extraction methods, it presents many drawbacks. First, it is poorly scalable because of the high investment in equipment and the high costs of energy required. Secondly, the cooking procedure at high temperatures may induce lipid oxidation in the products. Last but not least, this technique has only been observed to give a total lipid yield of 2.2% and does not extract all of the available oil from krill. For these reasons, mechanical separation can be used to initially obtain part of the krill oil, but also to produce krill meal, which can be subsequently treated with other techniques including supercritical fluid extraction and solvent extraction [80].

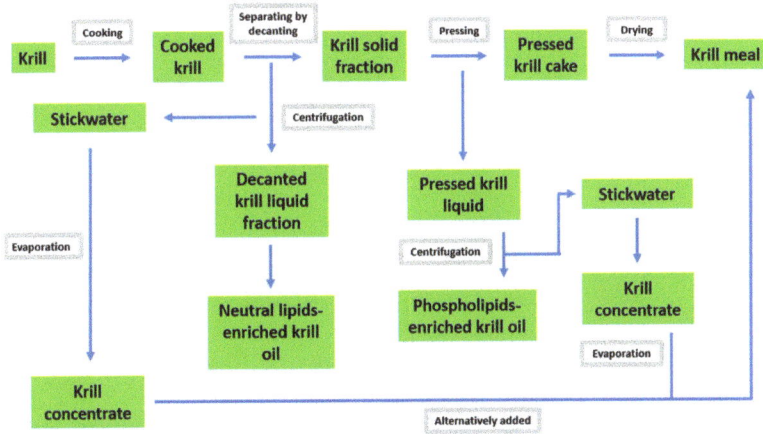

Figure 2. An overview of non-solvent extraction technique (Adapted from Katevas et al. [70]).

4.2. Unconventional Extraction Techniques

The supercritical fluid extraction method is an unconventional extraction technique that can be used for krill oil extraction and is known to be solvent-free [81]. It is considered environmentally friendly as it uses supercritical carbon dioxide, which is safe, non-toxic and chemically inert. Nevertheless, carbon dioxide is not an ideal molecule for the extraction of all the lipid content from krill as it fails to extract PLs [82]. For this reason, the addition of 5–20% of ethanol to supercritical carbon dioxide extraction has been tested and demonstrated to improve PL solubility and thus lipid recovery [83]. The use of this technique presents some issues, including its limited processing capacity, the high cost of the equipment and the risk of de-solvation by the liquid state of ethanol at 25 °C.

Subcritical fluid extraction with compressed butane and propane, performed at low temperature and pressure, is commonly used for oil extraction [84]. In a study conducted by Xie et al., the use of subcritical butane (30 °C, 0.3 to 0.8 MPa) gave results that are comparable to those of hexane in terms of yield and krill oil quality, although it was faster and the extraction process required less solvent [73]. In addition, in a study by Sun et al., subcritical butane extraction was proven to give the extract that was richest in astaxanthin and tocopherol, and the lowest in oxidation degree, compared to the solvent extraction technique [85]. However, even in this case, the high cost of equipment and limited processing capacity are the main issues for a successful scale-up process.

Enzyme-assisted extraction is a novel pre-treatment technique than can increase lipid yield, as it can release the bound molecules using specific enzymes (e.g., amylase, protease, glucanase, cellulase and pectinase) [86]. These enzymes can selectively enhance the extractability of lipid compounds, improving the breakdown of cell walls and destroying lipid bodies. The high quality of the extracted oil and the mild process conditions also make this technique attractive for the extraction of krill oil [75]. Bruheim et al., have obtained satisfactory results with enzyme-assisted extraction for krill oil. After an initial krill-disintegration process, the small particles were treated with water and heat and the hydrolytic enzymes were then added to hydrolyze the material and improve lipid extraction. Finally, the enzymes were deactivated and, after removal of the solid material, the PL-protein complex was separated and dried, and the krill oil was extracted [75]. Finally, in a study by Lee et al., a combination of an enzyme-assisted extraction process and an ultrahigh-pressure (10 to 300 MPa) reactor made krill easily liquefiable and ensured full contact with the proteases [87].

The high costs and longer hydrolysis times are still challenging for the use of this technique in large-scale industrial applications.

5. Bioavailability and Bioaccessibility of Krill Oil Omega-3

Several studies have investigated the effects of krill oil supplementation on health, and these effects appear to be superior to those of fish oil [88,89]. The superiority of krill oil has been attributed to the higher bioavailability of EPA and DHA, which are in the form of PL [90]. Nevertheless, most of the RCTs conducted to date did not use the same doses of EPA and DHA (for the same outcomes) from krill and fish oil and ignored the differences between the bioactive substances in fish and krill oil [91].

In fact, the minor components contained in krill oil, such as astaxanthin, alpha-tocopherol, vitamin A and flavonoids, can exert pleiotropic activities and have a positive impact on health, in addition to probably improving the bioaccessibility of EPA and DHA. In this regard, a study by Kohler et al., s reported that EPA and DHA from krill meal had lower bioavailability than krill oil, but the same as fish oil. This study underlines the potential role of minor lipophilic molecules in improving the bioaccessibility, and thus the bioavailability, of EPA and DHA from krill oil [92]. However, the mechanisms of action by which krill oil appears to be superior remain unknown and seem to be closely related to the extract in its entirety and the extraction method.

Long-term RCTs are needed to determine the differences in efficacy and performance of krill oil compared to fish oil. This information is currently incomplete and needs clarification, starting from the role of minor components in the extracts. In addition, EPA and DHA supplemented from fish and krill oils in comparative studies should be at the same dosages and ratio. In fact, in a study by Ramprasath et al., which reported the superiority of krill oil over fish oil (expressed as concentration of n-3 PUFA plasmatic levels), supplementation with EPA and DHA was 777 mg for the krill oil group and 664 mg for the fish oil group [91]. Ulven et al., have demonstrated a change in the EPA/DHA ratio after supplementation with 543 mg of krill oil and 864 mg of fish oil (EPA/DHA ratio: 1.74 for krill group and 1.12 for fish oil group) [12]. Weather this improvement of EPA/DHA ration is an advantage in terms of health effect it is yet to be fully demonstrated.

6. Krill and Metabolic Disorders

Dietary supplementation with omega-3 fatty acids has been demonstrated to be beneficial for the prevention and/or treatment of cardiovascular diseases (CVD) [93] and possibly other inflammatory and neurological disorders [94,95]. Moreover, increased consumption of EPA and DHA may also be of clinical significance in the prevention and reversal of insulin resistance [96].

The American Heart Association (AHA) recommends a daily intake of at least 1000 mg of omega-3 fatty acids to minimize risk factors associated with CVD, even for patients at high risk of developing CVD. Therefore, despite the great abundance of omega-3 fatty acids available in fish oil, the delivery of fatty acids and presence of astaxanthin in krill oil may provide superior health benefits and meet the AHA recommendations [97].

Krill oil is endowed with a unique chemical composition. Unlike fish oil, it is rich in omega-3 fatty acids present in the form of phospholipids rather than triglycerides. This may be biologically and therapeutically significant, since phospholipids are well-absorbed by the intestine and they are readily incorporated into cell membranes, suggesting that they could be endowed with a more favorable pharmacokinetic profile [98]. Moreover, supplementation with krill oil gives the advantage of not only supplying n-3 PUFAs, but also choline, which is an essential nutrient, since that it is needed in the synthesis of neurotransmitters (acetylcholine) and phospholipids and is important in the transport of lipids and reduction of homocysteine [23]. In addition, krill contains several endogenous antioxidants including astaxanthin (which is responsible for the deep red color), the preservation of krill oil against oxidation and it has potential health-promoting properties [99].

Maki and colleagues observed that a supplementation for four weeks with Antarctic krill oil (2 g/day) increased plasma concentration of EPA and DHA [100]. This suggests it could be used similar to the way fish and fish oil are used, as it is also rich in long-chain omega-3 polyunsaturated fatty acids which contains cardiovascular risk. In this context, supplementation with krill can also represent a promising approach to ameliorate obesity and obesity-associated diseases. To date, preclinical evidence has been collected on the positive impact of krill oil in conditions of metabolic disorders.

It has been also demonstrated that plasma EPA level was significantly greater following krill oil treatment when compared to fish oil treatment. Significant remodeling of the plasma lipidome was observed after four weeks of treatment with krill oil (containing 1.27 g/day of long-chain omega-3 polyunsaturated fatty acids) if compared to fish oil (containing 1.44 g/day of long-chain omega-3 polyunsaturated fatty acids), with a clear differentiation in their effects on different plasma lipids species. In particular the authors reported that more than 38% of the lipids species increased following krill treatment, while only 12% increased when fish oil was used as supplementation [101]. Similar results have been obtained in healthy women over a five hour postprandial period. Clear differences between krill oil and fish oil supplementations in the postprandial period were reported. The most noticeable changes were revealed in diacyl-phospholipids and ether-phospholipids [102].

Finally, subchronic toxicity and genotoxicity studies in rats confirm that krill oil is well-tolerated and seems to be safe with a daily supplementation of 5% [103].

In male Sprague Dawley rats who were fed a high-fat diet (HFD) for two weeks, the consumption of krill oil significantly reduced serum lipids, and the two highest krill oil doses (100 and 200 g/L) also significantly increased HDL levels [104].

In 2009 Cohn's group demonstrated that supplementation of krill oil to HFD mice for eight weeks, dose-dependently reduced hepatic triglycerides, cholesterol and serum, as well as total cholesterol and glucose. Unfortunately, this study was inconclusive regarding the putative mechanism. The peroxisome proliferator-activated receptor (PPAR)α which is supposed to be critical to promote β-oxidation at the liver level, did not significantly change which means it was not involved [105].

The intake of a powder isolated from Antarctic krill showed to ameliorate the hepatic metabolism in a transgenic mouse model of chronic inflammation, for expressing the human tumor necrosis factor-alpha (hTNFα) gene. Lower hepatic and plasma triacylglycerol levels, as well as hepatic gene expression of sterol regulatory element binding transcription factor 2 (SREBP2) and enzymes involved in cholesterol synthesis were found. In addition, genes involved in lipogenesis and glycerolipid synthesis were down-regulated and β-oxidation was promoted, confirming the capability of this product to increase the hepatic lipid catabolism and suppress lipidogenesis. Finally, krill powder reduced endogenous TNFα in the liver, indicating anti-inflammatory effects [106].

In 2020, Saito et al. evaluated the effects of 8-HEPE-concentrated material from Pacific krill on dyslipidemia and hepatic steatosis in low-density lipoprotein (LDL) receptor-deficient (LDLR-KO) mice. Very interestingly, they observed that over 18 weeks a supplementation of a typical western diet with Pacific krill (8-HEPE (100 mg/kg), but not EPA or DHA) improved the lipidic profile (reducing LDL and total cholesterol levels and increasing HDL levels) and reduced hepatic triglyceride levels [107]. This led to the hypothesis that eicosapentaenoic acid (EPA) and 8-hydroxyeicosapentaenoic acid (8 HEPE) have more positive effects on the metabolic syndrome by activating the peroxisome proliferator activated receptor (PPAR α) in the liver.

In addition, in dyslipidemic and diabetic non-human primates, the daily intake omega-3 phospholipids purified from krill showed a positive impact on CVD risk factors by reducing total cholesterol, LDL-cholesterol and triglycerides and increasing HDL-cholesterol, if used at the dose equal to 150 mg/Kg/day [108].

Runbland and colleagues reported a randomized control study carried out on 36 individuals who were divided in three groups: fish group, krill group and control group. For eight weeks, krill and control groups received capsules containing oil, while the fish group was invited to consume lean and fatty fishes based on dietary guidelines. As expected, the levels of EPA and DHA increased in the fish group and krill group, whereas docosapentaenoic acid (DPA) increased only in the krill group. However, the overall differences between the three intervention groups were significant for EPA ($p < 0.0001$), DPA ($p < 0.001$) and DHA ($p < 0.001$). In general, the authors observed a great variability among the participants, however a tendency towards a decrease in total lipids and triacylglycerols was observed in the fish and krill groups with the largest VLDL levels. In agreement with previous works in animal models, in which a down-regulation of the genes involved in gluconeogenesis has been demonstrated [109,110], as well as in clinical studies [111], they reported a significant reduction in fasting blood glucose in the krill group compared with the control group. This result is strongly predictive of a reduction of CVD risk [112].

In humans with borderline or high triglyceride levels (range between 150–499 mg/dL), the treatment with krill oil at the dose of 0.5, 1, 2, or 4 g/day for 6 and 12 weeks could be efficient to reduce triglycerides. Nevertheless, the great heterogeneity of the selected sample impeded to have a clear view of the real nutritional value [113].

Cicero et al., published a randomized cross-over clinical trial in which 25 moderately hypertriglyceridemic subjects (150–500 mg/dL) were treated with omega 3 ethyl ester (2000 mg/day) or krill oil (1000 mg/day) for four weeks. Only the krill oil treatment significantly improved HDL and apolipoprotein AI levels, compared to the values measured both at baseline ($p < 0.05$) and at end of treatment in the group supplemented with esterified omega 3 ($p < 0.05$). Both treatments were able to significantly reduce high-sensitivity C-reactive protein (hs-CRP) levels from the baseline ($p < 0.05$), but krill oil improved it more efficaciously than esterified omega 3 ethyl ester group ($p < 0.05$) [114].

A reduction in body weight because of krill oil supplementation in obesity models has been reported in some animal studies. Sun and colleagues observed that an Antarctic krill oil, extracted from dry krill using an innovative procedure of hot pump dehydration combined with freezing-drying, was endowed with anti-obesity effects in metabolic disorder conditions. In particular, supplementation for 12 weeks improved dyslipidemia, fatty liver and glucose metabolism in C57BL/6J mice fed with HFD. Krill oil also reduced body weight gain, reduced fat accumulation in adipose and liver tissue, lowered serum density of lipoprotein-cholesterol (LDL-C) content and ameliorated glucose tolerance. In addition, krill oil feeding also reduced oxidative damage in the liver [115].

In another study, rats were fed a control diet, an HFD or an HFD supplemented with 2.5% krill oil for 12 weeks. Krill oil significantly prevented increased body weight in the HFD group [105].

An improvement of insulin sensitivity and secretion after administration of krill oil (600 mg/day) has also been seen in an obesity model of castrated male New Zealand white rabbits [110]. Expression levels of key enzymes involved in the β-oxidation and lipogenesis were different after krill oil feeding for 8 weeks, compared to placebo, which ultimately led to decreased fasting blood glucose and improved glucose tolerance in the rabbits.

Further evidence suggested that omega-3 phospholipids of krill oil enhanced intestinal fatty acid oxidation and could contribute to the anti-steatotic effects in obese mice, meaning there could exist an axis microbiota-intestine-liver [116]. Indeed, omega-3 alleviated hepatic steatosis in various rodent models of obesity even in exacerbated hepatic steatosis conditions, in which an HFD was combined with thermoneutral animal housing (i.e., ambient temperature approximately 30 °C) [117].

Several authors highlighted that omega-3 supplemented by krill oil is even more effective, mainly phosphatidylcholine -rich phospholipids when compared to the same dose of the triacylglycerol form. It has been observed that omega-3 phospholipids contribute more effectively to improve glucose intolerance and insulin resistance in dietary obese mice when compared to their triacylglycerol form [116]. The reason for this is likely due to the amelioration of bioavailability; EPA and DHA present in fish and fish oil are almost exclusively in triacylglycerol form, while in krill oil up to 65% of EPA and DHA occur in phospholipids [118].

Krill oil was also found to directly influence cardiac remodeling and function in an experimental myocardial infarction (MI). In such experimental conditions, rats were randomized in krill oil or control groups for 14 days before the induction of MI. Seven weeks after the MI induction, the echocardiography showed a significant attenuation of left ventricular (LV) dilation in the group pre-treated with krill oil. Attenuated heart and lung hypertrophy and reduced mRNA levels encoded classical markers of LV stress, including matrix remodeling and inflammation [119].

Krill oil has been also associated with moderate improvement in endothelial dysfunction and HDL, two known CVD risk factors, in patients with type 2 diabetes. In 34 participants with type 2 diabetes, an improvement of their endothelial function and a reduction in blood C peptide levels and HOMA scores were reported after four weeks of supplementation with krill oil (1 g/day in PUFA) when compared to the olive oil group. There were differences in weight loss between krill oil and olive oil after 17 weeks, though if compared with their respective baseline measurements, the participants of each group had a statistically significant improvement in endothelium [120].

A close relationship between krill oil consumption and reduction of circulating levels of endocannabinoids 2-arachidonoylglycerol (2-AG) and N-arachidonoyl-ethanolamine (AEA) has been highlighted [116].

In obese subjects, the endocannabinoids are elevated in the blood and this phenomenon appears to be due to changes in expression of adipose tissue metabolizing enzymes. Moreover, endocannabinoids are made by enzymatic reactions from arachidonic acid; hence, the more omega-6 arachidonic acid (ARA) available, the more endocannabinoids can be made. On the other hand, an increased intake of omega-3 might help to counterbalance a disturbed omega-3 to omega-6 ratio and result in lower endocannabinoid levels that may positively affect membrane signaling and energy metabolism. Recently, Di Marzo and Silvestri brought to light the existence of a triangle among the lifestyle–gut microbiome–endocannabinoid system and its crucial role in the development of metabolic syndrome [121].

Interestingly, krill oil supplementation (dose ranging 1.25–5%) led to a significant decrease in AEA, as compared to controls [122]. According to previous preclinical evidence, Berge and colleagues demonstrated that besides a reduction of plasma triglycerides, supplementation with krill powder (4 g/day per os) contributed to a reduction in 11 obese men's anthropometric parameters and blood endocannabinoid (AEA and 2-AG), whose levels were correlated with high levels of triglycerides and were responsible for hyperactivity of the cannabinoid system which feeds metabolic dysfunction. Indeed, the endocannabinoid system is deeply involved in the regulation of the homeostasis of body composition by regulating food intake and energy expenditure; therefore, this could be another mechanism through which krill may have beneficial effects on metabolism [123]. According to a previous paper, a significant reduction of the 2-AG levels has been highlighted with 2 g/day of krill oil (providing 309 mg/day of EPA/DHA 2:1), although no significant effect on anthropometric parameters has been observed [124].

7. Krill and Inflammatory Bowel Diseases and Gut Microbiota

It is well known that obesity and its complications, such as insulin resistance, hyperlipidemia and atherosclerosis caused by HFD are often accompanied with alteration in gut microbiota, in particular an increase of pro-inflammatory/pathogenic bacteria. In 2017, Cui et al. observed that treatment with fish oil (600 µg/g/day), krill oil (600 µg/g/day) and their mixture (300 + 300 µg/g/day) for 12 weeks led to obesity alleviation, as well as gut microbiota modulation. In fact, they reported a decrease of body weight gain, adiposity index and liver index. They also reported an increase in the abundance of some positive phyla in the gut, including *Bacteroides* and *Lactobacilli* [125]. Likewise, Lu and colleagues demonstrated that supplementation with krill oil shifted the gut microbiota composition and that it was associated with the alleviation of hyperlipidemia. According to an experimental model, mice fed for 12 weeks with a high fat and high sugar diet showed obesity and hyperlipidemia. Treatment with a high dose (600 µg/g/day) of krill oil, but not with lower doses (100 µg/g/day or 200 µg/g/day) improved the microbiotic alteration and cardiometabolic parameters [126].

Krill oil treatments for seven weeks at different dosages (100, 200 and 600 mg/kg) decreased the abundance of tyrosine consumers and increased the abundance of *Lactobacillus* spp. and short-chain fatty acids producers [127].

Moreover, other research points out beneficial effects of krill supplementation against inflammatory bowel diseases (IBD), including ulcerative colitis and Crohn's disease, which share common symptoms such as bleeding, diarrhea and weight loss. In these cases, the integrity of the intestinal barrier layer and the gut microbiota play a critical role. In this regard, a mixture composed of krill oil plus probiotic *Lactobacillus reuteri* plus vitamin D has demonstrated to significantly improve clinical and histological scores, restore epithelial restitution and reduce proinflammatory cytokines in an experimental model of colitis induced by dextran sulphate sodium (DSS) treatment [128]. Of note, krill oil also appears to attenuate inflammation in an experimental model of ulcerative colitis in rats. In male rats submitted to treatment with dextran sulphate sodium (DSS), the supplementation with krill oil (5%) for 30 days preserved the colon length, which was significantly shortened in the DSS-treated compared to control animals, in line with oedema and inflammation in the colonial mucosa. Moreover, typical factors such as disease activity index (DAI) and TNF-α and IL-1β levels were positively affected by krill oil compared to DSS administration alone [129].

Suppression of the pro-inflammatory cytokines TNF and IL6 and the systemic levels of endotoxin, a marker of IBD, were also found. Recently innovative krill oil-entrapped liposomes were developed and their efficacy in an IBD model was demonstrated. The authors observed that liposomes were incorporated into the impaired enterocyte membrane, which contributed to re-establish the hydrophobic protective barrier in the inflamed/impaired region and decrease the permeation typical of IBD [130].

Liu and colleagues suggested that krill oil could contribute both to attenuating the inflammatory pathway and modulating gut microbiota through the reduction of Rickettsiales and several species of *Lactobacillus* [131].

8. Inflammation
Arthritic Diseases

Based on pre-clinical studies carried out on mice experimental models of inflammatory arthritis, krill oil was supposed to have a positive effect in reducing joint inflammation more so than fish oil. In a rodent model of rheumatoid arthritis, mice fed with a krill oil diet, in which EPA and DHA were 0.44 g/100 g of krill oil diet, exhibited a decreased infiltration of inflammatory cells at the joint level, and decreased hyperplasia at the synovial layer, compared to controls [132]. Moreover, in mice transgenic for human TNF-α, while the fish oil and krill oil had a similar effect on cholesterol levels, only krill oil reduced markers of fatty acid oxidation [133]. This is consistent with the observation that fish oil and krill oil are both rich in EPA and DHA, but only krill oil naturally contains antioxidants agents like astaxanthin [134].

In a previous randomized, double blind, placebo controlled clinical trials carried out on 90 patients affected by cardiovascular diseases and/or osteoarthritis and/or rheumatoid arthritis, the effect of krill oil on C-reactive protein (CRP) and on arthritic symptoms were evaluated. Patients received krill oil 300 mg/day or placebo for 30 days and CRP and osteoarthritis symptoms were recorded at baseline and at days 7, 14 and 30. Despite the short treatment, krill oil significantly reduced CRP levels even after 7 days (about 20% of CRP reduction versus an increase of about 16% in the placebo group), reaching a higher reduction (about 30% versus an increase of CRP levels of about 25% in the placebo arm) after 30 days. Moreover, krill oil significantly reduced symptoms such as pain by about 29%, stiffness by about 20% and functional impairment by about 23%, suggesting that a 300 mg daily dose of krill oil could represent a good strategy to counteract arthritic symptoms and inflammation period [135].

In a more recent randomized, double-blind, parallel-group, placebo-controlled study, 50 adult patients affected by mild knee pain received 2 g/day of krill oil or placebo for 30 days. After 30 days of treatment, patients treated with krill oil exhibited a significant reduction of knee pain both in sleeping and in standing and the range of motion in both knees was improved [136].

These promising pre-clinical and clinical studies led Laslett and co-workers to design and start a clinical trial named "KARAOKE" (Krill oil for OA of the knee), focused on the use of krill oil to improve knee osteoarthritis (OA). This study is currently ongoing and 260 Australian patients affected by knee OA characterized by pain, synovitis and effusion will be recruited and randomized to receive 2 g/day of krill oil or placebo every day for six months. Symptoms, functionality and knee structural abnormalities will be monitored at the beginning of the study and after 6 months using validated clinical methods and magnetic resonance imaging. In particular, the primary outcomes of this study are change in knee pain and in size of knee synovitis/effusion over 24 weeks. The secondary outcomes are improvement in knee pain over 4, 8, 12, 16 and 20 weeks [11].

9. Neuroprotection

9.1. Neurodegeneration and Alzheimer Disease

The astaxanthin content present in krill oil was evaluated as a peculiar feature which gives krill oil more antioxidant properties than fish oil. In particular, the first results demonstrated that astaxanthin was able to protect the human neuronal SH-SY5Y cell line from an oxidative stimulus via its ability to act as a mitochondria protective agent [137]. In the same neuronal cell line, astaxanthin induction increased expression of the antioxidant enzyme heme oxygenase-1 (HO-1) by activation of the ERK1/2 signal pathways. This mechanism could account for the neuroprotection induced by astaxanthin against the cellular apoptosis induced by beta-amyloid (Aβ25-35). This protection was abolished by the administration of a specific ERK inhibitor [138]. Finally, astaxanthin (250–1000 nM) in primary culture of cortical neurons prevents the H_2O_2-induced (50 μM) reduction of cell-viability, restores mitochondrial potential and inhibits apoptosis. In a rat model of focal cerebral ischemia, in vivo, astaxanthin which was administered intragastrically at 80 mg/kg twice (5 h and 1 h before the induction of cerebral ischemia), induced a significant protection against infarct volume, improving the neurological deficit [139].

Several pre-clinical studies investigated the role of krill oil on cognitive function. In particular, Lee and colleagues evaluated the potential improvement in memory and learning due to the administration of phosphatidylserine isolated from krill (PK) in aged rats through the Morris water maze experimental model. Their results demonstrated that the administration of PK 20 or 50 mg/kg/day for 7 days significantly improved the escape latency for finding the platform in the Morris water maze compared with rats which received the 50 mg/kg/day of phosphatidylserine isolated from soybean. Moreover, the treatment with PK also improved the loss of cholinergic immunoreactivity, muscarinic receptors and choline transporters typically observed in the hippocampus of aged rats, demonstrating a neuroprotective role for PK [140]. The examination of these results on different components naturally contained in krill oil, taken together with the presence of omega-3, led Barros and colleagues to hypothesize a perspective for the use of krill oil as a neuroprotective supplement [141].

After the above reported studies demonstrating the neuroprotective effect of krill oil, more specific studies on neurodegenerative diseases were carried out on recognized animal models. Among them, Choi and co-workers administered krill oil 80 mg/kg/day for one month to a mice model of Alzheimer obtained through lipopolysaccharide (LPS) injections, 250 µg/kg, seven times daily. The team found that krill oil induced a general reduction in oxidative and inflammatory markers. Krill oil administration prevented the LPS-induced expression of the inducible isoform of nitric oxide synthase (iNOS) and of cyclooxygenase-2 (COX-2), inhibited IkB degradation suppressing the NFkB pro-inflammatory signaling and induced a decrease of ROS levels and malondialdehyde levels. Moreover, krill oil also suppressed amyloid beta (1–42) peptide generation, demonstrating a multitarget mechanism on the three main aspects which support Alzheimer disease: oxidation, inflammation and amyloid beta production [142].

A recent study, carried out on a more specific animal model of neurodegenerative diseases, represented by the senescence-accelerated prone mouse strain 8 (SAMP8) mice, demonstrated that krill oil improved both cognitive function and anxiety. In particular, the administration of a diet enriched with 1% of krill oil for 12 weeks improved SAMP-8 performances tested through the Morris water maze, the open-field test and the Barnes maze test, resulting in reduction of memory deficit and learning improvement. Moreover, by examining the hippocampus it was clear that krill oil reduced β-amyloid Aβ42 accumulation. This effect was linked to a mechanism involving an increase in activity of glutathione peroxidase and superoxide dismutase and a contemporary decrease in malondialdehyde and 7,8-dihydro-8-oxoguanine levels [143]. Interesting findings about possible use of krill oil in prevention and treatment of Alzheimer disease were recorded by Kim and co-workers through the employment of a mouse model of Alzheimer obtained by injection of amyloid Aβ25-35 in mice. After the Aβ25-35 injection, mice developed cognitive impairments but the mice receiving an oral administration (gavage) of 100, 200 or 500 mg/kg/day of krill oil for 14 days showed shorter latency in the Morris water maze test, downregulation of Bax/Bcl-2 ratio in the brain and reduced levels of ROS, malondialdehyde and NO [89].

Despite the evidence obtained in pre-clinical studies, the clinical trials studying the effect of krill oil on human brain are very poor. In particular, a randomized, double-blind clinical trial was performed on 45 healthy elderly males (61–72 years-old), treated for 12 weeks with placebo (represented by medium-chain triglycerides), sardine-oil (abundant in n-3 polyunsaturated fatty acids-PUFAs- incorporated in triglycerides) or krill oil (abundant in n-3 PUFAs incorporated in phosphatidylcholine). The results of this study indicated that during the working memory task, both in the sardine and in the krill group the oxyhemoglobin concentrations in the cerebral cortex were significantly increased compared to the placebo group. In the calculation task, only the krill oil evoked an increase in oxyhemoglobin significantly different from the placebo group. Only the krill group showed a significantly lower differential value for P300 latency when compared to the placebo group [144,145].

9.2. Depression

The effect of krill oil supplementation was evaluated on cognition and depression-like behaviors both in pre-clinical and clinical studies.

One of the first studies in this field was carried out for seven weeks in rats, which received krill oil 0.2 g/rat/day, or imipramine 20 mg/kg/day (used as an anti-depressant reference drug) or placebo. At the end of the treatment, the cognitive abilities were tested by the Aversive Light Stimulus Avoidance Test (ALSAT) while the potential anti-depressant effect was tested by the Unavoidable Aversive Light Stimulus (UALST) and the Forced Swimming Test (FST). The results showed that krill oil treated rats had a significant ability to discriminate between the active and the inactive levers in the ALSAT test since the first day of training. Moreover, rats treated with krill oil and impramine exhibited significant improvement in behavior features such as lower levels in the UALST test since day three, and shorter immobility time in the FST test. The investigation also involved the expression of brain-derived neurotrophic factor (Bdnf) which was found to be upregulated in the hippocampus of krill oil treated rats [146].

Similar results were obtained by Zadeh-Ardabili and colleagues on mice treated with fish oil, krill oil, vitamineB12, imipramine or saline 5 mL/kg once per day for 14 days starting after one week of the Chronic Unpredictable Stress (CUS) paradigm overnight procedure. During CUS procedures, light was used to stress the mice overnight with an illumination of 10 W LED, 15 Hz for 12 hours for 3 weeks. The potential antidepressant effect of the treatments was tested by tail suspension test (TST) and FST. After animal sacrifice, the presence of oxidation markers was evaluated in the brain tissue. Both fish oil and krill oil significantly reduced the immobility factors and increased the time of climbing and swimming, similar to imipramine, when compared with the control group. Both the fish oil and the krill oil led to decreased malondialdehyde and hydrogen peroxide levels, decreased catalase activity, increased glutathione peroxidase levels and increased superoxide dismutase activities and glutathione levels in hippocampal tissue [147].

Another pre-clinical study, by Mendoza et al., investigated the role of krill oil on restraint stress in mice after reduced mobility. After two weeks of acclimation and handling, mice were immobilized for three weeks followed by a week dedicated to behavioral tests. During the four weeks of the study, the mice orally received PBS or cotinine (a nicotine-derivative) at 5 mg/kg, or cotinine plus krill oil 143 mg/kg. The results showed that cotinine alone reduced both the loss in cerebral synaptic density, memory deficits, anxiety and depression-like behaviors, but that the co-administration of cotinine plus krill oil was more effective than cotinine alone in reducing depression-like behaviors linked with reduced mobility. This confirms krill oil plays a role in depression mechanisms [148].

These encouraging pre-clinical data encouraged van der Wurff and colleagues to design and carry out a year long randomized, controlled, double-blind clinical trial on the effects of a krill oil supplementation on adolescent behaviors linked to learning, cognition, visual processing and mental well-being. The study included 264 adolescents between the ages of 13 and 15 years, who were divided in two cohorts. Cohort I started with 400 mg/day of EPA + DHA or placebo, and after three months the dose was increased to 800 mg of EPA + DHA per day. Cohort II started with 800 mg of EPA+DHA per day. The effects of these treatments were assessed by Omega-3 Index finger-prick blood measurements, Centre for Epidemiologic Studies Depression Scale evaluation and the Rosenberg Self Esteem questionnaire. The authors concluded that there was no evidence of an effect of krill oil in reducing depressive feelings or in inducing higher self-esteem. However, the authors reported that the results were affected by low adherence and drop-out, and for these reasons they suggest caution when interpreting the data [149,150].

10. Cancer

Only a few studies carried out with respect to krill oil and cancer cell lines are available. In a screening study carried out on several cancer cell lines such as cells derived from histiocytic lymphoma (U937), leukemia (K562, HL60), human hepatocarcinoma (SMMC-

7721), bone metastasis of pancreatic cancer (PC3) and breast cancer (MDA-MB-231, MCF-7), a general inhibition of cancer cells proliferation by krill oil was observed [151].

In a comparison with fish oil, EPA and DHA incubated in human osteosarcoma cells for 24, 48 and 72 h, found only krill oil induced a significant inhibition of cancer cells proliferation (23, 50 and 64% of inhibition, respectively). Fish oil did not change the proliferation observed in control cells except for an increase observed after 24 h. On the contrary, EPA and DHA promoted cell proliferation and cell migration [152].

Some researchers have focused their attention on human colorectal cancer cells, in particular, Jayathilake and co-workers treated HCT-15, SW-480 and Caco-2 cells for 48 h with free fatty acid (FFA) extract from krill oil and fish oil. Their results indicated that krill oil and fish oil extracts inhibited cell proliferation in a similar manner but only an increase in mitochondrial membrane potential and consequent cell apoptosis was only observed with krill oil [153]. The same research group further investigated the antiproliferative effect of free fatty acid extract (FFAE) of krill oil on other human (DLD-1, HT-29 and LIM-2405) and murine (CT-26) colorectal cancer cells, in comparison with EPA, DHA (after 24 and 48 h) and oxaliplatin (after 24 h). Osteosarcoma, with colorectal cancer FFAE of krill oil, EPA and DHE inhibited cell proliferation and ROS formation in a similar way to oxaliplatin. FFAE of krill oil also induced a significant increase in caspase 3 and 9 levels which are markers of apoptosis [154]. An investigation of potential mechanisms of action was then carried out on DLD-1 and HT-29 cell lines treated with FFAE of krill oil at 8 and 24 h. From the evaluation of epidermal growth factor receptor (EGFR) signaling, the results indicated that FFAE of krill oil, at 0.03 and 0.12 µL/100 µL, induced reduction in EGFR, pEGFR, pERK1/2 and pAKT expression without any changes in total ERK1/2 and AKT levels. The expression of the ligand PD-L1 was significantly inhibited by FFAE of krill oil [155].

11. Exercise Performance

Krill oil has been associated with improvement of exercise and antioxidant/anti-inflammatory markers and several clinical trials have been carried out. The first was a small double-blind study carried out on 17 members of the Polish National Rowing Team. The rowers were divided in two groups: one received 1 g/day of krill oil for six weeks and one received placebo. The parameter of athletes was tested before, after 1 min and after 24 h, the latter of which was deemed maximum effort whereby participants had rowed 2000 m. Exercise induced an increase in erythrocytes or serum levels of some markers collected from rowers, such as superoxide dismutase, TNF-α and thiobarbituric acid reactive substances (TBARS, a marker of lipid peroxidation). While the other parameters did not differ from control and krill oil supplemented group, during recovery time TBARS continued to increase in the control group while the krill oil supplemented group showed significantly lower levels of lipid peroxidation. This suggests that krill oil could reduce the effort-associated free radical mediated injuries [156].

The effects of krill oil were also investigated to see its ability to influence exercise performance and post-effort immune function. In a small randomized clinical trial, 37 young (25.8 ± 5.3 years) athletes were divided into two groups: one received 2 g/day of krill oil for six weeks and the other received a placebo. A cycling time test was performed before and at the end of the supplementation period, where blood samples were collected before supplementation and immediately after exercise, or after 1 or 3 h, or at rest. The results showed that after six weeks of supplementation, the levels of peripheral blood mononuclear cell IL-2 production and natural killer cell cytotoxic activity 3 h post-exercise were significantly increased in krill oil supplemented athletes [157]. On this basis, other authors investigated the ability of krill oil to increase the body mass and the potential mechanism action behind this effect. To investigate the mechanism of action, they used C2C12 rat myoblasts (skeletal muscle) treated with krill oil or phosphatidylcholine derived from soy or control and observed that only krill oil was able to stimulate the mTOR pathway. In the clinical part of the study, a double-blind, placebo-controlled clinical trial was performed on resistance trained athletes receiving 3 g/day of krill oil or placebo during the resistance training program of eight weeks. At the end of the study, no difference in comprehensive metabolic panel, complete blood count or urine analysis were recorded between the two groups. However, krill oil was able to induce a significant increase in the lean body mass from baseline of about 2.1% [158].

Moreover, a particular mixed formulation, named ESPO-572® composed of 75% PCSO-524®, which is green-lipped mussel oil and 25% krill oil, was effective in mitigation of exercise-induced muscle damage and cytokine-induced tissue degradation when administered for 26-day, 600 mg/day, in untrained men who underwent a running test [159]. As the levels of choline are known to maintain muscle function and exercise performance, a decrease in choline levels were recorded after high-resistance or high-intensity exercises. Storsve and colleagues performed a clinical trial to evaluate a possible protective effect by krill oil on this loss of choline. There were 47 triathletes placed randomly in two groups, one receiving 4 g/day of a particular formulation of krill oil named SuperbaBoost™ for five weeks before the race and another group receiving placebo. Blood samples were collected pre-, immediately post-race and one day after the race and the serum choline and the choline metabolites were evaluated. As expected, the choline levels significantly decreased after the race, but significantly higher choline levels were found in athletes of the krill oil group compared with athletes who received placebo. These results seem to suggest that a krill oil supplement could prevent choline levels from falling and could avoid impairment in exercise performance, especially during high-resistance efforts [160].

Table 3. Experimental studies in which krill supplementation has been tested. Primary endpoints have been reported, as well as design and duration of the studies. (TG = triglycerides).

Classification of Health Benefits	Model	Diets	Duration of Supplementation	Outcomes	References
Metabolic disorders	Sprague Dawley rats HFD	100 and 200 g/krill oil (KO)	2 weeks	↓ serum lipid levels	[104]
	HFD mice	1.25–2.5–5% KO	8 weeks	↓ liver TGs, cholesterol and serum cholesterol and glucose	[105]
	hTNFα over-expressing mice	Krill powder (4.3% of proteins)	8 weeks	↓ liver and plasma TGs, hepatic expression SREBP2, ↑ β-oxidation, ↓ inflammation	[106]
	LDLR-KO mice fed with a western diet + Pacific krill	8-HEPE (100 mg/kg)	18 weeks	↓ plasma LDL and total cholesterol, ↑ HDL, ↓ hepatic TG levels	[107]
	Dyslipidemic and diabetic non-human primates	150 mg/Kg/day		↓ plasma total and LDL-cholesterol, and TGs, ↑ HDL-cholesterol	[108]
	C57BL/6J mice fed with HFD	5% krill powder	12 weeks	↓ body weight gain, the fat accumulation in tissue adipose and liver, ↓ serum LDL, ↑ glucose tolerance. ↓ oxidative damage in liver	[114]
	Rats HFD	2.5% krill	12 weeks	↓ body weight gain	[109]
	Obesity model in castrated New Zealand white rabbits	600 mg/day	8 weeks	↑ insulin sensitivity and secretion, ↓ fasting blood glucose	[110]
	HFD combined with thermoneutral animal housing	KO (containing EPA ~13%, DHA ~8%)	24 weeks	↓ liver steatosis	[152]

Table 3. Cont.

Classification of Health Benefits	Model	Diets	Duration of Supplementation	Outcomes	References
	Randomized controlled study on 36 individuals	4 g/day	8 weeks	↑ EPA, DHA and DPA in krill group	[111]
	Human with borderline or high TG levels	0.5, 1, 2, or 4 g/day for	6 and 12 weeks	↓ plasma TGs	[112]
	Randomized cross-over clinical trial on 25 moderately hyperTGmic subjects	1000 mg/day	4 weeks	↑ plasma HDL and apolipoprotein AI levels	[113]
	11 obese men	4 g/day per os	24 weeks	↓ anthropometric parameters and blood AEA and 2-AG	[122]
	63 obese subjects	2 g/day	4 weeks	↓ 2-AG levels, no significant effect on antropometric	[123]
Pretection against myocardial infarct	MI and euthanasia after 7 days	KO containing 0.47 g/100 g EPA + DHA	14 days of pretreatment with KO before MI	↓ heart and lung hypertrophy, and and inflammation	[118]
Vascular function	34 participants with type 2 diabetes	1 g/day in PUFA	4 weeks	↑ endothelial function ↓ blood C peptide levels and HOMA scores	[119]
Gut microbiota and IBD	ICR mice fed with HFD	fish oil (600 µg/g/day), KO (600 µg/g/day) and their mixture (300 + 300 µg/g/day	12 weeks	↓ obesity, ↑ positive phyla (i.e., *Bacteroides* and *Lactobacilli*)	[124]
	Obesity and hyperlipidemia induced by HFD+ high sugar diet	100, 200, 600µg/g/day	12 weeks	↑ microbiotic alteration and cardiometabolic parameters	[125]
		100, 200 and 600 mg/kg	7 weeks	↑ abundance of *Lactobacillus* spp. and short-chain fatty acids producers	[126]
	Dextran sulfate sodium (DSS)-induced colitis in mice	mixture of KO, *Lactobacillus reuteri* and vitamin	4 weeks	↑ clinical and histological scores, restore epithelial restitution, ↓ proinflammatory cytokines	[110]
	DSS-induced colitis in mice	5%	4 weeks	↓ disease activity index and TNF-α and IL-1β levels	[128]

Table 3. Cont.

Classification of Health Benefits	Model	Diets	Duration of Supplementation	Outcomes	References
	DSS-induced colitis in mice	KO-entrapped liposomes (containing 42% w/w phospholipids, ≥26.5 w/w% total Omega-3, ≥8.5% w/w DHA, ≥14.5% w/w EPA, and 0.125±0.025 w/w% astaxanthin)	8 weeks	↓TNF and IL6 and the systemic levels of endotoxin, ↑ hydrophobic protective barrier	[129]
	C. rodentium infected mice	1.5 g KO	4 weeks	↓ inflammatory pathway, ↓of Rickettsiales and several species of Lactobacillus	[130]
Arthritic disease	Mice experimental models of inflammatory arthritis	KO diet, in which EPA + DHA were 0.44 g/100 g of KO diet	2 months	↓ infiltration of inflammatory cells and hyperplasia at synovial layer	[132]
	hTNF-α over-expressing mice		6 weeks	↓ markers of fatty acid oxidation	[133]
	Randomized, double blind, placebo controlled clinical trials on 90 patients with CVD and/or osteoarthritis and/or rheumatoid arthritis	300 mg/day		↓ CRP levels and pain (about 29%), stiffness (about 20%) and functional impairment (about 23%).	[134]
	Randomized, double-blind, parallel-group, placebo-controlled study, 50 patients with mild knee pain	2 g/day	30 days	↓ knee pain, ↑ motion of both the knees	[135]
	260 Australian patients affected by knee OA	2 g/day	6 months (ongoing)	↑ knee pain and in size of knee synovitis/effusion	[11]
Neurodegeneration	Human neuronal SH-SY5Y cell line			↓ oxidative stress and mitochondrial protection	[137]
	Aged rats	20, 50 mg/kg/day	7 days	↑ cholinergic trasmission, muscarinic receptors and choline transporters	[139]
	LPS-induced mice model of Alzheimer	80 mg/kg/day	4 weeks	↓ iNOS, COX-2, NFkB, ROS and malondialdehyde levels, amyloid beta (1–42) peptide	[141]

Table 3. *Cont.*

Classification of Health Benefits	Model	Diets	Duration of Supplementation	Outcomes	References
	Senescence-accelerated prone mouse strain 8 (SAMP8)	1% of KO	12 weeks	↑ cognitive function and the anxiety, ↓ memory deficit and learning, ↓ β-amyloid Aβ42 accumulation	[142]
	Amyloid Aβ25-35-induced mouse model of Alzheimer	100, 200 or 500 mg/Kg/day	14 days	↓ latency in the Morris water maze test, ↓ Bax/Bcl-2 ratio in the brain and ↓ levels of ROS, malondialdehyde and NO	[143]
	Randomized, double-blind clinical trial on 45 healthy elderly males (61–72 years-old)	sardine-oil, KO or placebo	12 weeks	↑ cognitive capacity	[144]
		KO 0.2 g/rat/day, or imipramine 20 mg/kg/day	7 weeks	↑ cognitive abilities, in behaviour features and Bdnf	[145]
		KO or vitamine B12 or imipramine or saline 5 mL/kg	14 days	↓ malondialdehyde and hydrogen peroxide levels, catalase activity, ↑ glutathione peroxidase levels, superoxide dismutase activities and glutathione levels	[146]
	Immobility-induced murine depression model	PBS, or cotinine (a nicotine-derivative) 5 mg/kg, or cotinine plus KO 143 mg/kg	4 weeks	↓ depression-like behaviours	[147]
	Randomized, controlled, double-blind clinical trial on 264 adolescent (13–15 years)	cohort I: 400 mg/day of EPA + DHA or placebo, and after 3 months increased the dose to 800 mg/day of EPA + DHA. cohort II: 800 mg/day of EPA + DHA	1 year	no evidence about an effect on depressive feelings, low adherence	[148,149]
Cancer	Several human and murine colorectal cancer cells	0.03 and 0.12 μL/100 μL	24–48 h	↓ cell proliferation, ↓ expression of EGFR, pEGFR, pERK1/2 and pAKT	[154]
Exercise performance	Double-blind on 17 rowers members of the Polish National Rowing Team	1 g/day of KO	6 weeks	↑ erythrocytes or serum levels of superoxide dismutase, TNF-α and thiobarbituric acid	[155]
	Randomized clinical trial on 37 young athletes	2 g/day of KO	6 weeks	↑ levels of peripheral blood mononuclear cell IL-2 production and natural killer cell cytotoxic activity, 3 h post-exercise	[156]

Table 3. Cont.

Classification of Health Benefits	Model	Diets	Duration of Supplementation	Outcomes	References
	Double-blind, placebo-controlled clinical trial	3 g/day of KO or placebo during the resistance training	8 weeks	↑ in the lean body mass (about 2.1% vs. baseline)	[157]
		ESPO-572® (75% of PCSO-524® and 25% KO) 600 mg/day	26 days	↑ mitigation of exercise-induced muscle damage and cytokine-induced tissue degradation	[158]
	47 triathletes randomized supplemented before the race.	4 g/day of a KO (Superba Boost™)	5 weeks	↑ exercise performance, especially during high-resistance efforts	[159]

12. Discussion and Future Perspectives

Considering the increased market of n-3 PUFA containing dietary supplements, supported by increased clinical evidence, there is a constant search for new n-3 PUFA sources and formulations [13].

Krill oil possesses several health benefits in clinical practice, in particular in cardiovascular disease risk factor management and in neurological diseases and inflammation [161]. It is commercialized in both the nutraceutical and pharmaceutical market in different dosage forms including soft gels, gummies, capsules and tablets.

However, despite many activities and functionalities that have been attributed to krill oil, the molecular pathways of actions are still in part unclear because few studies of pharmacodynamic are available and few have provided detailed information about molecular mechanisms of krill components such as astaxanthin, vitamin A, tocopherols, flavonoids, and minerals [162]. Most published RCTs do not provide any information regarding krill oil composition (except for the EPA and DHA content) [93]. In this regard, further studies are necessary to emphasize the relationship between krill oil components, mechanisms of action, health benefits and diversifying the different composition of krill oils for specific applications.

The importance of knowing the actions of the active components of krill oil is fundamental for the future development of new extraction techniques which could give rise to new chemical extract compositions for certain pathological conditions. To date, solvent and non-solvent extraction, super and subcritical fluid extraction and enzyme-assisted pre-treatment extraction represent the main technologies used for krill oil extraction, each of which have both advantages and disadvantages [163].

Among the active ingredients contained in krill oil, EPA and DHA constitute the main title of the products studied in clinical trials. EPA and DHA from krill oil are attached to phospholipids and to phosphatidylcholine. This composition promotes the efficiency of absorption of fatty acids into the blood when compared with omega-3 from fish oil [4]. However, the minor components contained in krill oil such as astaxanthin, alpha-tocopherol, vitamin A and flavonoids could exert pleiotropic activities and improve the bioaccessibility of EPA and DHA, even if data need to be clarified. Many studies on krill rarely detail the concentration in minor components, so it is hard to estimate their contribution to the final observed effects.

Krill oil products can be associated with other nutritional supplements to provide more benefits. Alvarez-Ricartes et al. demonstrated the efficacy of krill oil in addition to cotinine in the treatment of depressive symptoms in posttraumatic stress disorder people [164]. A study by Costanzo et al. found an association of krill oil with *Lactobacillus reuteri*, and vitamin D showed to reduce gut inflammation, reducing gut dysbiosis as well as increasing the epithelial restitution [135].

Currently, supplementation with krill oil is considered safe and well tolerated. Side effects are minimal or absent, and may include bloating, diarrhea and flatulence [165]. However, the available evidence is limited and further long-term RCTs, including many people, are needed to confirm both safety and efficacy of this nutraceutical. In addition, a cost/benefit analysis is necessary to better understand the implication of krill oil supplementation on health.

In conclusion, preliminary clinical data suggest that krill oil represent a valid supplement in the treatment of several conditions including CVDs, osteoarthritis, premenstrual syndrome and dysmenorrhea. Innovative technologies applied to improve krill oil purification and concentration could improve its cost-efficacy ratio.

Author Contributions: Conceptualization, A.F.G.C. and A.C.; methodology, A.F.G.C. and A.C.; writing—original draft preparation, A.C., G.C., V.C., A.M., L.T., A.F.G.C.; writing—review and editing, A.C., G.C., V.C., A.M., L.T., A.F.G.C.; supervision, A.F.G.C. All authors have read and agreed to the published version of the manuscript.

Funding: This research received no external funding.

Institutional Review Board Statement: Not applicable.

Informed Consent Statement: Not applicable.

Data Availability Statement: Not applicable.

Acknowledgments: We acknowledge Elisa Grandi for her support in the paper preparation.

Conflicts of Interest: The authors declare no conflict of interest.

References

1. Nicol, S.; Endo, Y. Krill fisheries: Development, management and ecosystem implications. *Aquat. Living Resour.* **1999**, *12*, 105–120. [CrossRef]
2. Commission for the Conservation of Antarctic Marine Living Resources (CCAMLR). Krill Fisheries and Sustainability. Available online: https://www.ccamlr.org/en/fisheries/krill-fisheries-and-sustainability (accessed on 23 May 2021).
3. Nicol, S.; Foster, J.; Kawaguchi, S. The fishery for Antarctic krill—Recent developments. *Fish Fish.* **2011**, *13*, 30–40. [CrossRef]
4. Cicero, A.F.; Colletti, A. Krill oil: Evidence of a new source of polyunsaturated fatty acids with high bioavailability. *Clin. Lipidol.* **2015**, *10*, 1–4. [CrossRef]
5. Grantham, G.J. *The Southern Ocean: The Utilization of Krill*; Southern Ocean Fisheries Survey Programme GLO/SO/7/3; Food and Agriculture Organization: Rome, Italy, 1977; pp. 1–61.
6. Ramprasath, V.R.; Eyal, I.; Zchut, S.; Jones, P.J. Enhanced increase of omega-3 index in healthy individuals with response to 4-week n-3 fatty acid supplementation from krill oil versus fish oil. *Lipids Health Dis.* **2013**, *12*, 178. [CrossRef]
7. Cicero, A.F.G.; Ertek, S.; Borghi, C. Omega-3 polyunsaturated fatty acids: Their potential role in blood pressure prevention and management. *Curr. Vasc. Pharmacol.* **2009**, *7*, 330–337. [CrossRef] [PubMed]
8. Cicero, A.F.G.; De Sando, V.; Parini, A.; Borghi, C. Polyunsaturated fatty acids application in internal medicine: Beyond the established cardiovascular effects. *Arch. Med. Sci.* **2012**, *8*, 784–793. [CrossRef] [PubMed]
9. Zheng, J.-S.; Hu, X.-J.; Zhao, Y.-M.; Yang, J.; Li, D. Intake of fish and marine n-3 polyunsaturated fatty acids and risk of breast cancer: Meta-analysis of data from 21 independent prospective cohort studies. *BMJ* **2013**, *346*, f3706. [CrossRef] [PubMed]
10. Saravanan, P.; Davidson, N.C.; Schmidt, E.B.; Calder, P. Cardiovascular effects of marine omega-3 fatty acids. *Lancet* **2010**, *376*, 540–550. [CrossRef]
11. Laslett, L.L.; Antony, B.; Wluka, A.E.; Hill, C.; March, L.; Keen, H.I.; Otahal, P.; Cicuttini, F.M.; Jones, G. KARAOKE: Krill oil versus placebo in the treatment of knee osteoarthritis: Protocol for a randomised controlled trial. *Trials* **2020**, *21*, 1–14. [CrossRef] [PubMed]
12. Ulven, S.M.; Kirkhus, B.; Lamglait, A.; Basu, S.; Elind, E.; Haider, T.; Berge, K.; Vik, H.; Pedersen, J.I. Metabolic Effects of Krill Oil are Essentially Similar to Those of Fish Oil but at Lower Dose of EPA and DHA, in Healthy Volunteers. *Lipids* **2010**, *46*, 37–46. [CrossRef]
13. Kim, M.G.; Yang, I.; Lee, H.S.; Lee, J.-Y.; Kim, K. Lipid-modifying effects of krill oil vs fish oil: A network meta-analysis. *Nutr. Rev.* **2020**, *78*, 699–708. [CrossRef]
14. Ulven, S.M.; Holven, K.B. Comparison of bioavailability of krill oil versus fish oil and health effect. *Vasc. Health Risk Manag.* **2015**, *11*, 511–524. [CrossRef]

15. Ahmmed, M.K.; Ahmmed, F.; Tian, H.; Carne, A.; Bekhit, A.E. Marine omega-3 (n-3) phospholipids: A comprehensive review of their properties, sources, bioavailability, and relation to brain health. *Compr. Rev. Food Sci. Food Saf.* **2019**, *19*, 64–123. [CrossRef]
16. Phleger, C.F.; Nelson, M.M.; Mooney, B.D.; Nichols, P.D. Interannual and between species comparison of the lipids, fatty acids and sterols of Antarctic krill from the US AMLR Elephant Island survey area. *Comp. Biochem. Physiol. Part B* **2002**, *131*, 733–747. [CrossRef]
17. Xie, D.; Gong, M.; Wei, W.; Jin, J.; Wang, X.; Wang, X.; Jin, Q. Antarctic Krill (*Euphausia superba*) Oil: A Comprehensive Review of Chemical Composition, Extraction Technologies, Health Benefits, and Current Applications. *Compr. Rev. Food Sci. Food Saf.* **2019**, *18*, 514–534. [CrossRef]
18. Gang, K.-Q.; Wu, Z.-X.; Zhou, D.-Y.; Zhao, Q.; Zhou, X.; Lv, D.-D.; Rakariyatham, K.; Liu, X.-Y.; Shahidi, F. Effects of hot air drying process on lipid quality of whelks Neptunea arthritica cumingi Crosse and Neverita didyma. *J. Food Sci. Technol.* **2019**, *56*, 4166–4176. [CrossRef]
19. Bottino, N.R. Lipid composition of two species of antarctic krill: *Euphausia superba* and *E. crystallorophias*. *Comp. Biochem. Physiol. Part B* **1975**, *50*, 479–484. [CrossRef]
20. Han, X.; Liu, D. Detection and analysis of 17 steroid hormones by ultra-high-performance liquid chromatography-electrospray ionization mass spectrometry (UHPLC-MS) in different sex and maturity stages of Antarctic krill (*Euphausia superba* Dana). *PLoS ONE* **2019**, *14*, e0213398. [CrossRef]
21. Xie, D.; Jin, J.; Sun, J.; Liang, L.; Wang, X.; Zhang, W.; Wang, X.; Jin, Q. Comparison of solvents for extraction of krill oil from krill meal: Lipid yield, phospholipids content, fatty acids composition and minor components. *Food Chem.* **2017**, *233*, 434–441. [CrossRef]
22. Lim, C.W.; Kim, B.H.; Kim, I.-H.; Lee, M.-W. Modeling and optimization of phospholipase A1-catalyzed hydrolysis of phosphatidylcholine using response surface methodology for lysophosphatidylcholine production. *Biotechnol. Prog.* **2014**, *31*, 35–41. [CrossRef]
23. Burri, L.; Johnsen, L. Krill Products: An Overview of Animal Studies. *Nutrients* **2015**, *7*, 3300–3321. [CrossRef] [PubMed]
24. Clarke, A. The biochemical composition of krill, Euphausia superba Dana, from South Georgia. *J. Exp. Mar. Biol. Ecol.* **1980**, *43*, 221–236. [CrossRef]
25. WHO, Food and Agriculture Organization of the United Nations. *Codex Standard for Fish Oils. Codex Alimentarius Commission*; Codex Standard 329-2017; WHO: Geneva, Switzerland; Food and Agriculture Organization of the United Nations: Quebec, QC, Canada, 2017.
26. Paluchova, V.; Vik, A.; Cajka, T.; Brezinova, M.; Brejchova, K.; Bugajev, V.; Draberova, L.; Draber, P.; Buresova, J.; Kroupova, P.; et al. Triacylglycerol-Rich Oils of Marine Origin are Optimal Nutrients for Induction of Polyunsaturated Docosahexaenoic Acid Ester of Hydroxy Linoleic Acid (13-DHAHLA) with Anti-Inflammatory Properties in Mice. *Mol. Nutr. Food Res.* **2020**, *64*, e1901238. [CrossRef] [PubMed]
27. Kołakowska, A. The influence of sex and maturity stage of krill (*Euphausia superba* Dana) upon the content and composition of its lipid. *Pol. Polar Res.* **1991**, *12*, 73–78.
28. Li, D.-M.; Zhou, D.-Y.; Zhu, B.-W.; Chi, Y.-L.; Sun, L.-M.; Dong, X.-P.; Qin, L.; Qiao, W.-Z.; Murata, Y. Effects of krill oil intake on plasma cholesterol and glucose levels in rats fed a high-cholesterol diet. *J. Sci. Food Agric.* **2013**, *93*, 2669–2675. [CrossRef] [PubMed]
29. Siriwardhana, N.; Kalupahana, N.S.; Moustaid-Moussa, N. Health benefits of n-3 polyunsaturated fatty acids: Eicosapentaenoic acid and docosahexaenoic acid. *Adv. Food Nutr. Res.* **2012**, *65*, 211–222.
30. Skubic, C.; Vovk, I.; Rozman, D.; Križman, M. Simplified LC-MS Method for Analysis of Sterols in Biological Samples. *Molecules* **2020**, *25*, 4116. [CrossRef]
31. Tocher, D.R.; Betancor, M.B.; Sprague, M.; Olsen, R.E.; A Napier, J. Omega-3 Long-Chain Polyunsaturated Fatty Acids, EPA and DHA: Bridging the Gap between Supply and Demand. *Nutrients* **2019**, *11*, 89. [CrossRef] [PubMed]
32. Chang, N.W.; Huang, P.C. Effects of the ratio of polyunsaturated and monounsaturated fatty acid to saturated fatty acid on rat plasma and liver lipid concentrations. *Lipids* **1998**, *33*, 481–487. [CrossRef]
33. Rincón-Cervera, M.Á.; González-Barriga, V.; Romero, J.; Rojas, R.; López-Arana, S. Quantification and Distribution of Omega-3 Fatty Acids in South Pacific Fish and Shellfish Species. *Foods* **2020**, *9*, 233. [CrossRef]
34. Murru, E.; Banni, S.; Carta, G. Nutritional Properties of Dietary Omega-3-Enriched Phospholipids. *BioMed Res. Int.* **2013**, *2013*, 1–13. [CrossRef] [PubMed]
35. Schuchardt, J.P.; Schneider, I.; Meyer, H.; Neubronner, J.; Von Schacky, C.; Hahn, A. Incorporation of EPA and DHA into plasma phospholipids in response to different omega-3 fatty acid formulations—A comparative bioavailability study of fish oil vs. krill oil. *Lipids Health Dis.* **2011**, *10*, 145. [CrossRef]
36. Šimat, V.; ElAbed, N.; Kulawik, P.; Ceylan, Z.; Jamroz, E.; Yazgan, H.; Čagalj, M.; Regenstein, J.M.; Özogul, F. Recent Advances in Marine-Based Nutraceuticals and Their Health Benefits. *Mar. Drugs* **2020**, *18*, 627. [CrossRef] [PubMed]
37. Takaichi, S.; Matsui, K.; Nakamura, M.; Muramatsu, M.; Hanada, S. Fatty acids of astaxanthin esters in krill determined by mild mass spectrometry. *Comp. Biochem. Physiol. Part B* **2003**, *136*, 317–322. [CrossRef]
38. Sun, W.; Shi, B.; Xue, C.; Jiang, X. The comparison of krill oil extracted through ethanol–hexane method and subcritical method. *Food Sci. Nutr.* **2019**, *7*, 700–710. [CrossRef] [PubMed]

39. Molino, A.; Rimauro, J.; Casella, P.; Cerbone, A.; Larocca, V.; Chianese, S.; Karatza, D.; Mehariya, S.; Ferraro, A.; Hristoforou, E.; et al. Extraction of astaxanthin from microalga Haematococcus pluvialis in red phase by using generally recognized as safe solvents and accelerated extraction. *J. Biotechnol.* **2018**, *283*, 51–61. [CrossRef] [PubMed]
40. Grynbaum, M.D.; Hentschel, P.; Putzbach, K.; Rehbein, J.; Krucker, M.; Nicholson, G.; Albert, K. Unambiguous detection of astaxanthin and astaxanthin fatty acid esters in krill (*Euphausia superba* Dana). *J. Sep. Sci.* **2005**, *28*, 1685–1693. [CrossRef]
41. Alessandri, J.M.; Goustard, B.; Guesnet, P.; Durand, G. Docosahexaenoic acid concentrations in retinal phospholipids of piglets fed an infant formula enriched with long-chain polyunsaturated fatty acids: Effects of egg phospholipids and fish oils with different ratios of eicosapentaenoic acid to docosahexaenoic acid. *Am. J. Clin. Nutr.* **1998**, *67*, 377–385. [CrossRef]
42. Araujo, P.; Zhu, H.; Breivik, J.F.; Hjelle, J.I.; Zeng, Y. Determination and Structural Elucidation of Triacylglycerols in Krill Oil by Chromatographic Techniques. *Lipids* **2013**, *49*, 163–172. [CrossRef] [PubMed]
43. Souchet, N.; Laplante, S. Seasonal and geographical variations of sterol composition in snow crab hepatopancreas and pelagic fish viscera from Eastern Quebec. *Comp. Biochem. Physiol. Part B* **2007**, *147*, 378–386. [CrossRef]
44. Bruheim, I.; Cameron, J. Flowable Concentrated Phospholipid Krill Oil Composition. U.S. Patent 20170020928 Al, 26 January 2017.
45. Dunlap, W.C.; Fujisawa, A.; Yamamoto, Y.; Moylan, T.J.; Sidell, B.D. Notothenioid fish, krill and phytoplankton from Antarctica contain a vitamin E constituent (α-tocomonoenol) functionally associated with cold-water adaptation. *Comp. Biochem. Physiol. Part B* **2002**, *133*, 299–305. [CrossRef]
46. Sampalis, F.; Bunea, R.; Pelland, M.F.; Kowalski, O.; Duguet, N.; Dupuis, S. Evaluation of the effects of Neptune Krill Oil on the management of premenstrual syndrome and dysmenorrhea. *Altern. Med. Rev.* **2003**, *8*, 171–179. [PubMed]
47. Peng, Y.; Ji, W.; Zhang, D.; Ji, H.; Liu, S. Composition and content analysis of fluoride in inorganic salts of the integument of Antarctic krill (*Euphausia superba*). *Sci. Rep.* **2019**, *9*, 7853. [CrossRef] [PubMed]
48. Dawson, M.I.; Xia, Z. The retinoid X receptors and their ligands. *Biochim. Biophys. Acta* **2012**, *1821*, 21–56. [CrossRef] [PubMed]
49. Wang, Y.; Nakajima, T.; Gonzalez, F.J.; Tanaka, N. PPARs as Metabolic Regulators in the Liver: Lessons from Liver-Specific PPAR-Null Mice. *Int. J. Mol. Sci.* **2020**, *21*, 2061. [CrossRef]
50. Ma, X.; Wang, D.; Zhao, W.; Xu, L. Deciphering the Roles of PPARgamma in Adipocytes via Dynamic Change of Transcription Complex. *Front. Endocrinol.* **2018**, *9*, 473. [CrossRef] [PubMed]
51. Youssef, J.; Badr, M. Role of Peroxisome Proliferator-Activated Receptors in Inflammation Control. *J. Biomed. Biotechnol.* **2004**, *2004*, 156–166. [CrossRef] [PubMed]
52. Zhang, W.; Chen, R.; Yang, T.; Xu, N.; Chen, J.; Gao, Y.; Stetler, R.A. Fatty acid transporting proteins: Roles in brain development, aging, and stroke. *Prostaglandins Leukot. Essent. Fat. Acids* **2018**, *136*, 35–45. [CrossRef]
53. Marechal, L.; Laviolette, M.; Rodrigue-Way, A.; Sow, B.; Brochu, M.; Caron, V.; Tremblay, A. The CD36-PPARgamma Pathway in Metabolic Disorders. *Int. J. Mol. Sci.* **2018**, *19*, 1529. [CrossRef]
54. Monsalve, F.A.; Pyarasani, R.D.; Delgado-Lopez, F.; Moore-Carrasco, R. Peroxisome Proliferator-Activated Receptor Targets for the Treatment of Metabolic Diseases. *Mediat. Inflamm.* **2013**, *2013*, 1–18. [CrossRef]
55. Korbecki, J.; Bobiński, R.; Dutka, M. Self-regulation of the inflammatory response by peroxisome proliferator-activated receptors. *Inflamm. Res.* **2019**, *68*, 443–458. [CrossRef]
56. Son, S.-E.; Kim, N.-J.; Im, D.-S. Development of Free Fatty Acid Receptor 4 (FFA4/GPR120) Agonists in Health Science. *Biomol. Ther.* **2021**, *29*, 22–30. [CrossRef]
57. Si, T.-L.; Liu, Q.; Ren, Y.-F.; Li, H.; Xu, X.-Y.; Li, E.-H.; Pan, S.-Y.; Zhang, J.-L.; Wang, K.-X. Enhanced anti-inflammatory effects of DHA and quercetin in lipopolysaccharide-induced RAW264.7 macrophages by inhibiting NF-κB and MAPK activation. *Mol. Med. Rep.* **2016**, *14*, 499–508. [CrossRef] [PubMed]
58. Oh, D.Y.; Talukdar, S.; Bae, E.J.; Imamura, T.; Morinaga, H.; Fan, W.Q.; Li, P.; Lu, W.J.; Watkins, S.M.; Olefsky, J.M. GPR120 Is an Omega-3 Fatty Acid Receptor Mediating Potent Anti-inflammatory and Insulin-Sensitizing Effects. *Cell* **2010**, *142*, 687–698. [CrossRef] [PubMed]
59. Liu, T.; Zhang, L.; Joo, D.; Sun, S.C. NF-kappaB signaling in inflammation. *Signal Transduct. Target Ther.* **2017**, *2*, 17023. [CrossRef] [PubMed]
60. Calder, P.C. Omega-3 polyunsaturated fatty acids and inflammatory processes: Nutrition or pharmacology? *Br. J. Clin. Pharmacol.* **2013**, *75*, 645–662. [CrossRef] [PubMed]
61. Encarnacion, M.M.D.; Warner, G.M.; Cheng, J.; Gray, C.E.; Nath, K.A.; Grande, J.P. n-3 Fatty acids block TNF-α-stimulated MCP-1 expression in rat mesangial cells. *Am. J. Physiol. Physiol.* **2011**, *300*, F1142–F1151. [CrossRef] [PubMed]
62. Wang, Y.; Huang, F. N-3 Polyunsaturated Fatty Acids and Inflammation in Obesity: Local Effect and Systemic Benefit. *BioMed Res. Int.* **2015**, *2015*, 1–16. [CrossRef] [PubMed]
63. Magee, P.; Pearson, S.; Whittingham-Dowd, J.; Allen, J. PPARgamma as a molecular target of EPA anti-inflammatory activity during TNF-alpha-impaired skeletal muscle cell differentiation. *J. Nutr. Biochem.* **2012**, *23*, 1440–1448. [CrossRef]
64. Mosser, D.M.; Zhang, X. Interleukin-10: New perspectives on an old cytokine. *Immunol. Rev.* **2008**, *226*, 205–218. [CrossRef]
65. Tiedge, M.; Lortz, S.; Munday, R.; Lenzen, S. Complementary action of antioxidant enzymes in the protection of bioengineered insulin-producing RINm5F cells against the toxicity of reactive oxygen species. *Diabetes* **1998**, *47*, 1578–1585. [CrossRef] [PubMed]
66. Chen, Q.; Tao, J.; Xie, X. Astaxanthin Promotes Nrf2/ARE Signaling to Inhibit HG-Induced Renal Fibrosis in GMCs. *Mar. Drugs* **2018**, *16*, 117. [CrossRef] [PubMed]

67. Landon, R.; Gueguen, V.; Petite, H.; Letourneur, D.; Pavon-Djavid, G.; Anagnostou, F. Impact of Astaxanthin on Diabetes Pathogenesis and Chronic Complications. *Mar. Drugs* **2020**, *18*, 357. [CrossRef]
68. Solinas, G.; Becattini, B. JNK at the crossroad of obesity, insulin resistance, and cell stress response. *Mol. Metab.* **2017**, *6*, 174–184. [CrossRef] [PubMed]
69. Feng, W.; Wang, Y.; Guo, N.; Huang, P.; Mi, Y. Effects of Astaxanthin on Inflammation and Insulin Resistance in a Mouse Model of Gestational Diabetes Mellitus. *Dose-Response* **2020**, *18*, 1559325820926765. [CrossRef]
70. Katevas, D.S.; Toro Guerra, R.R.; Chiong Lay, M. Solvent-Free Process for Obtaining Phospholipids and Neutral Enriched Krill Oils. U.S. Patent 8865236 B2, 6 March 2014.
71. Beaudoin, A.; Martin, G. Method of Extracting Lipids from Marine and Aquatic Animal Tissues. U.S. Patent 6800299 B1, 5 October 2004.
72. Yoshitomi, B.; Shigematsu, Y. Process for Making Dried Powdery and Granular Krill. U.S. Patent 20030113432 A1, 16 June 2003.
73. Xie, D.; Mu, H.; Tang, T.; Wang, X.; Wei, W.; Jin, J.; Wang, X.; Jin, Q. Production of three types of krill oils from krill meal by a three-step solvent extraction procedure. *Food Chem.* **2018**, *248*, 279–286. [CrossRef]
74. Ronen, L.; Ran, N.; Ben-Dror, G. Krill Oil Preparations with Optimal Mineral and Metal Composition, Low Impurities and Low and Stable TMA Levels. US Patent 20170354694 Al, 14 December 2017.
75. Bruheim, I.; Griinari, M.; Ervik, J.R.; Remoy, S.R.; Remoy, E.; Cameron, J. Method for Processing Crustaceans to Produce Low Fluoride/Low Trimethyl Amine Products Thereof. U.S. Patent 20160345616 Al, 2 June 2016.
76. Gigliotti, J.C.; Davenport, M.P.; Beamer, S.K.; Tou, J.C.; Jaczynski, J. Extraction and characterisation of lipids from Antarctic krill (*Euphausia superba*). *Food Chem.* **2011**, *125*, 1028–1036. [CrossRef]
77. Yin, F.-W.; Liu, X.-Y.; Fan, X.-R.; Zhou, D.-Y.; Xu, W.-S.; Zhu, B.-W.; Murata, Y.-Y. Extrusion of Antarctic krill (*Euphausia superba*) meal and its effect on oil extraction. *Int. J. Food Sci. Technol.* **2014**, *50*, 633–639. [CrossRef]
78. Khan, L.M.; Hanna, M.A. Expression of oil from oilseeds—A review. *J. Agric. Eng. Res.* **1983**, *28*, 495–503. [CrossRef]
79. Larsen, P.M.; Fey, S.J.; Breuning, J.; Ludvigsen, B. A Method for the Extraction of Lipid Fractions from Krill. WO Patent 2007080514 A2, 15 January 2007.
80. Tilseth, S.; Høstmark, Ø. New Method for Making Krill Meal. U.S. Patent 20150050403 A1, 16 January 2015.
81. Friedrich, J.P.; Pryde, E.H. Supercritical CO_2 extraction of lipid-bearing materials and characterization of the products. *J. Am. Oil Chem. Soc.* **1984**, *61*, 223–228. [CrossRef]
82. Yamaguchi, K.; Miki, W.; Toriu, N.; Kondo, Y.; Murakami, M.; Konosu, S. The composition of carotenoid pigments in the Antarctic krill (*Euphausia superba*). *Nippon Suisan Gakkaishi* **1983**, *49*, 1411–1415. [CrossRef]
83. Bruheim, I.; Tilseth, S.; Mancinelli, D. Bioeffective Krill Oil Compositions. U.S. Patent 9889163 B2, 13 February 2018.
84. Liu, H.-M.; Wang, F.-Y.; Li, H.-Y.; Wang, X.-D.; Qin, G.-Y. Subcritical Butane and Propane Extraction of Oil from Rice Bran. *Bioresources* **2015**, *10*, 4652–4662. [CrossRef]
85. Sun, D.; Cao, C.; Li, B.; Chen, H.; Cao, P.; Li, J.; Liu, Y. Study on combined heat pump drying with freeze-drying of Antarctic krill and its effects on the lipids. *J. Food Process. Eng.* **2017**, *40*, e12577. [CrossRef]
86. Domínguez, H.; Núñez, M.; Lema, J. Enzymatic pretreatment to enhance oil extraction from fruits and oilseeds: A review. *Food Chem.* **1994**, *49*, 271–286. [CrossRef]
87. Lee, S. Krill Oil and Method for Manufacturing the Same. U.S. Patent 8624046 B2, 7 January 2014.
88. Bunea, R.; El Farrah, K.; Deutsch, L. Evaluation of the effects of Neptune Krill Oil on the clinical course of hyperlipidemia. *Altern. Med. Rev.* **2004**, *9*, 420–428.
89. Konagai, C.; Yanagimoto, K.; Hayamizu, K.; Han, L.; Tsuji, T.; Koga, Y. Effects of krill oil containing n-3 polyunsaturated fatty acids in phospholipid form on human brain function: A randomized controlled trial in healthy elderly volunteers. *Clin. Interv. Aging* **2013**, *8*, 1247–1257. [CrossRef]
90. Laidlaw, M.; Cockerline, C.A.; Rowe, W.J. A randomized clinical trial to determine the efficacy of manufacturers' recommended doses of omega-3 fatty acids from different sources in facilitating cardiovascular disease risk reduction. *Lipids Health Dis.* **2014**, *13*, 99. [CrossRef]
91. Salem, N.; Kuratko, C.N. A reexamination of krill oil bioavailability studies. *Lipids Health Dis.* **2014**, *13*, 1–6. [CrossRef]
92. Köhler, A.; Sarkkinen, E.; Tapola, N.; Niskanen, T.; Bruheim, I. Bioavailability of fatty acids from krill oil, krill meal and fish oil in healthy subjects–a randomized, single-dose, cross-over trial. *Lipids Health Dis.* **2015**, *14*, 1–10. [CrossRef]
93. Harris, W.S.; Miller, M.; Tighe, A.P.; Davidson, M.H.; Schaefer, E.J. Omega-3 fatty acids and coronary heart disease risk: Clinical and mechanistic perspectives. *Atherosclerosis* **2008**, *197*, 12–24. [CrossRef]
94. Cleland, L.G.; James, M.J.; Proudman, S.M. The Role of Fish Oils in the Treatment of Rheumatoid Arthritis. *Drugs* **2003**, *63*, 845–853. [CrossRef] [PubMed]
95. Boudrault, C.; Bazinet, R.P.; Ma, D.W. Experimental models and mechanisms underlying the protective effects of n-3 polyunsaturated fatty acids in Alzheimer's disease. *J. Nutr. Biochem.* **2009**, *20*, 1–10. [CrossRef]
96. Fedor, D.; Kelley, D.S. Prevention of insulin resistance by n-3 polyunsaturated fatty acids. *Curr. Opin. Clin. Nutr. Metab. Care* **2009**, *12*, 138–146. [CrossRef] [PubMed]
97. Kris-Etherton, P.M.; Harris, W.S.; Appel, L.J. American Heart Association. Nutrition Committee. Fish consumption, fish oil, omega-3 fatty acids, and cardiovascular disease. *Circulation* **2002**, *106*, 2747–2757. [CrossRef] [PubMed]

98. Cohn, J.S.; Wat, E.; Kamili, A.; Tandy, S. Dietary phospholipids, hepatic lipid metabolism and cardiovascular disease. *Curr. Opin. Lipidol.* **2008**, *19*, 257–262. [CrossRef] [PubMed]
99. Hussein, G.; Nakagawa, T.; Goto, H.; Shimada, Y.; Matsumoto, K.; Sankawa, U.; Watanabe, H. Astaxanthin ameliorates features of metabolic syndrome in SHR/NDmcr-cp. *Life Sci.* **2007**, *80*, 522–529. [CrossRef] [PubMed]
100. Maki, K.C.; Reeves, M.S.; Farmer, M.; Griinari, M.; Berge, K.; Vik, H.; Hubacher, R.; Rains, T.M. Krill oil supplementation increases plasma concentrations of eicosapentaenoic and docosahexaenoic acids in overweight and obese men and women. *Nutr. Res.* **2009**, *29*, 609–615. [CrossRef]
101. Sung, H.H.; Sinclair, A.J.; Huynh, K.; Smith, A.A.T.; Mellett, N.A.; Meikle, P.J.; Su, X.Q. Krill Oil Has Different Effects on the Plasma Lipidome Compared with Fish Oil Following 30 Days of Supplementation in Healthy Women: A Randomized Con-trolled and Crossover Study. *Nutrients* **2020**, *12*, 2804. [CrossRef]
102. Sung, H.H.; Sinclair, A.J.; Huynh, K.; Smith, A.T.; Mellett, N.A.; Meikle, P.J.; Su, X.Q. Differential plasma postprandial lipidomic responses to krill oil and fish oil supplementations in women: A randomized crossover study. *Nutrients* **2019**, *65*, 191–201. [CrossRef]
103. Robertson, B.; Burri, L.; Berge, K. Genotoxicity test and subchronic toxicity study with Superba™ krill oil in rats. *Toxicol. Rep.* **2014**, *1*, 764–776. [CrossRef]
104. Zhu, J.-J.; Shi, J.-H.; Qian, W.-B.; Cai, Z.-Z.; Li, D. Effects of Krill Oil on serum lipids of hyperlipidemic rats and human SW480 cells. *Lipids Health Dis.* **2008**, *7*, 30. [CrossRef] [PubMed]
105. Tandy, S.; Chung, R.W.S.; Wat, E.; Kamili, A.; Berge, K.; Griinari, M.; Cohn, J.S. Dietary Krill Oil Supplementation Reduces Hepatic Steatosis, Glycemia, and Hypercholesterolemia in High-Fat-Fed Mice. *J. Agric. Food Chem.* **2009**, *57*, 9339–9345. [CrossRef] [PubMed]
106. Bjørndal, B.; Vik, R.; Brattelid, T.; Vigerust, N.F.; Burri, L.; Bohov, P.; Nygård, O.; Skorve, J.; Berge, R.K. Krill powder increases liver lipid catabolism and reduces glucose mobilization in tumor necrosis factor-alpha transgenic mice fed a high-fat diet. *Metabolism* **2012**, *61*, 1461–1472. [CrossRef] [PubMed]
107. Saito, M.; Ishida, N.; Yamada, H.; Ibi, M.; Hirose, M. 8-HEPE-Concentrated Materials from Pacific Krill Improve Plasma Cholesterol Levels and Hepatic Steatosis in High Cholesterol Diet-Fed Low-Density Lipoprotein (LDL) Receptor-Deficient Mice. *Biol. Pharm. Bull.* **2020**, *43*, 919–924. [CrossRef]
108. Hals, P.-A.; Wang, X.; Xiao, Y.-F. Effects of a purified krill oil phospholipid rich in long-chain omega-3 fatty acids on cardiovascular disease risk factors in non-human primates with naturally occurring diabetes type-2 and dyslipidemia. *Lipids Health Dis.* **2017**, *16*, 11. [CrossRef] [PubMed]
109. Ferramosca, A.; Conte, A.; Burri, L.; Berge, K.; De Nuccio, F.; Giudetti, A.M.; Zara, V. A Krill Oil Supplemented Diet Suppresses Hepatic Steatosis in High-Fat Fed Rats. *PLoS ONE* **2012**, *7*, e38797. [CrossRef]
110. Ivanova, Z.; Bjørndal, B.; Grigorova, N.; Roussenov, A.; Vachkova, E.; Berge, K.; Burri, L.; Berge, R.; Stanilova, S.; Milanova, A.; et al. Effect of fish and krill oil supplementation on glucose tolerance in rabbits with experimentally induced obesity. *Eur. J. Nutr.* **2015**, *54*, 1055–1067. [CrossRef]
111. Rundblad, A.; Holven, K.B.; Bruheim, I.; Myhrstad, M.C.; Ulven, S.M. Effects of krill oil and lean and fatty fish on cardiovascular risk markers: A randomised controlled trial. *J. Nutr. Sci.* **2018**, *7*, e3. [CrossRef]
112. Berge, K.; Musa-Veloso, K.; Harwood, M.; Hoem, N.; Burri, L. Krill oil supplementation lowers serum triglycerides without in-creasing low-density lipoprotein cholesterol in adults with borderline high or high triglyceride levels. *Nutr. Res.* **2014**, *34*, 126–133. [CrossRef]
113. Cicero, A.F.; Rosticci, M.; Morbini, M.; Cagnati, M.; Grandi, E.; Parini, A.; Borghi, C. Lipid-lowering and anti-inflammatory effects of omega 3 ethyl esters and krill oil: A randomized, cross-over, clinical trial. *Arch. Med. Sci.* **2016**, *3*, 507–512. [CrossRef]
114. Sun, D.; Zhang, L.; Chen, H.; Feng, R.; Cao, P.; Liu, Y. Effects of Antarctic krill oil on lipid and glucose metabolism in C57BL/6J mice with high fat diet. *Lipids Health Dis.* **2017**, *16*, 218. [CrossRef]
115. Sistilli, G.; Kalendova, V.; Cajka, T.; Irodenko, I.; Bardova, K.; Oseeva, M.; Zacek, P.; Kroupova, P.; Horakova, O.; Lackner, K.; et al. Krill Oil Supplementation Reduces Exacerbated Hepatic Steatosis Induced by Thermoneutral Housing in Mice with Diet-Induced Obesity. *Nutrients* **2021**, *13*, 437. [CrossRef] [PubMed]
116. Kroupova, P.; Van Schothorst, E.M.; Keijer, J.; Bunschoten, A.; Vodicka, M.; Irodenko, I.; Oseeva, M.; Zacek, P.; Kopecky, J.; Rossmeisl, M.; et al. Omega-3 Phospholipids from Krill Oil Enhance Intestinal Fatty Acid Oxidation More Effectively than Omega-3 Triacylglycerols in High-Fat Diet-Fed Obese Mice. *Nutrients* **2020**, *12*, 2037. [CrossRef] [PubMed]
117. Rossmeisl, M.; Pavlisova, J.; Bardova, K.; Kalendova, V.; Buresova, J.; Kuda, O.; Kroupova, P.; Stankova, B.; Tvrzicka, E.; Fiserova, E.; et al. Increased plasma levels of palmitoleic acid may contribute to beneficial effects of Krill oil on glucose homeostasis in dietary obese mice. *Biochim. Biophys. Acta* **2020**, *1865*, 158732. [CrossRef] [PubMed]
118. Fosshaug, L.E.; Berge, R.K.; Beitnes, J.O.; Berge, K.; Vik, H.; Aukrust, P.; Gullestad, L.; Vinge, L.E.; Oie, E. Krill oil attenuates left ventricular dilatation after myocardial infarction in rats. *Lipids Health Dis.* **2011**, *10*, 245. [CrossRef] [PubMed]
119. Lobraico, J.M.; DiLello, L.C.; Butler, A.D.; Cordisco, M.E.; Petrini, J.R.; Ahmadi, R. Effects of krill oil on endothelial function and other cardiovascular risk factors in participants with type 2 diabetes, a randomized controlled trial. *BMJ Open Diabetes Res. Care* **2015**, *3*, e000107. [CrossRef]
120. Di Marzo, V.; Silvestri, C. Lifestyle and Metabolic Syndrome: Contribution of the Endocannabinoidome. *Nutrients* **2019**, *11*, 1956. [CrossRef] [PubMed]

121. Piscitelli, F.; Carta, G.; Bisogno, T.; Murru, E.; Cordeddu, L.; Berge, K.; Tandy, S.; Cohn, J.S.; Griinari, M.; Banni, S.; et al. Effect of dietary krill oil supplementation on the endocannabinoidome of metabolically relevant tissues from high-fat-fed mice. *Nutr. Metab.* **2011**, *8*, 51. [CrossRef] [PubMed]
122. Berge, K.; Piscitelli, F.; Hoem, N.; Silvestri, C.; Meyer, I.; Banni, S.; Di Marzo, V. Chronic treatment with krill powder reduces plasma triglyceride and anandamide levels in mildly obese men. *Lipids Health Dis.* **2013**, *12*, 78. [CrossRef]
123. Banni, S.; Carta, G.; Murru, E.; Cordeddu, L.; Giordano, E.; Sirigu, A.R.; Berge, K.; Vik, H.; Maki, K.C.; Di Marzo, V.; et al. Krill oil significantly decreases 2-arachidonoylglycerol plasma levels in obese subjects. *Nutr. Metab.* **2011**, *8*, 7. [CrossRef]
124. Cui, C.; Li, Y.; Gao, H.; Zhang, H.; Han, J.; Zhang, D.; Li, Y.; Zhou, J.; Lu, C.; Su, X. Modulation of the gut microbiota by the mixture of fish oil and krill oil in high-fat diet-induced obesity mice. *PLoS ONE* **2017**, *12*, e0186216. [CrossRef]
125. Lu, C.; Sun, T.; Li, Y.; Zhang, D.; Zhou, J.; Su, X. Modulation of the Gut Microbiota by Krill Oil in Mice Fed a High-Sugar High-Fat Diet. *Front. Microbiol.* **2017**, *8*, 905. [CrossRef]
126. Jiang, Q.; Lu, C.; Sun, T.; Zhou, J.; Li, Y.; Ming, T.; Bai, L.; Wang, Z.J.; Su, X. Alterations of the Brain Proteome and Gut Microbiota in d-Galactose-Induced Brain-Aging Mice with Krill Oil Supplementation. *J. Agric. Food Chem.* **2019**, *67*, 9820–9830. [CrossRef] [PubMed]
127. Costanzo, M.; Cesi, V.; Palone, F.; Pierdomenico, M.; Colantoni, E.; Leter, B.; Vitali, R.; Negroni, A.; Cucchiara, S.; Stronati, L. Krill oil, vitamin D and Lactobacillus reuteri cooperate to reduce gut inflammation. *Benef. Microbes* **2018**, *9*, 389–399. [CrossRef] [PubMed]
128. Grimstad, T.; Bjørndal, B.; Cacabelos, D.; Aasprong, O.G.; Janssen, E.A.; Omdal, R.; Svardal, A.; Hausken, T.; Bohov, P.; Portero-Otin, M.; et al. Dietary supplementation of krill oil attenuates inflammation and oxidative stress in experimental ulcerative colitis in rats. *Scand. J. Gastroenterol.* **2011**, *47*, 49–58. [CrossRef] [PubMed]
129. Kim, J.-H.; Hong, S.-S.; Lee, M.; Lee, E.-H.; Rhee, I.; Chang, S.-Y.; Lim, S.-J. Krill Oil-Incorporated Liposomes as an Effective Nanovehicle to Ameliorate the Inflammatory Responses of DSS-Induced Colitis. *Int. J. Nanomed.* **2019**, *14*, 8305–8320. [CrossRef] [PubMed]
130. Liu, F.; Smith, A.D.; Solano-Aguilar, G.; Wang, T.T.Y.; Pham, Q.; Beshah, E.; Tang, Q.; Urban, J.F., Jr.; Xue, C.; Li, R.W. Mechanistic insights into the attenuation of intestinal inflammation and modulation of the gut microbiome by krill oil using in vitro and in vivo models. *Microbiome* **2020**, *8*, 83. [CrossRef] [PubMed]
131. Ierna, M.; Kerr, A.; Scales, H.; Berge, K.; Griinari, M. Supplementation of diet with krill oil protects against experimental rheu-matoid arthritis. *BMC Musculoskelet. Disord.* **2010**, *11*, 136. [CrossRef]
132. Vigerust, N.F.; Bjørndal, B.; Bohov, P.; Brattelid, T.; Svardal, A.; Berge, R.K. Krill oil versus fish oil in modulation of inflammation and lipid metabolism in mice transgenic for TNF-α. *Eur. J. Nutr.* **2013**, *52*, 1315–1325. [CrossRef]
133. Tou, J.C.; Jaczynski, J.; Chen, Y.-C. Krill for Human Consumption: Nutritional Value and Potential Health Benefits. *Nutr. Rev.* **2007**, *65*, 63–77. [CrossRef]
134. Deutsch, L. Evaluation of the Effect of Neptune Krill Oil on Chronic Inflammation and Arthritic Symptoms. *J. Am. Coll. Nutr.* **2007**, *26*, 39–48. [CrossRef] [PubMed]
135. Suzuki, Y.; Fukushima, M.; Sakuraba, K.; Sawaki, K.; Sekigawa, K. Krill Oil Improves Mild Knee Joint Pain: A Randomized Control Trial. *PLoS ONE* **2016**, *11*, e0162769. [CrossRef] [PubMed]
136. Liu, X.; Osawa, T. Astaxanthin Protects Neuronal Cells against Oxidative Damage and Is a Potent Candidate for Brain Food. *Forum Nutr.* **2009**, *61*, 129–135. [CrossRef] [PubMed]
137. Wang, H.-Q.; Sun, X.-B.; Xu, Y.-X.; Zhao, H.; Zhu, Q.-Y.; Zhu, C.-Q. Astaxanthin upregulates heme oxygenase-1 expression through ERK1/2 pathway and its protective effect against beta-amyloid-induced cytotoxicity in SH-SY5Y cells. *Brain Res.* **2010**, *1360*, 159–167. [CrossRef] [PubMed]
138. Lu, Y.-P.; Liu, S.-Y.; Sun, H.; Wu, X.-M.; Li, J.-J.; Zhu, L. Neuroprotective effect of astaxanthin on H_2O_2-induced neurotoxicity in vitro and on focal cerebral ischemia in vivo. *Brain Res.* **2010**, *1360*, 40–48. [CrossRef]
139. Lee, B.; Sur, B.-J.; Han, J.-J.; Shim, I.; Her, S.; Lee, H.-J.; Hahm, D.-H. Krill phosphatidylserine improves learning and memory in Morris water maze in aged rats. *Prog. Neuro. Psychopharmacol. Biol. Psychiatry* **2010**, *34*, 1085–1093. [CrossRef]
140. Barros, M.P.; Poppe, S.C.; Bondan, E.F. Neuroprotective Properties of the Marine Carotenoid Astaxanthin and Omega-3 Fatty Acids, and Perspectives for the Natural Combination of Both in Krill Oil. *Nutrients* **2014**, *6*, 1293–1317. [CrossRef]
141. Choi, J.Y.; Jang, J.S.; Son, D.J.; Im, H.-S.; Kim, J.Y.; Park, J.E.; Choi, W.R.; Han, S.-B.; Hong, J.T. Antarctic Krill Oil Diet Protects against Lipopolysaccharide-Induced Oxidative Stress, Neuroinflammation and Cognitive Impairment. *Int. J. Mol. Sci.* **2017**, *18*, 2554. [CrossRef]
142. Li, Q.; Wu, F.; Wen, M.; Yanagita, T.; Xue, C.; Zhang, T.; Wang, Y. The Protective Effect of Antarctic Krill Oil on Cognitive Function by Inhibiting Oxidative Stress in the Brain of Senescence-Accelerated Prone Mouse Strain 8 (SAMP8) Mice. *J. Food Sci.* **2018**, *83*, 543–551. [CrossRef]
143. Kim, J.H.; Meng, H.W.; He, M.T.; Choi, J.M.; Lee, D.; Cho, E.J. Krill Oil Attenuates Cognitive Impairment by the Regulation of Oxidative Stress and Neuronal Apoptosis in an Amyloid β-Induced Alzheimer's Disease Mouse Model. *Molecules* **2020**, *25*, 3942. [CrossRef]
144. Andraka, J.M.; Sharma, N.; Marchalant, Y. Can krill oil be of use for counteracting neuroinflammatory processes induced by high fat diet and aging? *Neurosci. Res.* **2020**, *157*, 1–14. [CrossRef]

145. Wibrand, K.; Berge, K.; Messaoudi, M.; Duffaud, A.; Panja, D.; Bramham, C.R.; Burri, L. Enhanced cognitive function and antidepressant-like effects after krill oil supplementation in rats. *Lipids Health Dis.* **2013**, *12*, 6. [CrossRef] [PubMed]
146. Zadeh-Ardabili, P.M.; Rad, S.K.; Rad, S.K.; Movafagh, A. Antidepressant-like effects of fish, krill oils and Vit B12 against exposure to stress environment in mice models: Current status and pilot study. *Sci. Rep.* **2019**, *9*, 19953. [CrossRef]
147. Mendoza, C.; Perez-Urrutia, N.; Alvarez-Ricartes, N.; Barreto, G.E.; Pérez-Ordás, R.; Iarkov, A.; Echeverria, V. Cotinine Plus Krill Oil Decreased Depressive Behavior, and Increased Astrocytes Survival in the Hippocampus of Mice Subjected to Restraint Stress. *Front. Neurosci.* **2018**, *12*, 952. [CrossRef]
148. Van der Wurff, I.S.; von Schacky, C.; Berge, K.; Kirschner, P.A.; de Groot, R.H. A protocol for a randomised controlled trial in-vestigating the effect of increasing Omega-3 index with krill oil supplementation on learning, cognition, behaviour and visual processing in typically developing adolescents. *BMJ Open* **2016**, *6*, e011790. [CrossRef] [PubMed]
149. Van der Wurff, I.; von Schacky, C.; Bergeland, T.; Leontjevas, R.; Zeegers, M.; Kirschner, P.; de Groot, R. Effect of one year krill oil supplementation on depressive symptoms and self-esteem of Dutch adolescents: A randomized controlled trial. *Prostaglandins Leukot. Essent. Fat. Acids* **2020**, *163*, 102208. [CrossRef] [PubMed]
150. Zheng, W.; Wang, X.; Cao, W.; Yang, B.; Mu, Y.; Dong, Y.; Xiu, Z. E-configuration structures of EPA and DHA derived from Euphausia superba and their significant inhibitive effects on growth of human cancer cell lines in vitro. *Prostaglandins Leukot. Essent. Fat. Acids* **2017**, *117*, 47–53. [CrossRef]
151. Xiao, S.U.; Tanalgo, P.; Bustos, M.; Dass, C.R. The Effect of Krill Oil and n-3 Polyunsaturated Fatty Acids on Human Osteosarcoma Cell Proliferation and Migration. *Curr. Drug Targets* **2018**, *19*, 479–486. [CrossRef]
152. Jayathilake, A.G.; Senior, P.V.; Su, X.Q. Krill oil extract suppresses cell growth and induces apoptosis of human colorectal cancer cells. *BMC Complement. Altern. Med.* **2016**, *16*, 328. [CrossRef]
153. Jayathilake, A.G.; Kadife, E.; Luwor, R.B.; Nurgali, K.; Su, X.Q. Krill oil extract suppresses the proliferation of colorectal cancer cells through activation of caspase 3/9. *Nutr. Metab.* **2019**, *16*, 53. [CrossRef]
154. Jayathilake, A.G.; Veale, M.F.; Luwor, R.B.; Nurgali, K.; Su, X.Q. Krill oil extract inhibits the migration of human colorectal cancer cells and down-regulates EGFR signalling and PD-L1 expression. *BMC Complement. Med. Ther.* **2020**, *20*, 1–15. [CrossRef] [PubMed]
155. Skarpańska-Stejnborn, A.; Pilaczyńska-Szcześniak, L.; Basta, P.; Foriasz, J.; Arlet, J. Effects of Supplementation with Neptune Krill Oil (Euphasia Superba) on Selected Redox Parameters and Pro-Inflammatory Markers in Athletes during Exhaustive Exercise. *J. Hum. Kinet.* **2010**, *25*, 49–57. [CrossRef]
156. Da Boit, M.; Mastalurova, I.; Brazaite, G.; McGovern, N.; Thompson, K.; Gray, S.R. The Effect of Krill Oil Supplementation on Exercise Performance and Markers of Immune Function. *PLoS ONE* **2015**, *10*, e0139174. [CrossRef] [PubMed]
157. Georges, J.; Sharp, M.H.; Lowery, R.P.; Wilson, J.M.; Purpura, M.; Hornberger, T.A.; Harding, F.; Johnson, J.H.; Peele, D.M.; Jäger, R. The Effects of Krill Oil on mTOR Signaling and Resistance[tnq_nbsp] Exercise: A Pilot Study. *J. Nutr. Metab.* **2018**, *2018*, 1–11. [CrossRef]
158. Barenie, M.J.; Freemas, J.A.; Baranauskas, M.N.; Goss, C.S.; Freeman, K.L.; Chen, X.; Dickinson, S.L.; Fly, A.D.; Kawata, K.; Chapman, R.F.; et al. Effectiveness of a combined New Zealand green-lipped mussel and Antarctic krill oil supplement on markers of exercise-induced muscle damage and inflammation in untrained men. *J. Diet Suppl.* **2020**, 1–26. [CrossRef]
159. Storsve, A.B.; Johnsen, L.; Nyborg, C.; Melau, J.; Hisdal, J.; Burri, L. Effects of Krill Oil and Race Distance on Serum Choline and Choline Metabolites in Triathletes: A Field Study. *Front. Nutr.* **2020**, *7*, 133. [CrossRef]
160. Ibrahim, S.H.; Hirsova, P.; Malhi, H.; Gores, G.J. Animal Models of Nonalcoholic Steatohepatitis: Eat, Delete, and Inflame. *Dig. Dis. Sci.* **2015**, *61*, 1325–1336. [CrossRef]
161. Cicero, A.F.G.; Morbini, M.; Borghi, C. Do we need 'new' omega-3 polyunsaturated fatty acids formulations? *Expert Opin. Pharmacother.* **2015**, *16*, 285–288. [CrossRef]
162. Kwantes, J.M.; Grundmann, O. A Brief Review of Krill Oil History, Research, and the Commercial Market. *J. Diet. Suppl.* **2014**, *12*, 23–35. [CrossRef]
163. Wang, L.; Yang, F.; Rong, Y.; Yuan, Y.; Ding, Y.; Shi, W.; Wang, Z. Effects of different proteases enzymatic extraction on the lipid yield and quality of Antarctic krill oil. *Food Sci. Nutr.* **2019**, *7*, 2224–2230. [CrossRef]
164. Alvarez-Ricartes, N.; Oliveros-Matus, P.; Mendoza, C.; Perez-Urrutia, N.; Echeverria, F.; Iarkov, A.; Barreto, G.E.; Echeverria, V. Correction to: Intranasal Cotinine Plus Krill Oil Facilitates Fear Extinction, Decreases Depressive-Like Behavior, and Increases Hippocampal Calcineurin a Levels in Mice. *Mol. Neurobiol.* **2018**, *55*, 7961. [CrossRef] [PubMed]
165. Van Der Wurff, I.S.; Von Schacky, C.; Bergeland, T.; Leontjevas, R.; Zeegers, M.P.; Jolles, J.; Kirschner, P.A.; De Groot, R.H. Effect of 1 Year Krill Oil Supplementation on Cognitive Achievement of Dutch Adolescents: A Double-Blind Randomized Controlled Trial. *Nutrients* **2019**, *11*, 1230. [CrossRef] [PubMed]

MDPI
St. Alban-Anlage 66
4052 Basel
Switzerland
Tel. +41 61 683 77 34
Fax +41 61 302 89 18
www.mdpi.com

Marine Drugs Editorial Office
E-mail: marinedrugs@mdpi.com
www.mdpi.com/journal/marinedrugs

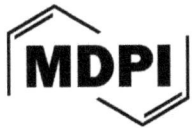

www.ingramcontent.com/pod-product-compliance
Lightning Source LLC
LaVergne TN
LVHW070708100526
838202LV00013B/1047